Short Notes for Dental PG Entrance Examinations

Second Edition

Including Review for UG Students

Basic Sciences Volume 1

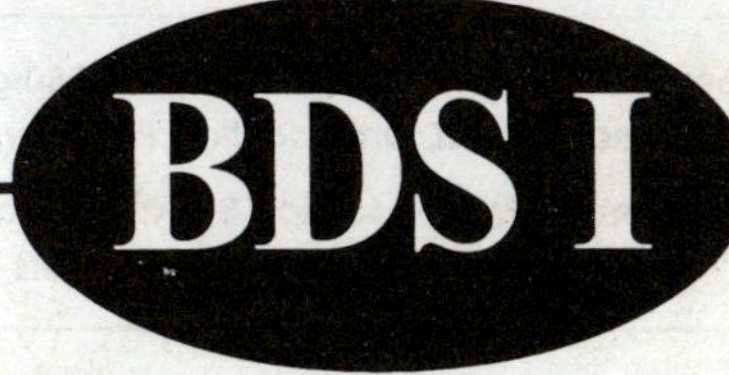

Volumes in the Series

Short Notes for **Dental PG Entrance Examinations**

Second Edition

Basic Sciences	
• **Volume 1**	**BDS I**
• **Volume 2**	**BDS II**
• **Volume 3**	**BDS III**

Clinical Sciences	
• **Volume 4**	**Operative Dentistry, Endodontics, Oral Surgery, Local Anaesthesia, Orthodontics, Pedodontics**
• **Volume 5**	**Periodontics, Prosthodontics, Basic Radiology Self-Assessment Paper, Model Test Papers**

Short Notes for Dental PG Entrance Examinations

Second Edition

Including Review for UG Students

Basic Sciences Volume 1

SANDEEP GOYAL MDS (Orthodontics)
Professor
Department of Orthodontics and Dentofacial Orthopedics
ITS College of Dental Sciences and Research
Murad Nagar, UP

Edited by
Sonia Goyal MDS (Oral and Maxillofacial Surgery)
Associate Professor, Department of Oral and Maxillofacial Surgery
ITS College of Dental Sciences and Research, Murad Nagar, UP

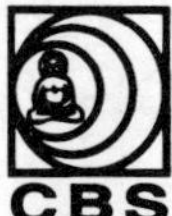

CBS Publishers & Distributors Pvt Ltd
New Delhi • Bangalore • Pune • Cochin • Chennai

Second Edition

Short Notes for Dental PG Entrance Examinations

Volume 1

First Edition : 2003
Second Edition : 2010

ISBN : 978-81-239-1798-6

Published by Satish Kumar Jain and produced by Vinod K. Jain for
CBS Publishers & Distributors Pvt Ltd
4819/XI Prahlad Street, 24 Ansari Road, Daryaganj,
New Delhi 110 002, India.
Fax: 011-23243014 e-mail: cbspubs@vsnl.com; delhi@cbspd.com
Website: www.cbspd.com

Branches

- **Bangalore:** Seema House 2975, 17th Cross, K.R. Road, Banasankari 2nd Stage, Bangalore 560 070
  Fax: 080-26771680 e-mail: cbsbng@gmail.com
- **Pune:** Shaan Brahmha Complex, Basement, Appa Balwant Chowk,
  Budhwar Peth, next to Ratan Talkies, Pune 411 002
  Fax: 020-24464059 e-mail: pune@cbspd.com
- **Cochin:** 36/14 Kalluvilakam, Lissie Hospital Road, Cochin-682018, Kerala
  e-mail: cochin@cbspd.com
- **Chennai:** 20, West Park Road, Shenoy Nagar, Chennai 600030.
  email: chennai@cbspd.com

Printed at Somya Printers, Delhi-110053

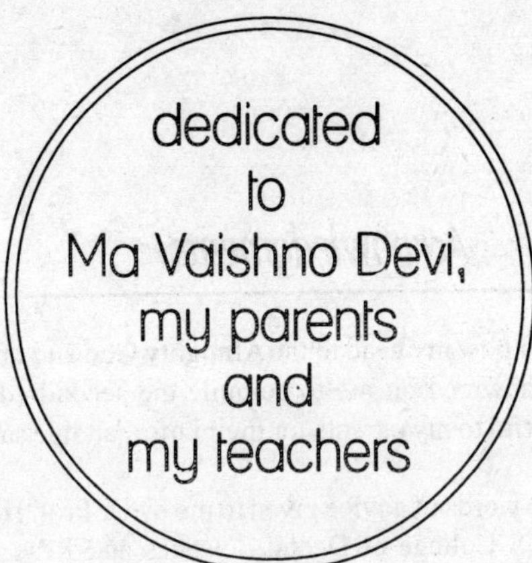
dedicated
to
Ma Vaishno Devi,
my parents
and
my teachers

Acknowledgments

At the very outset, I bow my head to the Almighty God and my Guruji for all the grace showered on me to compile the second edition of the book. I am also thankful to my parents for their unforgettable sacrifices and choicest blessings.

I acknowledge the words of advice given to me by Dr Prof. Hari Parkash, Director General, ITS College of Dental Sciences and Research, Murad Nagar.

I place on record my deep gratitude towards my mentors and guides, my respected teachers during my postgraduation, Dr D N Kapoor, the then Professor and Head; Dr V P Sharma, Professor; Dr Pradeep Tandon, Professor, Department of Orthodontics and Dentofacial Orthopedics, Faculty of Dental Sciences, KGMC, Lucknow, for all their blessings, ideas and inspiration.

Prof P B Sood, Principal, ITS College of Dental Sciences and Research, Murad Nagar, has always been a constant source of insipiration and advice.

Dr Sanjay Tiwari, Professor and Head, Department of Endodontics, and Principal, GDC, PGIMS, Rohtak, for all his good wishes, the support, stimulating criticism and magnanimous help during my UG/PG days and afterwards.

My wife Dr Sonia Goyal MDS (oral and maxillofacial surgery), for her support, constant advice, contribution and editing the text, and all the pains she took during the compilation of the project.

Mr S K Jain and Mr Y N Arjuna of CBS Publishers & Distributors Pvt Ltd and their team of professionals for their best suggestions and help in getting this work published in the present form.

Last but not the least, I acknowledge all my family members and friends for their best wishes to boost my morale.

Sandeep Goyal MDS

Preface to the Second Edition

We thank all our readers for their overwhelming support and inputs for the first edition of our series **Short Notes for PG Dental Entrance Examinations**. However, with the increasing competition and increasing base of knowledge, a strong requirement for the improvement has been felt.

In the second edition, we have tried to incorporate a few new topics which will be helpful to postgraduate aspirants. We have now compiled the basic subjects and clinical subjects separately. This will help those undergraduate students also who aspire to compete for postgraduate entrance examination in the future. This edition will help and guide them to build their knowledge base from the very beginning of their dental career and will be helpful in their regular BDS examinations and also *viva voce* examinations.

We have included MCQs in this new edition for the side-by-side exercise and testing the skills and growth of their knowledge base. The book in the second edition has now been split into five volumes, considering the valuable additions made in the text as well new sections of MCQs which have been selectively added to strengthen the inherent appeal of this title amongst the potential readers. Basic Sciences are covered in Vols 1–3 and Clinical Sciences in Vols 4 and 5.

We request our readers to continue sending their suggestions to us for future improvements for the benefit of their friends, juniors and other future dental surgeons.

In the end, we again emphasize that all the aspirants should synergize their knowledge by reading standard theory books to smoothly sail through the ocean of entrance examination, since our volumes may not be complete in every aspect.

Sandeep Goyal MDS
Sonia Goyal MDS
goyalsandeep2000@rediffmail.com
goyalsandeep2000@gmail.com

Preface to the First Edition

There has been a marked increase in competition in dental PG entrance examinations, which have become tougher in recent times. A proper guidance to the aspirants is, therefore, necessary for making their preparations.

The trend of today being MCQ-based, the aspirants just memorise the MCQs from the books available in the market without going into the depth of the statement, leading to errors during the examination. Also, a series of MCQs currently available in the market unfortunately contain 50 to 60% repetition of the questions, and the answers to many questions given in the answer key are also misleading and confusing for the students.

Most of the students do not want to undertake a detailed study of the subjects for their preparation and hence look for the easiest method to get through in the examinations which they consider to be present in the MCQ books.

In my view, MCQ books are for practice only. Your basic knowledge is tested through MCQs and they help to churn your mind, but you should not read them blindly thinking that they will be repeated in the examinations as such. The paper setters change the statements and options of the MCQs for better judgement of the student, therefore, only those students who have a strong basic knowledge can easily analyze and correlate the statement and the option. Also, for some of those students who read the textbooks and do not make notes but rather underline the text or write in the textbooks only, revision becomes very confusing and time-consuming.

This book has been compiled with an idea in mind to provide handy information in the form of a ready-reckoner to the aspirants. This volume covers eight important subjects, and other subjects will be included in the latter volume(s). The motive of compiling information in this manner is to bring important points of each topic together so that a student while reading the topics can revise all the key points immediately and at one stretch.

I have tried with the best possible efforts to tabulate and alphabetically arrange most of the important information so as to make it easy for the students to search for the required topic. The book speaks about the points to be stressed in the form of lists, like the most common terms, syndromes, synonyms, etc.

This book gives the students the guidelines and information about the topics most often asked in the examinations. However, they are advised to go for **further detailed reading from standard textbooks to supplement and reinforce their knowledge.**

I have attempted my best to include almost 80 to 90% of the important information on the covered subjects. However, the readers must study additionally and add their own points on the topics for their benefit.

No project can be completed and improved upon without **feedback,** constructive criticism and healthy suggestions. It is my humble request to all the readers and students to send me their suggestions and points/ topics to be added in further editions of the book, to make it more informative and useful for their younger friends and students. It is promised that these suggestions will be suitably incorporated in the future editions and all the contributors will be suitably acknowledged. My e–mail address is goyalsandeep2000@sify.com. Wishing you all the success in your examinations.

Sandeep Goyal MDS

Suggested Readings

Since we do not claim this book to be complete in all the respects, we advise the students to further supplement their information by going through other standard textbooks on particular topics. We are providing below a list of some books for reference for the students.

	Author	Textbook on
1.	Monheim's	Local anesthesia
2.	Malamed's	Local anesthesia
3.	Graber's	Orthodontics – an art or science
4.	Profitt's	Orthodontics
5.	Grossman's	Endodontics
6.	Cohen's	Endodontics, i.e. pathways to the pulp
7.	Ingle's	Endodontics
8.	Gupta	Removable Partial Prosthodontics
9.	Orban's	Dental and oral histology
10.	Ten cate's	Oral histology
11.	Shafer's	Oral pathology
12.	Stone's	Oral pathology
13.	Burkitt's	Oral medicine
14.	Sikri	Dental Radiology, 4/e
15.	Sikri	Conservative Dentistry
16.	Goaz /White	Radiology
17.	Singh	Embryology
18.	Garg	Histology, 4/e

Standard books of MCQs which should be read definitely:

- ❑ Series of NDBs, i.e. national dental board papers, available upto L – series in I and II volumes.
- ❑ Rudman's
- ❑ Boucher's
- ❑ Steele's
- ❑ Gardiner's
- ❑ Cawson's
- ❑ Reed's Vols I & II
- ❑ Arco's Vols I & II

Besides these books, the students should always refer to the MCQ books available in the market for practice but they should not get confused.

Contents of Volume 1

Contents of Volumes 2 and 3

VOLUME 2 BDS II

VOLUME 3 BDS III

Abbreviations Used in the Book

- AD — autosomal dominant
- A. — artery
- Ag/Ab/ — antigen/antibody
- Aka — also known as
- Alv. — alveolar
- Ant./post. — anterior/posterior
- As — arsenic
- Ass. — associated
- B/W — between
- Bact. — bacteria
- BCC — basal cell ca.
- C/E — clinical exam.
- Ca. — carcinoma
- Ch. — chronic/characteristics
- Chr. — chromosomes
- Cp. — compared
- CT — connective tissue
- Def. — deficiency
- Dev. — develop/developmental
- Dis — disease/distance as per the case
- D/D — differential diagnosis
- Enz. — enzyme
- Epith. — epithelium/-al
- ECA/ICA — external/internal carotid A
- H/E — histology examination
- IU — intrauterine
- LAP — lymphadenopathy
- LN — lymph nodes
- LO — lateral oblique
- M. — muscles
- Mm — mucous membrane
- MO/m.o. — malocclusion
- Md/mand — mandibular
- Memb. — membrane
- MNGC — multinucleated giant cells
- MNP/LNP — median/lateral nasal process

❑ Mo.	months
❑ Mx/max	maxillary
❑ n.m.	neuromuscular
❑ O/F	oral features
❑ Org./orgs.	organisms
❑ OTM	orthodontic tooth movement
❑ OMV	occipito-mental view
❑ OFD	object – film dis.
❑ PO	presence of
❑ PA	periapical/posteroanterior
❑ PNS	para nasal sinus
❑ Pt.	patient
❑ PDL	periodontal ligament
❑ R/G	radiograph
❑ R/L	radiolucent
❑ R/O	radiopaque
❑ REE	reduced enamel epith
❑ Reqd.	required
❑ SCC	squamous cell ca.
❑ SG	salivary gland
❑ S/S	signs and symptoms
❑ SMV	submento-vertex view
❑ Synd	syndrome
❑ TFD	target-film distance
❑ TOD	target – object dis.
❑ Vit.	vitamin

How to Prepare for the Entrance Examinations

This is my personal experience for PG entrance preparation and a time-tested method as many of my friends who have followed this method have been successful in the exams.

1. You have to believe in that hard work and luck go side by side.
2. Keep at least 6–8 months for preparation, which should be free from any sort of disturbance and forget about your surroundings.
3. Devote at least 8–10 hrs/day for the studies.
4. Divide your time and make a time bound schedule.
5. Pick important subjects first depending on the numbers of questions asked in the examinations. The subjects to be studied and stressed during entrance preparation are : general anatomy; dental materials; dental histology; pharmacology; oral pathology; fluorides; endodontics; periodontology; local anaesthesia; pedodontics; basics of all the clinical subjects.
6. Make your daily routine and diligently follow it.
7. Read MCQs two times from NDBs and any other standard book available on a particular subject. This will give you an idea about the style of MCQs and the part of the topic from which the question has been picked from the text, e.g. many MCQs are taken from the legends written below the figures in the book especially dental histology, periodontology, orthodontics.
8. Pick up a standard textbook which you have read during UG days. Read the topics and make notes separately and underline the important points. This will help you to strengthen your knowledge on that topic. Then take other subjects and follow the same pattern.
9. Read only relevant parts of the non-clinical subjects. Stress on anatomy, embryology, dental histology, pharmacology and physiology during the preparation.

10. All the topics and subjects should be covered in the time that at least two months are left for revision before the examination which you are preparing for.
11. When you have finished all the subjects, pick the MCQs books and read the 2–3 times. Any problem can be referred to your notes/textbooks.
12. Mark difficult MCQs in the book with different colors and read them carefully everytime.
13. 15 days before exams, read the notes on all the subjects, followed by one more revision of MCQs.
14. Discussion with your friends is a very important part of preparation. It gives an insight into the topics and more informations.
15. Take all the exams as far as possible; it tells you the trend; your standing and reshuffles your knowledge.

If you follow these rules, I can guarantee you 100% success in the examinations.

Syllabus

Given below is brief outline of the syllabus and topics the students should follow during preparation which should be supplemented by other topics for better knowledge.

Subjects	Topics	Books advised
Anatomy	♦ Head and neck — complete ♦ Brain — basics	Chaurasia's
Embryology	♦ Basics ♦ Pharyngeal arches ♦ Fetal circulation ♦ Fate of germ layers ♦ Development of oral cavity and face	I B Singh
Histology	♦ Basics ♦ Cell structure, cell division ♦ All glands and appendages, spleen, liver, etc. ♦ Skin, epithelium, A, V, N, M, CT	I B Singh
Dental materials	Complete	Skinners
Physiology	♦ Basics ♦ Blood, GIT, CVS, respiration, endocrinology	Chatterjee
Biochemistry	Basic concepts, enzymes, DNA/RNA, Krebs's cycle, HMP, etc. cycles carbohydrate/ lipid/ protein structure and metabolism, vitamins, minerals, energy requirements, etc.	Rama Rao, Harper's

Subjects	**Topics**	**Books advised**
Dental histology	Complete	Orbans
Dental anatomy	Basics, difference in morphology of molars, premolars, canines, mand lateral incisors, etc., occlusion, TMJ, alveolar bone	Wheeler's
Microbiology	Basics, sterilisation, structure of bacteria and virus, immunity, Ag–Ab reactions, *Strept.*, *Staph., Clostridia, Mycobacterium,* HIV, Hepatitis virus	Ananthnarayan
Pathology	Basics only, neoplasia definitions, blood pathology (Do not waste much time on it.)	Robins
Pharmacology	Basic concepts, pharmacokinetics and dynamics, dental pharmacology, antibiotics, analgesics, LA/GA, sympathomimetic/lytic drugs, cholinergics/adrenergic, etc., briefly about CVS, CNS, antiepileptic, etc. Mechanism of action of all the drugs, MCQs	K D Tripathi
Oral pathology	Complete	Shafer's
Surgery/ medicine	Basics only, HT, TB, DM, infections, etc.	Any book
PCD	Fluorides, epidemiology, definitions, indices;	
Orthodontics	Basics, growth, ceph, diagnosis, appliances, wire properties, tissue reactions, forces, anchorage, tooth movements	Graber's, Proffit's

Subjects	Topics	Books advised
Local anesthesia	Complete	Monheim's, Malamed
Oral surgery	Basics; sterilisation, sutures, grafts, fascial infections, maxillary sinus, TMJ, salivary glands, fractures and x-rays	Kruger's, Killey's
Operative	Basics, cavity preparation, classification, cariolgy, instruments, cements and restorative materials, differences between cavity of silver, gold, porcelain, etc.	Sturdevant, Marzouk
Endodontics	Complete book	Grossman, Weine
Pedodontics	Complete book	Mcdonald's, Finn's
Periodontics	Complete book	Glickmann's
Radiography	Brief, basics	Any standard book
Prosthodontics	Basics of CD/impressions; materials, occlusions, jaw relations, implants, TMJ, movements, immediate dentures, etc.	Boucher's Fenn Winkler's
	Basics of FPD preparations, finish lines, crown preparations, principles, gingival retraction, impression, casting, etc.	Shillinburg Dykema
	Basics of RPD, DR, IR, connectors, classification of RPDs, diagnosis and Rx plan, surveyor, etc.	McCracken's Steward

BDS I

1

Anatomy

A. Parasympathetic ganglia associated with trigeminal N.

Divn. and position	Ganglion	Source of preganglionic fibres	Main effecter organ
I. Ophthalmic (Nasociliary N)	Ciliary	Oculomotor =Inferior division	1. Muscle of accommodation (ciliary M.) 2. Sphincter of pupil
II. Maxillary (Trunk of N)	Pterygo-palatine	Facial = Greater petrosal N. (through pterygoid canal)	Lacrimal gland
III. Mandibular	Submandibular (lingual N)	Facial=Chorda Tympanic (through petrotympanic fissure)	1 Submandibular gland 2 Sublingual
	OTIC (medial pterygoid N)	9th N = Lesser petrosal N. (through F-ovale)	• Parotid gland

B. Main sensory branches of the 5th N.

Divn.	**Internal Br.**	**Intermediate**	**External**
Ophthalmic	Nasociliary	Frontal	Lacrimal
Maxillary	Pterygopalatine	Infraorbital	Zygomatic
Mandibular	Buccal N and Lingual N.	Inferior alveolar	Auriculo-temporal

C. Communication between extracranial and intracranial veins

I Venous emissaries

Parietal	**Superior sagittal sinus** with a branch of superficial temporal V.
Mastoid	**Sigmoid sinus** with a branch of occipital V.
Condylar	Terminal part of **sigmoid sinus** with one of the deep occipital or cervical V.
Occipital	**Confluence of sinuses** with an occipital V.
Sphenoid	**Cavernous sinus** with pterygoid plexus of Vs.
Zuckerkandl's V through foramen cecum	Superior sagittal sinus with nasal V; in children only
ICA plexus	**Cavernous sinus** with pterygoid plexus of Vs.
Frontal diploic	Drains in **superior sagittal sinus** and one of the frontal V.
Ant. Temporal diploic	Into **sphenoparietal sinus** and middle temporal V.
Post. Temporal diploic	Into **sigmoid sinus** and an occipital V.
Occipital	**Transverse sinus** and branch of occipital V.
Ophthalmic V.	**Cavernous sinus** and facial Vs.
Sup.Ophthalmic V.	With **angular V**. (facial V.)
Inferior Ophthalmic V.	With infraorbital V. or inferior palpebral V. (facial V.)
Inferior Ophthalmic V.	With retromandibular. V. via pterygoid plexus of Vs.

IMPORTANT EXCEPTIONS

- All **infrahyoid Ms.** are supplied by **Ansa cervicalis** (C1,2,3), i.e. branch of cervical plexus except **thyrohyoid**, which is supplied by C1 through 12th N.
- All ms. of **soft palate** are supplied by **pharyngeal plexus (cranial XIth)** except **tensor veli palatini**, which is supplied by mandibular N.
- All ms. of **pharynx** are supplied by **pharyngeal plexus** except **stylopharyngeus** which is supplied by 9th N.
- All ms. of **tongue** are supplied by **12th / HYPOGLOSSAL N** except **palatoglossus,** which is supplied by pharyngeal plexus (cranial accessory through vagus N) of Ns.
- All **intrinsic m. of larynx** are supplied by inferior or **recurrent laryngeal N** except **cricothyroid,** which is supplied by external laryngeal N.
- All ms. of **mastication** are supplied by 5th N (mandibular).
- All ms. of **eyeball** (is SR/IR/MR/LPS/IO) by 3rd N except LR 6 and SO4.
- Ms. of mastication receive major blood supply from pterygoid (2nd) PART OF MAXILLARY A.
- Mandibular N (Vth N) supplies motor fibers to **8 muscles** = M,M,T,L,DGA, TVP, Tensor tympani, MH (derived from Ist branchial ARCH).
- Only M. of orbit which arises **from outer orbit** = I.O.
- Only M. of orbit which **gets trapped** on orbital fracture and causes diplopia = I.O.
- Sensory nerve supply of face is through 5th N except at the **angle of jaw**, which is supplied by GREAT AURICULAR N. (C2,3).
- **SENSORY N supply of tongue** is

  Anterior 2/3rd = lingual N (branch of 5th N)

  Posterior 1/3rd = 9th N.

  Posterior most part = vagus N (th, internal laryngeal N)

MUSCLES

Muscle	Nerve supply	
Buccinator	Facial N	
Cricothyroid	External laryngeal	
Diaphragm	Phrenic N	C3,4,5
Digastric, anterior belly	Mandibular	
Digastric, posterior belly	Facial	
Frontal belly	Temporal br of 7th	
Lateral rectus	Abducent /6th	LR – 6
Levator palpebrae superioris	Oculomotor	
Mylohyoid	Trigeminal	
Occipital belly of occipitofrontalis	Posterior auricular branch of facial N	
Orbicularis oculi	Facial N	
Palatoglossus	Cranial accessory th. Vagus N	
Platysma	Facial N	
Stapedius	Facial N	
Sternomastoid	Spinal accessory	
Stylohyoid	Facial N	
Stylopharyngeus	Glossopharyngeal	
Superior oblique	Trochlear/ 4th	SO – 4
Tensor palati	Mandibular	
Tensor tympani	Mandibular	
Trapezius	Spinal accessory	

Muscles

- Most important muscle in **jaw protrusion** = lateral pterygoid m esp **inferior head**, it is attached to the pterygoid fovea on the condylar neck and joint capsule. Its superior head is attached to the articular disc and used for **power stroke**. This muscle esp inferior head, produces **pterygoid response** during treatment with myofunctional appliances.
- Most important muscle in **jaw retrusion** = temporalis
- **Sole opener** of rima glottidis = posterior crico = arytenoid
- **Sole protruder** of tongue = genioglossus
- Only muscle having **no attachment** from tendinous ring = inferior oblique muscle
- **Smallest muscle** of the body = stapedius
- **Longest muscle** of the body = sartorius
- **Boxer's muscle** = serratus anterior
- Climbing m = latissimus dorsi
- Locking m = popliteus
- Largest joint = knee joint

P-sympathetic fibres = in 3,7,9,10 Ns. and S2,3,4 (cranio-sacral)

Superior salivatory nucleus = supply for submandibular and sublingual glands

Inferior salivatory nucleus = supply for parotid gland

Sensations of **pain and temperature** carried by = Lateral spinothalamic tract.

- Pain mediator in PULP = Substance- P
- Pain mediator in rest body = Bradykinin

Lateral wall of nose

1. Sphenoethmoidal recess = Sphenoidal sinus opens here
2. Superior meatus = **Posterior ethmoidal** sinus opens here
3. Middle meatus = **Anterior and middle ethmoidal** sinus open here, **frontal** and **maxillary sinus** open here
4. Inferior meatus = Nasolacrimal duct.

Nerve supply of

1. **Lacrimal gland**	• Preganglionic through **N of pterygoid canal** • Postganglionic p-sympathetic fibres from **pterygopalatine ganglion**.
2. **Parotid gland**	• P-sympathetic fibres of **lessser petrosal N** relay in OTIC gang. • Postganglionic fibres supply to parotid gland through **auriculotemporal N**
3. **Thyroid gland**	• Mainly from middle cervical ganglion (vasoconstrictor)
4. **Submandibular gland**	• Preganglionic fibres through **chorda tympani N** (7th N) relay in submandibular gang. • Postganglionic fibres are secretomotor to SMG/SLG/anterior lingual glands.

- ♦ **Lacrimal N** = sensory, secretomotor (through **greater petrosal N**)
- ♦ **Greater petrosal N** - branch from 7th N
  - Gustatory - Does not relay in pterygopalatine ganglion
  - P-sympathetic – postganglionic fibres go to lacrimal gland.
- ♦ **N. of pterygoid canal** = Deep petrosal N (sympathetic) + greater petrosal N.
- ♦ **Deep petrosal N** (sympathetic) has post ganglionic fibres of superior cervical symp. ganglion; branches of symp. plexus around ICA.
- ♦ **Lesser petrosal N** (p-symp.) → preganglionic fibres of tympanic branch of 9th N.

Fibres relay in OTIC ganglion.

Postganglionic fibres supply PAROTID gland through auriculotemporal N.

Plexuses formed from —

♦ Cervical	Ventral rami of upper 4 cervical nerves
♦ Brachial	Ventral rami of lower 4 cervical nerves and part of ramus of ventral T1 N
♦ Lumbar	Ventral rami of first 3 lumbar nerves and part of 4th N
♦ Sacral	Lumbosacral trunk, ventral rami of 1,2,3 sacral nerves
♦ Coccygeal	Part of ventral ramus of S4, ventral ramus of S5 and coccygeal N

Nerves formed by

Lesser occipital	C2
Greater auricular	C2,3
Phrenic	C3,4,5
Musculocutaneous	C5,6,7
Median	C5,6,7,8, T1
Axillary	C5,6
Radial	C5,6,7,8, T1
Femoral	L2,3,4

Branches of the nerves

Trigeminal	Ophthalmic Maxillary Mandibular
Ophthalmic	Lacrimal Frontal = supratrochlear, supraorbital Nasociliary

Branches of the nerves (*Contd.*)

Maxillary	Meningeal branch Pterygopalatine ganglionic branch Zygomatic Posterior, middle and anterior Superior alveolar Palpebral; nasal; superior labial branch
Mandibular Also see p. 20, 26	Meningeal/nervous spinosus; Medial pterygoid; Deep temporal; bucccal; masseteric; Auriculotemporal; lingual; inferior alveolar and mylohyoid
Facial; lower facial ms have unilateral cortical represen-tation through opposite pyramidal tract; **upper facial ms have bilateral cortical representations**.	Chorda tympani; posterior auricular; lesser petrosal with otic ganglion; Temporal; zygomatic; buccal; marginal mandibular; cervical Nervus intermedius = is sensory com-ponent of 7th N.

Mental foramen at birth

- Mental Foramen opens below the sockets of premolars near lower border.
- Mandibular canal near lower border.
- Obtusegonial angle (≥140°), coronoid is longer and above the level of condyle

In adults - Mental F. midway between U/L borders.

- Mandibular canal runs parallel to mylohyoid line.
- Angle= 110–120°, ramus vertical.

In old age - Mental F. and mandibular canal close to Alveolar border/ ridge

- ≥140°, ramus oblique.

In injury to inferior alveolar N = Area supplied by mental N is **insensitive**

- Patient can not feel glass on the injured side, while drinking.

Hyoid

- Lies at **C3 level**, develops from cartilages of **2nd and 3rd branchial arches**
- Lesser cornu and (U) half of body = 2nd arch
- Greater cornu and (L) half of body = 3rd arch
- Ossifies from **6 centres** - 2 for body; 1 each for 4 cornus.

Centre of ossification appear - Just before birth = for greater cornu

- Shortly after birth = for body
- At puberty = for lesser cornu

Attachment of lesser cornu is fibrous throughout life.

Cervical vertebrae: 1,2,7 are atypical (Atlas, axis)

Stylohyoid = is **perforated by tendon of DG** muscle.

Sphenomandibular = remnant of Meckle's cartilage.

2 roots of auriculotemporal N = encircle the MMA.

CONTENTS OF THE FORAMINA

Carotid canal	ICA; sympathetic plexus
F of Luschka	Opening of lateral recess of 4th ventricle
F of Magendie	Median aperture in roof of 4th ventricle
F of Monro/ interventricular F	Opening of lateral ventricle into 3rd ventricle
F of Scarpa	Incisor formen in the mouth
F of Vesalli	Has Vs communicating the cevernous sinus to pterygoid plexus
F. ovale	Mandibular N; accessory meningeal A; lesser petrosal N; emissary V (**MALE**)

CONTENTS OF THE FORAMINA (*Contd.*)

F. rotundum	Maxillary N
F. spinosum; i.e. 3 M's	Middle meningeal A; meningeal branch of mandibular N; posterior trunk of middle meningeal V
Jugular canal	9th,10th,11th Ns; IJV; inferior petrosal sinus etc; sigmoid sinus;
Mandibular notch	Masseteric N and vessels
Optic canal	Optic N; ophthalmic A
Petrotympanic fissure	Chorda tympani N
Stylomastoid F	Facial N

GLANDS

Bartholin's	In labia majora
Brunner's	In duodenum
Cowper's	In bulbous part of urethra
Krause's	Are accessory lacrimal glands
Meibomian glands	Highly developed sebaceous glands of tarsal plate
Molar mucus gland	In buccopharyngeal fascia around parotid duct
Moll's glands	Modified sweat glands at the edge of the eyelid in the skin
Montgomery's	In the areola of breast
Zeis's	Differentiated sebaceous follicles in eyelashes in skin

DUCTS

Bellini	Straight collecting tubules of kidney
Rivinus/Bartholin's duct	of sublingual gland
Santorini	Accessory pancreatic duct
Stensen's	Of parotid gland
Wharton's	Of submandibular gland
Wirsung	Pancreatic duct

VARIOUS RECEPTORS

Nociceptors = pain

Chemoreceptors = chemical

Exteroceptors = fine touch

Proprioceptors = stretch reflex

Proprioceptors in ms spindles are = *annulospiral* endings and flower sprayed endings; for muscle tone.

And in golgi tendon organs = are *pacinian* corpuscles

Meissner's corpuscles	Touch
Pacinian corpuscles	Pressure
Free nerve endings	Pain
Krause's end bulbs	Cold
Ruffini's end organs	Heat
Organs of Corti	Sound
Rods and cones in retina	Vision
Utricle	Position of head wrt pull of gravity
Schnedeirian membrane	Olfaction

PARASYMPATHETIC GANGLIA OF HEAD AND NECK REGION

Ganglion	Trigeminal association, i.e. topographical connections	Parasymp./ motor /functional connections	Nucleus	Main Glands supplied
Ciliary	Ophthalmic div	Inferior div of 3rd N	Edinger–Westphal nucleus	——
Pterygopalatine	Maxillary div	Facial N; greater petrosal N	Superior salivatory	Lacrimal
Submandubular	Mandibular div th. Lingual N	Facial N through Chorda tympani	Superior salivatory	Submandibular, sublingual
Otic	Mandibular div	Glossopharyngeal th lesser petrosal N	Inferior salivatory	Parotid

LOCATION OF VARIOUS GANGLIA

Ganglion	Location
Gasserian / semilunar ganglion	Of 5th cranial nerve trunk
Ciliary ganglion	On ophthalmic N
Sphenopalatine ganglion	On maxillary N
Otic ganglion	On mandibular N
Submaxillary / Langley's ganglion	On lingual N
Geniculate ganglion	On facial N
Stellatelion	By union of 1st thoracic and lower cervical gang

COMPARISON B/W CAROTID SINUS AND CAROTID BODY

Carotid sinus	Carotid body
Baroceptor	Chemoceptor
Sensitive to BP changes	Stimulated by low O_2 tensions
Controls blood flow to brain	Regulates cardiac and respiratory rates
Supplied by 9th N	Supplied by 9th N

NERVOUS SYSTEM

Parasympathetic outflow = is **cranio-sacral,** i.e. 3, 7, 9, 10 cranial Ns and S2, 3, 4 spinal Ns.

Sympathetic outflow = is **thoraco-lumbar,** i.e. T 1 – 12, and L1, 2, 3 spinal Ns.

SALIVARY GLANDS

Gland	Duct	Status	Origin	Nerve	Artery
Parotid	Stensen	Serous	Ectoderm	Auriculo-temporal	Superior temporal
Submandibular	Wharton	Mixed; mainly serous	Endoderm	Facial	Facial
Sublingual	Rivinus ducts/ Bartholine's	Mainly mucus	Endoderm	Facial	Lingual and submental A.
Von – ebner's	Open in groove of circumvellate papillae	Serous			
Glands of Blandin and Nuhn	—	Mucous	—	—	—

CRANIAL NERVES

Nerves	**Attachments**
1, 2	Forebrain
3, 4	Mid brain
5–8	Pons
9–12	Medulla
Only cranial nerve coming from **dorsal side** of brainstem	Trochlear
Thinnest cranial nerve	Trochlear
Thickest cranial nerve	6th nerve
Longest intracranial course	6th N
Longest intracranial canal course	7th N
Musician's N	Ulnar
Saturday night palsy	Radial N
Labourer's N	Median N
Vidian N / N of pterygoid canal	Greater + deep petrosal Ns
Jacobson's N	Tympanic br of 9th N
Thickest cutaneous N	Greater occipital N / C2
Longest nerve	Sciatic N
Optic nerve	Is actually a tract of brain, carries with it the meningeal sheaths; so intracranial pressure of CSF is directly reflected in subarachnoid space of 2nd N;

Exit through cranium: of various cranial nerves is

I	Cribriform plate of ethmoid
II	Optic canal
III,IV,VI	Superior orbital fissure
Ophthalmic, V1	Superior orbital fissure
Maxillary, V2	Foramen rotundum
Mandibular, V3	Foramen ovale
VII	Stylomastoid foramen
VIII	________________
IX, X, XI	Jugular foramen
XII	Hypoglossal canal

Glands

- Zeis's glands = sebaceous glands of eyelashes
- Moll's glands = sweat glands in eyelids
- Mebomian's glands = sebaceous glands of tarsal plate
- Lacrimal glands = are serous glands

CONTENTS OF CAROTID SHEATH

1. CCA and ICA (**medially**)
2. IJV (**laterally**)
3. Vagus N (in **middle**) (longest cranial N)
4. Ansa cervicalis (in **anterior wall** of sheath)
5. Sympathetic chain (**posteriorly**)

CCA can be compressed against carotid tubercle, i.e. at anterior tubercle of transverse process of C6 which lies at cricoid level.

CAVERNOUS SINUS

1. In **lateral wall** = 3rd N, 4th N, ophthalmic N, maxillary N, trigeminal ganglion
2. In the **centre** = ICA, 6th N

STYLOID APPARATUS: has 3 muscles and 2 ligaments attached

- Stylohyoid muscle = reinforces DGP m.
- Styloglossus muscle
- Stylopharyngeus muscle = passes b/w ECA and ICA; enters pharynx b/w superior and middle constrictor ms; inserted on thyroid C.
- Stylohyoid ligament
- Stylomandibular ligament

Originate	From	Nerve supply
Styloid process; SHm; SH lig	2nd branchial arch	7th
SP m	3rd brachial arch	9th
SG m	Occipital myotomes	12th
SM lig	Deep fascia of neck	

Movements at the joints

1. Atlanto-occipital joint = nodding, i.e. **yes movement,** i.e. up - down
2. Atlanto-axial joint = negating, i.e. **no movements,** i.e. sideways rotatory
3. TMJ = upper compartment = gliding; lower compartment = rotatory movements

Lymphatics

1. Main LN of tongue= JUGULO – OMOHYIOD
2. Main LN of tonsil = JUGULO – DIGASTRIC
3. Thoracic duct drains in = left subclavian vein
4. Right lymphatic duct drains in = right subclavian vein

NOMENCLATURE

Supra-sternal space of BURNS	Sternal head of SCM m; jugular venous arch; lymph nodes; interclavicular ligament
Ligament of BERRY	Is suspensory ligament of thyroid gland, formed from pre-tracheal fascia.
Vidian N	Also ka nerve of pterygoid canal. It is formed by greater petrosal N and deep petrosal N
Waldeyer's ring of lymphatics	2 palatine tonsils + 1 pharyngeal tonsil + 1 lingual tonsil
Sinus of Morgagni	It is the gap b/w base of skull and upper border of superior constrictor m; the **contents of** this space are auditory tube; levator palati m; ascending palatine A.
Little's area	Lies in anterior part of septum, which is an anastomosis b/w superior labial A and spheno-palatine A.
Spaces of Fontanna	Thro' it, aqueous humor is drained from anterior chamber into anterior ciliary Vs.

OPENINGS INTO LATERAL WALL OF NOSE

♦ In spheno-ethmoidal recess	Sphenoid sinus
♦ In superior meatus; **smallest**	Posterior ethmoidal sinus
♦ In middle meatus	Middle ethmoidal sinus, Anterior ethmoidal sinus, Maxillary sinus, Frontal sinus
♦ In inferior meatus; **largest** meatus	Nasolacrimal duct through valve of Hasner

LEVELS

♦ Pharynx, 5" long	Upto C6 level
♦ Oesophagus, 10 – 15" long	From C6 to T 10 level
♦ CCA	Upto C4 (upper border of thyroid C)
♦ Trachea, 4 – 6" long	From C6 (lower border of cricoid C)
♦ Larynx	C3 – C6 level
♦ Spinal cord	Cord ends at lower border of L1vertebra; spinal dura at lower border of S2 vertebra

Arterial branches

1. Right CCA = branch of brachio-cephalic A
2. Left CCA = branch of arch of aorta

Nerves

1. Buccal N = **only sensory branch** of anterior trunk of mandibular N. (5th cranial N)
2. Mylohyoid N = has **all motor fibres of posterior div.** of mandibular N.

BRAIN

Cavities in brain

♦ Lateral ventricle	in cerebrum (in forebrain)
♦ Third ventricle	in diencephalon (in forebrain)
♦ Cerebral aqueduct	in mid brain
♦ 4th ventricle .	in hind brain

- foramen of Monro = opening of lateral ventricles in 3rd ventricle
- foramen of Luschka and F. of Magendie = drain CSF from 4th ventricle to sub-arachnoid space.
- Corpus callosum = joins the 2 cerebral hemispheres
- Vermis = joins the 2 cerebellar hemispheres
- In cerebrum =

  The precentral gyrus = is motor

  The postcentral gyrus = is sensory
- **Circle of Willis** = has *2 unpaired arteries,* i.e. ANTERIOR COMMUNICATING A and BASILAR A.
- **Vital centres,** i.e. respiratory and vasomotor, are situated in the **floor of 4th ventricle**, formed by medulla (the medullary depression in GA leads to death of the patient).
- OLFACTION is the only sensory path which directly reaches the cerebral cortex without passing through diencephalon (thalamus).
- **Sylvian sulcus** = divides frontal from parietal lobe.
- **Spinal cord** =

  Dorsal horn = sensory

  Ventral horn = motor

  Lateral horn = has preganglionic cell bodies of ANS i.e. (T1 – L2, S2 – 4.)
- Pure sensory nerves = 1, 2, 8 cranial Ns
- Pure motor nerves = 4, 6, 11, 12 nerves
- Mixed nerves = 3, 5, 7, 9, 10, nerves

PATHWAYS

1. LATERAL spino-thalamic tract = pain and temperature
2. Cell bodies of mechanoreceptors of PDL = in mesencephalic nucleus of 5th nerve
3. Primary sensory neurons nucleus of termination of pain pathway of tooth is in = spinal nucleus of 5th N

Quick revision points

- Sensation of pain and temperature are carried by = lateral spino-thalamic tracts.
- **Post-central gyrus** of cerebral cortex recognises **painful stimuli from teeth**; it is located in parietal lobe.
- General **sensory area** of brain is = posterior central gyrus.
- **Body temperature** is regulated by = hypothalamus.
- ANS regulation by = hypothalamus.
- Spinal cord is the only structure in CNS necessary for = simple reflex / reflex actions.
- Destruction of **cerebellum** causes loss of = voluntary muscular coordination.
- Cell bodies of **primary sensory neurons of mechano-receptors in PDL** are found in = **mesencephalic nucleus of 5th nerve,** i.e. proprioception.
- Primary sensory neurons nucleus of termination involved in pain from maxillary 7th tooth = is in spinal nucleus of 5th nerve, i.e. pain and temp.
- Preganglionic **parasympathetic fibres** pass through = superior orbital fissure and petro-tympanic fissure = i.e. 3rd nerve and chorda tympani nerve.
- Cerebellum = functions to modify the pattern of muscular response in reflex and **voluntary** contractions.
- Dorsal column system / ventral spino-thalamic tract = transmits touch, pressure, vibrations.
- Parkinsonism = i.e. patient has **resting tremors** = associated with basal ganglia deficit.
- **Intentional tremors** = if focal deficit in cerebellum.
- Destruction of ventro-medial nuclei which has **satiety centre** of hypothalamus = leads to obesity, i.e. increased food intake.
- Neuroectoderm / NCC = plays role in **dentin formation**; sympathetic ganglia neurons; **adrenal medulla**;
- Calcium trigger the contraction of muscles by binding to = troponin.

- TMJ = **fibrocartilge,** i.e. is not hyaline; forms articular disc; cover articular surfaces of head of condyle and articular tubercle of the temporal bone. It is a true synovial, ginglymo-arthroidal joint.
- Most imp muscle in jaw protrusion = lateral pterygoid.
- Most imp muscle in jaw retraction = temporalis.
- Muscles of tongue are = 9 pairs, i.e. 4 intrinsic and 5 extrinsic.
- Philtrum formed by = globular process.
- **Main mass of tongue** by = genioglossus
- **Waldeyer ring** has = palatine; lingual; and pharyngeal/ adenoid tonsils
- All salivary glands are = compound, racemose type.
- **Horner's syndrome** = constriction of pupils; ptosis; decreased sweating.
- 5th N = has no parasympathetic fibres.
- Only 3, 7, 9, 10 Ns have = parasympathetic fibres.
- **Betz cells** are = only in cerebral cortex.
- 5, 7, 9, 10, 11 Ns = special visceral efferent nuclei; are associated with pharyngeal arches.
- Nerves of branchiomeric segmentation = 5, 7, 9, 10, 11, 12 Ns, i.e. branchial arches I, II, III, IV, V, VI respectively.
- Somatic motor Ns = 3, 4, 6, 12 Ns + ventral roots of spinal nerves.
- **Phagocytes** of CNS = microglia cells.
- **Sensory ganglia** = on dorsal nerve roots of spinal Ns and 5, 7, 8, 9, 10 Ns.
- Nerves of special senses = 1, 2, 8 Ns are **entirely sensory** nerves.
- **Pure motor** nerves = 4, 6, 11, 12 Ns.
- Nerves of **somatic sensations** = 3, 4, 6, 12 Ns.
- Sympathetic nerves = thoraco-lumbar nerves, i.e. T1 – L 2.
- Parasympathetic nerves = cranio-sacral nerves, i.e. 3, 7, 9, 10 Ns + S 2- 4.
- Sensory ganglia are pseudo-unipolar type, except on 8th nerve which is bipolar.

Sympathetic nervous system

- Vasomotor = to blood vessels
- Sudomotor = to sweat glands
- Pilomotor = to errector pili ms. of hair follicles.

Exteroceptive receptors

1. Free nerve endings for pain, touch, esp in hair follicles.
2. Meissner's corpuscles for touch receptors
3. Pacini corpuscles pressure receptors
4. Krause/bulbous corpuscles controversial, regarded as regenerating or degenerating terminals of nerve fibres; are associated with cold.
5. Tactile discs of Merkel found in stratum spinosum.

Proprioceptive receptors

1. **Golgi tendon organs** = activated by pull upon the tendon during active contraction of muscles.
2. **Muscles spindles** = have intrafusal fibres; annulospiral endings are primary and flower spray endings are secondary; **maintain the tone of skeletal muscles**; it provides informations to brain about the extent and rate of stretching of muscles.

- Proprioception/mechanoceptor from head = in mesencephalic nucleus of 5th nerve.

Inferior oblique muscle of the eye = only muscle which **does not attach to** tendinous ring/ Tenon's capsule/ **annulus of Zinn.**

Transitional area of the lip has no glands so also ka **dry red area** of the lip.

Superior thyroid artery = is branch of **ECA**.

Inferior thyroid artery = is branch of thyrocervical trunk.

Berry's aneurysm = is related to circle of Willis.

There are no lymphatics in CNS.

CT sheath around the muscle as whole = ka epimysium.

CT sheath around the nerve fibre as whole = ka endoneurium.

GLANDS

- Parotid gland = ectodermal in origin
- Submandibular; sublingual; thyroid; parathyroid; thymus = are endodermal.
- Hassall's bodies in thymus = are vestiges of epithelium

Gland	Duct	Status	Salient features
Submandibular	Wharton's	Mixed	
Sublingual	Bartholin's	Mucus	
Parotid	Stensen's	Pure serous	
Von-Ebner's	In circumvallate papillae	Serous	
Other minor SGs		Mucous	Also labial, lingual glands
Glands of Blandin and Nuhn			Minor SGs in anterior tongue

Openings in sphenoid bone = forms **a crescent** which has

1. Superior orbital fissure
2. Foramen rotundum (FROS)
3. Foramen ovale
4. Foramen spinosum; they are arranged from anteriorly to posteriorly.

Parietal, frontal, maxilla, nasal bones are = entirely intramembranous.

Nasal conchae = are entirely endochondral.

Branches of maxillary nerve

1. Middle meningeal N.
2. Zygomatic N = Zygomatico-facial; Zygomatico-temporal N.

3. Pterygopalatine = orbital; posterior superior lateral nasal; medial septal; greater palatine; middle palatine; posterior palatine;
4. Posterior superior alveolar N
5. Infra orbital N = middle superior alveolar N; anterior superior alveolar N.
6. Terminal = lateral nasal; inferior palpebral N; superior labialis.

Branches of mandibular N

1. Undivided N = nervus spinosus; N to medial pterygoid M.
2. Anterior div = lateral pterygoid m; masseteric; temporal; long buccal; (**MOTOR**).
3. POSTERIOR DIV = auriculo-temporal N; lingual; inferior alveolar N; **(SENSORY)**.

BRANCHES OF FACIAL N

1. Branches in facial canal = greater petrosal N; (i.e. to pterygo-palatine ganglion); nerve to stapedius; chorda tympani N.
2. Branches which exit from stylomandibular foramen = posterior auricular; digastric; stylohyoid.
3. Terminal branches = temporal; zygomatic; buccal; marginal mandibular; cervical in a fan-shaped pattern.

Darwin's tubercle = i.e. auricular tubercle; on pinna of the ear.

NASION: Where internasal and frontonasal sutures meet.

PTERION: Frontal, parietal, temporal, sphenoid meet in (H-shape) suture (4 bones).

INION: Most prominent point on at occipital protuberance.

SCALP

Scalp = 5 layers, i.e. skin, CT; aponeurosis; loose areolar tissues; and periosteum.

2nd layer = provides proper medium for passage of BVs and Ns.

Wounds of scalp bleed profusely = because torn vessels are prevented from retracting by fibrous fascia.

Evulsed parts of scalp should not be cut away because = due to large blood supply.

3rd layer is freely movable on 5th = because of 4th layer, which is loose areolar tissue.

- 4th layer extends into eyelids (**frontalis has no bony attachments**). It is **Dangerous area of scalp** because of emissary Vs.

  Black eye may result by haemorrhage (**subaponeurotic space**).

  OCCIPITOFRONTALIS M.: Both bellies inserted in aponeurosis.

  Occipital ms = supplied by posterior auricular br of 7th **N**.

  Frontal ms = supplied by temporal br of 7th **N**.

- **Arterial supply** =

  Anterior to auricle = br of ECA and ICA, i.e. superficial temporal; supraorbital and supratrochlear (of ophthalmic A).

  Posterior to auricle = br of ECA, i.e. occipital and posterior auricular A.

VENOUS drainage

a. Supratrochlear + supraorbtial → Angular V → Facial V

b. Superficial temporal V. + Maxillary V → RMV

c. Anterior division of RMV + facial v → common facial v. → drains in ***IJV.***

d. Posterior division of RMV + posterior auricular v. → EJV → drains in subclavian v.

e. Occcipital v → drains in subocccipital venous plexus.

   Parietal emissary v → Drains in superior sagittal sinus

   Mastoid emissary → drains in sigmoid sinus.

   Occipital diploic V - drains in transverse sinus or in occipital V.

Lymphatic drainage

1. Anterior scalp = preauricular / parotid LN
2. Posterior scalp = posterior auricular / mastoid and occipital LN
3. Part of forehead above the root of the nose = submandibular LN.

Nerves = by 10 nerves per side, i.e. 4 sensory and 1 motor, in front and behind the auricle per side each.

Motor N = 7th N; temporal br (anterior to auricle); posterior auricular branch (posterior to auricle).

Sensory = branches of 5th N (anterior scalp), $C_{2,3,}$ C_2,C_3 (Posterior scalp).

FACE

MILIAN'S SIGN: Inflammation of subcutaneous tissues (cellulitis) stops short of auricle, but infections of skin (*erysipelas*) spread to whole external ear.

Wounds of scalp do not gape; but of face tend to gape.

All facial muscles are inserted in skin.

Facial muscles - S/C muscle, develop from mesoderm of 2nd arch, supplied by 7th N, remnants of **penniculus carnosus**

- Primary function of facial ms = to regulate facial opening.

Infranuclear lesion of 7th N = Bell's palsy, whole face paralysed, and drawn to normal side.

Supra nuclear lesion of 7th N = Only lower part paralysed.

At **pterygomandibular raphe** = Middle fibres of buccinator and superior constrictor ms. are attached.

Motor N of face = 7th N

Sensory N of face = 5th N; (**Cervical C2,3 plexus supplies only angle of the jaw** through anterior division of great auricular N.)

- Upper division of transverse (anterior) cutaneous N. of neck (C2,3) supplies lower margin of lower jaw.
- External acoustic meatus by V(1) N(mandibular) branch

Development = face develops by **3 processes** which corresponds to 3 div of 5th N., i.e. fronto-nasal; maxillary; mandibular; the **philtrum is supplied by max N**.

Cutaneous innervations = of 5th Ns are curved in postero-superior directions, i.e. in the direction of brain growth.

<u>**Port wine stains**</u>, i.e. congenital cutaneous nevi = involve accurately the **areas supplied by one / more div of 5th N.**

Facial A.= br of ECA; arises just above the tip of greater cornu of hyoid bone and terminates at medial angle of eye by supplying the LACRIMAL SAC and <u>anastomosing with dorsal nasal branch of ophthalmic A.(of ICA).</u>

- At **medial angle of eye = Anastomosis between ECA and ICA**. spread of infection to cranium.

<u>Transverse Facial A</u> = branch of superficial temporal a., Supplies PAROTID GLAND, duct, masseter, and overlying skin.

VEINS = drain in common facial V and RMV. Arranged as W-shape.

Largest V of face = facial V.

- Communicate with covernous sinus through ophthalmic V. brs.
- Joins with pterygoid plexus through Deep Facial V.
- **Dangerous Area of face** = (U) lip + (L) part of nose.

Lymphatics of face = 3 areas

1. **Preauricular**/parotid LNs = greater part of forehead, lateral halves of eyelid; conjunctiva; lateral part of cheeks; parotid area.
2. **Submandibular** LNs = middle, i.e. central strip of forehead; external nose; U lip; lateral part of L lip; medial ½ of eyelid; medial part of cheek; greater part of L jaw.
3. **Submental** LN = central part of L lip and chin.

Zeis's glands = sebaceous glands of cilia -in skin

Mole's glands = sweat glands of eye skin - in skin

Tarsal glands = open near the inner lip of free edge of eyelid.

Stye/ hordeolum = inflammation of Zeis glands.

Chalazion = inflammation of tarsal glands.

Lacrimal gland = serous; lies in antero-lateral part of roof of orbit. It is of J shape by tendon of levator M.

Nasolacrimal duct = open in inferior meatus of nose through **valve of Hasner** as opening.

SIDE OF NECK

Greater supraclavicular space = lies above and behind the middle 3rd of clavicle.

Lesser supraclavicular space = lies b/w sternal and clavicular part of SCM ms. overlies IJV.

Skin of neck supplied by 3 dermatomes - C2, C3, C4

- ♦ C1 has no cutaneous distribution
- ♦ C5,6,7,8 and T1 form brachial plexus
- ♦ C4 adjoins T2 dermatome at 2nd costal cartilage.

1. **Investing layer** = splits to enclose 2 glands, i.e. parotid gland and SMG, to enclose 2 ms. - SCM, trapezeus; forms 2 pulleys - to bind DG and omohyoid ms.

   Suprasternal space of Burns has = sternal head of SCM; jugular venous arch; lymph nodes; interclavicular ligament.

2. **Pretracheal fascia** = It encloses and suspends THYROID GLAND, forms suspensory ligament of thyroid gland (**ligament of Berry**) - attach to larynx.

3. **Carotid Sheath** - contains CCA, ICA, IJV, Vagus N

   - Vagus N lies posteriorly in between vein and arteries
   - Ansa cervicalis - in Ant. wall of C.sheath
   - Cervical symp. chain = behind the sheath
   - CCA / ICA - medially / IJV laterally /vagus (posteriorly).

EJV is formed by **union of posterior auricular V and posterior div of RMV** and opens in SCV. Oblique JV connects EJV and IJV at middle 3rd of anterior border of SCM m. Right atrial pressure is reflected in it as it has no valves.

Posterior triangle is subdivided **by inferior belly of omohyoid**.

3 trunks of brachial plexus emerge b/w = scalenus anterior and S. medius ms.

Left supraclavicular LNs (**Virchow's** or scalene LN) = aka **signal nodes**.

Torticollis or wry neck = is due to spasm of ms supplied by spinal accessory N, i.e. SCM and trapezius.

SCM - Motor = spinal accessory N

sensory = ventral ramis of C2 (3) - proprioceptive

BACK OF NECK

Skin - by dorsal rami of C2 (great occipital N)

- by dorsal rami of C3 (3rd occipital N)
- by dorsal rami of C4
- Dorsal ramus of C1 does not divide in medial and lateral branches and is distributed to ms bounding the suboccipital triangle of neck.
- Each dorsal ramus (i.e. posterior primary ramus) - gives medial brs. and lateral brs., both supply intrinsic ms. of back.

Greater occipital N = Large medial branch of dorsal ramus of C2

- **Thickest cutaneous** N. of body
- Supplies scalp and semispinalis capitis

CONTENTS OF VERTEBRAL CANAL

- Spinal cords ends at (lower) border of L1
- Spinal dura ends at (lower) border of S2
- Arachnoid dura ends at (lower) border of S2,
- Subarachnoid space - lumbar puncture = L3-L4 vertebral region
- SPINAL PIA mater - continued as FILUM TERMINALE
- Filum terminale = is 20 cm long; mainly of pia mater;
- Total no. of vertebrae in the vertebral column = 33 ($C_7T_{12}L_5S_5C_4$)
- Total no. of inter-vertebral discs = 23 – 24
- Total no. of spinal Ns = 31 Pairs

SPINAL CORD: Occupies upper 2/3 of vertebral canal

- From (U) border of C1 to (L) border of L1 or U border of L2. 18 inches / 45 cm long.
- 31 pairs of spinal Nerves - C8, T12, L5, S5, C1

CRANIAL CAVITY

Dura/pachymeninx = thickest; has 2 layers, i.e. endosteal and meningeal (protective) ; the endosteal layer has venous sinuses; the meningeal layer forms 4 folds, i.e. falx cerebri; falx cerebelli; tentorium cerebelli; and diaphragma-sellae, to divide the cranial cavity in different compartments.

Subarachoid space = has CSF in it.

Falx cerebri – has 3 sinuses, i.e.

- Straight sinus - at posterior end, along median plane,
- Superior sagittal sinus - along the upper margin
- Inferior sagittal sinus - along the lower margin in posterior 2/3 part.

Tentorium cerebelli: forms the roof of posterior cranial fossa; it forms trigeminal / Meckel's cave; it has 2 **sinuses.**

- Transverse sinus
- Superior petrosal sinus.

Falx cerebelli: encloses the **occipital sinus**.

Diaphragma sellae: forms the roof of hypophyseal fossa.

Nerve supply of dura: by 5, 9, 10 Ns; C 1,2,3 Ns.

Vault = by ophthalmic N.

DIFFERENCE B/W EXTRADURAL AND SUBDURAL HEMORRHAGE

Extradural	**Subdural**
Less common	More
Arterial ; **MMA** is involved	Venous
Late S/S of compression appear	Quick
Lucid interval is present	Absent
Paralysis first appears in face and marches down.	Haphazard
No blood in CSF is seen	Present

SINUSES : 15 in no.,

Paired	**Unpaired**
Cavernous; significant for eye surgeon	Superior sagittal; for neuro-physician
Superior petrosal sinus	Inferior sagittal
Inferior petrosal	Straight
Transverse	Occipital
Sigmoid; for ENT surgeon	Anterior intercavernous
Sphenoparietal	Posterior intercavernous
Petrosquamous	Basilar plexus of Vs.
MM veins	

1. Cavernous sinus: structures passing through lateral wall of the sinus: from upward to downwards are

1. 3rd nerve = superior and inferiors; pass through superior orbital fissure's tendinous ring.
2. 4th nerve = superficial to 3rd nerve.
3. Ophthalmic N = has L,F,N branches.
4. Maxillary N.
5. Trigeminal ganglion.

Structures **passing through center** of the sinus are

1. ICA + venous and sympathetic plexus.
2. 6th N = inferolateral to ICA.

Draining channels in cavernous sinus =

1. in transverse sinus = through superior petrosal sinus
2. in IJV = through inferior petrosal sinus and venous plexus of ICA.
3. **Facial V** = has 2 direct connections with cavernous sinus; through superior ophthalmic Vs ; and through deep facial V to pterygoid plexus; important as it may cause spread of infection to the cranial from face.

4. To pterygoid plexus = through emissary Vs passing through F. ovale; F. lacerum; sphenoidal foramen.

2. Superior sagittal sinus: **largest** sinus; continues as **right transverse** sinus;

3. Confluence of sinuses : lies on right side; continues as right transverse sinus; receives the CSF;

4. Inferior saggital sinus: ends by joining greater cerebral V and forms **straight sinus**.

5. Straight sinus: lies in the junction of F. cerebri and T. cerebelli; inferior saggital sinus and greater cerebral V form it; **continues as left transverse** sinus;

6. Transverse sinus: continues as **sigmoid sinus**;

7. Sigmoid sinus: continues as **superior bulb of IJV**; internal auditory Vs drains in it. Grooves mastoid part of temporal bone.

8. Lateral sinus: sigmoid sinus + transverse sinus.

9. Occipital sinus: **smallest**; ends in the confluence of sinuses.

10. Sphenoparietal sinus: lies along posterior free margins of lesser wing of sphenoid; drains in anterior part of cavernous sinus.

11. Superior petrosal sinus = drains cavernous sinus into transverse sinus; receives tympanic Vs; crosses 5th N anteriorly.

12. Inferior petrosal sinus: lies in petro-occipital fissures; drains cavernous sinus into IJV (superior bulb);

13. Basilar plexus of Vs = connects 2 inferior petrosal sinus; communicates with inferior petrosal sinuses;

14. Petrosquamous sinus = drains in transverse sinus.

Pituitary gland

Adenohypophysis: develops as upward growth of Rathke's pouch from **ectodermal** roof of stomodeum.

Anterior lobe = largest.

Intermediate lobe = remnants of lumen of Rathke's pouch; releases MSH.

Tuberal lobe = upward extension of anterior lobe.

Neurohypophysis: develops as downward growth **from floor of diencephalone**

Posterior lobe = smaller than anterior lobe. Has large no. of non-myelinated fibres as **hypothalamo-hypophyseal tract**; and modified neuroglial cells/pituicytes.

Infundibular stem = contains neural connections of posterior lobe with hypothalamus.

	Cells	**Hormones**
Acidophils / alpha cells/ 43 %	Somatotrophs	GH, STH
	Mammotrophs; prolactin cells	Lactogenic H
	Corticotrophs	ACTH
Basophils/ beta cells/ 7 %	Thyrotrophs	TSH
	Gonadotrophs	FSH
	Luteotrophs	LH / ICSH
Posterior lobe These 2 hormones are actually secreted by hypothalamus.	Vasopressin / ADH Oxytocin	On kidney tubules Promotes contraction of uterine and mammary smooth ms.

Arterial supply = Anterior lobe is exclusively by portal vessels arising from capillary tufts formed by superior hypophyseal A, a branch of ICA.

Portal vessels carry hormone releasing factors from hypothalamus to anterior lobe.

Acidophilic adenoma = causes **gigantism**; acromegaly.

Basophilic adenoma = causes **Cushing's syndrome**

Chromophobes adenoma = hypopituitarism

Posterior lobe damage = diabetes insipidus.

TRIGEMINAL GANGLION: aka semilunar/**Gasserian ganglion**. Lies in trigeminal Impression on apex of petrous temporal bone.

- Sensory; homologous to dorsal nerve root gang; all such ganglia are made of pseudounipolar nerve cells having a T-shape arrangement of processes.
- Central process = for sensory root
- Peripheral process = forms **3 divs of the 5th nerve**;
- Large sensory root = both attached to pons
- **Small motor root** = joins mandibular N at F. ovale.
- Blood supply = by ICA, MMA, etc.

Middle Meningeal A

- Branch of 1st part of maxillary A in infratemporal fossa.
- Chief source of **extradural hemorrhage** mainly its frontal branch; which after crossing **pterion** lies closely to **motor area** of brain. Its parietal br lies 4 cm above pterion.
- Passes through a loop formed by **2 roots of auriculotemporal nerve**.

Cranial Ns	Exit / Passes through
I	Cribriform plate of ethmoid
II	Optic canal with ophthalmic A
III, IV	Posterior part of roof of cavernous sinus
V	Crosses apex of petrous temporal beneath superior petrosal sinus
VI	Lower part of posterior wall of cavernous sinus; runs below petrosphenoidal ligament.
VII, VIII	Thro' internal acoustic meatus with labyrinthine vessels
IX, X, XI	Pierces dura at jugular F and pass through it.
XII	Thro' hypoglossal canal

ICA: CCA divides at the level of **upper border of thyroid C**. It has 4 parts, i.e.

1. Cervical = in carotid sheath; has no branches.
2. Petrous = in carotid canal of petrous temporal bone;
3. Cavernous
4. Cerebral = ophthalmic br supplies to orbit; rest branches supply to brain.

Petrous, cavernous, cerebral branches form **S–shaped** figure ka **carotid siphon**.

Greater petrosal N + deep petrosal N = **N of pterygoid canal.**

Nerve	Br of	Nature	Relays in	Supply
Greater petrosal N.	7th N, geniculate gang	p-symp gang.	Pterygopalatine and mucosal	Lacrimal gland glands of nose, palate, pharynx
Deep petrosal N	Superior Cervical gang; C 1 – 4 nerves; ICA	Symp	Thro' Pterygopalatine gang.	
Lesser petrosal N, through F. ovale	9th N	p-symp	Otic gang	Parotid gland through auri-culotemporal N.
External petrosal N	7th N; geniculate MMA gang;	Symp		

CONTENTS OF THE ORBIT

- Long axis of each orbit passes backward and medially; so **medial walls are parallel** to each other.
- Orbital fascia = is continuous with dura mater and sheath of optic N.
- Bulbar fascia has following parts:

1. **Tenon's capsule** = extends from the optic N to sclero-corneal junction.

2. Tubular sheath = covers each orbital ms.
3. Medial check ligament = from the sheath of MR; attached to lacrimal bone.
4. Lateral check ligament = from the sheath of LR; attached to zygomatic bone.

- **Suspensory lig. of Lockwood** = part of Tenon's capsule is thickened to form it; lies as **hammock** below the eyeball. It is formed by the union of margins of sheaths of IR and IO with medial and lateral check ligaments.
- **Extraocular ms** = 4 recti ms originate from common tendinous ring; ring encloses optic canal and middle part of superior orbital fissure.
- **3 involuntary ms** = superior tarsal elevates the eyelid; inferior tarsal depresses lower eyelid. Orbitalis bridges the inferior orbital fissure.
- Distal tendons = of **MR is shortest**; of LR is longest.
- SO passes through a pulley attached to trochlear fossa of frontal bone.
- Recti are inserted in sclera, posterior to **limbus**.
- Obliqui are inserted in sclera b/w SR and LR, behind equator of eyeball.
- **Levator palpebrae superioris** = its superior lamella is inserted in anterior surface of superior tarsus and skin; its inferior lamella is inserted in upper margin of superior tarsus.
- Nerve supply = SO – 4th ; LR – 6th ; rest 5 ms by 3rd N.

SUPERIOR ORBITAL FISSURE: divided in 3 parts by **tendinous ring of Zinn**;

1. Lateral part = LFT nerves; superior ophthalmic V, etc.
2. Middle part = 3rd as superior and inferior rami, 6th, nasociliary Ns.
3. Medial part = inferior ophthalmic V; symp plexus around ICA.

- Optic canal = contains optic N and ophthalmic A (A. lies in common dural sheath with optic N, infero-lateral to it).

- Ophthalmic A = is a br of ICA, terminates near medial angle of eye by dividing into supratrochlear and dorsal nasal branch
- Optic N = covered by 3 meningeal layers; has no neurilemmal sheath/ schwann cells; so it cannot regenerate
- Developmentally, optic N and retina are **direct prolongation of brain**.

Blood supply of nasal cavity is by =

- Upper part = by ICA (i.e. by br of ophthalmic A)
- Lower part = by ECA branches.

Oculomotor N = is **somatic motor** nerve; like 4, 6, 12 Ns and ventral root of spinal nerves, it supplies to all ms of eye except SO, LR. Its superior ramus supplies to SR and LPS ms; and inferior ramus supplies to MR, IR, IO ms. Nerve to IO is longest and gives off motor root to ciliary ganglion and enter IO on its posterior border.

Trochlear nerve = the **only cranial N** which emerges **on dorsal aspect** of brain stem. Lies in lateral part of cavernous sinus b/w 3rd N and ophthalmic N.

Ophthalmic N = branches are lacrimal N which is its smallest terminal br; supplies to lacrimal gland; conjunctiva and upper eyelid. Frontal br is largest terminal branch; nasociliary br is the 3rd branch (LFN).

Sympathetic nerve of orbit = arise from ICA plexus; dilator pupillae m. of iris is supplied through long ciliary br of nasociliary nerve via ophthalmic N.

ANTERIOR TRIANGLE OF NECK

- Isthmus of thyroid gland = against 2 – 4th tracheal rings.
- Transverse process of C 4 vertebra = at upper border of thyroid C.
- Transverse process of C 6 vertebra = cricoid C.
- Anterior tubercle of transverse process of C 6 = largest and is ka **carotid tubercle of Chassaignac**.
- **Platysma** = lies in superficial fascia; is a subcutaneous m.; releases pressure of skin over subjacent superficial vs; all superficial Ns, vs, in this area lie deep to this muscle.

- Anterior jugular V = lies in **suprasternal space of Burns**; R and L are joined by jugular arch; it drains in EJV.
- Structures lying superficial to mylohyoid ms = superficial part of SMGland with facial V and submental LNs superficial to it; and facial A deep to it.
- Structures lying **superficial to hyoglossus** ms = central tendon of DG m; bifurcated tendon of stylohyoid; 12th N.
- **Suspensory ligament of Berry** = is formed by false capsule of thyroid gland and it suspends the gland to the cricoid C;
- **Thyrohyoid membrane** = pierced by internal laryngeal and superior laryngeal vessels;
- **Cricothyroid** m = supplied by external laryngeal N.
- **All infrahyoid** ms (SH, ST, OH) are supplied by ANSA CERVICALIS except thyrohyoid m which is supplied by C 1 through 12th N.
- Anterior triangle is divided in 4 parts by = DG supplemented by SH m and superior belly of OH.
- 4 supra hyoid ms = DG, stylohyoid; mylohyoid; geniohyoid.
- 4 infra hyoid ms = sternohyoid; sternothyroid; thyrohyoid; omohyoid.

Submental triangle = has 2 – 4 submental LNs in superficial fascia which drain the

1. Superficial tissues below the chin.
2. **Central part of lower lip.**
3. Adjacent gums.
4. Anterior part of floor of mouth.
5. **Tip of the tongue**
6. Its efferents go to submand. LNs.

STRUCTURES PASSING B/W ECA and ICA: 6 structures

1. Styloglossus
2. Stylopharyngeus
3. 9th N

4. Pharyngeal br of 10th N
5. Styloid process
6. Part of parotid gland.

SUBMANDIBULAR LNs: lie below the deep cervical fascia; on the surface of SMG. Its **efferents go to JO mainly** and JD LNs partly. They drain the:

- **center of forehead**
- nose with frontal, maxillary, ethmoidal sinuses
- inner canthus of the eye
- **upper lip** and anterior part of cheek with gum / teeth.
- **Outer part of upper lip** with gum / teeth (excluding incisors)
- **Anterior 2/3rd part of tongue** and floor of mouth (excluding tip of tongue)
- Efferents from **submental LNs**.

Deep cervical LNs are found in carotid triangle along the IJV as

1. JD = **below posterior belly of DG m.**
2. JO = **above the inferior belly of OH m.**

COMMON CAROTID A.

- Right CCA = branch of **brachiocephalic**; **begins in neck** behind right sternoclavicular joint.
- Left CCA = branch of **arch of aorta**; **begins in thorax**.
- R and L CCAs run in carotid sheath in front of lower 4 cervical transverse processes;
- At **upper border of thyroid C** = ECA and ICA are formed.
- **Carotid sinus** =at the beginning of ICA; 9th N and sympathetic N; baroreceptor; regulates BP in cerebral As.

Carotid body

- Behind the bifurcation of CCA;
- Supplied mainly by **9th N; 10th N** and sympathetic N.

- Develops from **mesoderm of 3rd** branchial arch.
- **Chemoreceptor** = controls O_2 / CO_2 level in blood.
- Other chemoreceptors found at the arch of aorta, ductus arteriosus; and right SCA = supplied by 10th N.

ECA

1. Begins at the upper border of thyroid C; opposite the **disc b/w C3 and C4**.
2. Terminates behind the neck of mandible in 2 branches = maxillary and superficial temporal.
3. Lies below the anterior border of SCM m.
4. Deep to ECA are = ICA; 6 structures b/w ECA and ICA; 2 structures deep to ICA are superior laryngeal N and superior cervical sympathetic ganglion.
5. 8 **branches** = (S L F O P A S M)

Direction	**Branches**	**Imp points**
Anterior = 3	Superior thyroid; lingual; facial	
Posterior = 2	Occipital; posterior auricular	
Medial = 1	Ascending pharyngeal	**The only medial branch**
Terminal = 2	Maxillary; superficial temporal	

1. Superior thyroid A = *1st anterior branch*, arises **below the level of greater cornu** of hyoid. Its relation to external laryngeal N/ cricothyroid m is important and it should be ligated nearest to the thyroid gland to avoid injury to nerve.
2. Lingual = arises **opposite the tip of greater cornu of hyoid**; is divided in 3 parts by hyoglossus m. it forms a lingual loop in carotid triangle which **permits free movement of hyoid** bone. During tongue removal, its first part is ligated before any branching occurs to tongue or tonsils.

3. Facial A = arises just **above the tip of the greater cornu** of hyoid. It has a tortuous course to allow **for free movement of pharynx, mandible**, lip, cheek, etc. its cervical part grooves posterior border of SMG.

Branches	**Supply to**	**Imp points**
Ascending palatine	Soft palate	Pass b/w styloglossus and stylopharyngeus ms.
Tonsillar	Tonsil	Is its **main artery**.
Glandular	SMG, LNs	
Submental	SLG, submental triangle	

4. Posterior auricular A = is the 2nd posterior branch; arises just above the DGP m; its stylomastoid branch supplies to middle ear; facial N; semicircular canal; mastoid antrum and air cells;
5. Maxillary A = **larger terminal** branch; begins behind the neck of the mandible; under cover of the parotid gland;
6. Superficial temporal A = behind the neck of the mandible; its anterior branch joins the supraorbital and supratrochlear branches of ophthalmic A (ICA); it gives transverse facial A.

ANSA CERVICALIS: aka ansa hypoglossi;

1. It is formed by C1, 2, 3,
2. Lies in the **anterior wall of carotid sheath**, at the level of lower part of larynx.
3. Supplies infrahyoid ms *except thyrohyoid* which is supplied by C1 through 12th N.
4. **Superior root** supplies to = superior belly of OH
5. **Ansa cervicalis** to = SH, ST, OH-Inferior
6. Thyrohyoid, geniohyoid ms = by separate branch of C 1 th 12th N.

MUSCULAR TRIANGLE

- Infrahyoid ms form the floor of the triangle; i.e. sternohyoid, sternothyroid, thyrohyoid; omohyoid;
- All ms are derived from **longitudinal rectus sheet**.
- Arranged in 2 layers, i.e. superficial layer (of SH, OH); and deep layer (ST, TH)
- All ms are supplied by **ventral rami of C1,2,3 nerves / ansa cervicalis**.
- **Omohyoid ms** = arises by inferior belly and inserted by superior belly; the **central tendon is at the level of CRICOID C**; superior belly is supplied by superior root of ansa cervicalis; inferior belly by ansa cervicalis.

PAROTID GLAND

- Development = from **ectoderm**; i.e. from buccal epithelium.
- Is **largest** salivary gland; is inverted pyramid shape; **pure serous** gland; enclosed in splitted cervical fascia.
- It is **separated from SMG by stylomandibular-ligament** (which is formed by deep lamina of the cervical fascia).
- At **apex of the gland** = cervical br of 7th N and the 2 divisions of RMV emerge.
- Its antero-medial border = is related to emerging branches of 7th N.; is grooved by posterior border of ramus.
- At the **anterior border**, following structures emerge from it = parotid duct; branches of facial N; transverse facial vessels; accessory parotid gland.
- **Structures within the parotid gland** = from mesial to lateral side are = ECA, RMV, facial nerve; (RMV is formed within the gland by joining of the superficial temporal and maxillary Vs).
- **Parotid duct** = opens opposite the crown of max 2nd molars.
- Parotid abscess = best evacuated by Hilton's method / horizontal incision.

Nerve supply

1. P-sympathetic = secretomotor. The preganglionic fibres from **inferior salivatory nucleus** via 9th **N** to otic ganglion. Post-ganglionic fibres from otic ganglion via **auriculotemporal N**.
2. Sympathetic = vasomotor; from the plexus around ECA.
3. Sensory = auriculotemporal N.
4. Parotid fascia = by greater auricular N / C2.

Lymphatics = in parotid/preauricular LNs which goes to upper deep cervical LNs.

They drain = temple/side of scalp; lateral surface of auricle; external acoustic meatus; middle ear; parotid gland; upper part of cheek; part of eyelid; orbit.

FACIAL N: also supplies to stapedius / DGP/ stylohyoid / platysma/ facial ms.

- It is the nerve of **2nd branchial arch**.
- It is motor to face, i.e. ms of 2nd arch = branchial efferent / branchiomotor
- **Secretomotor**/p-sympathetic / general visceral efferent to = SMG; SLG; lacrimal glands, minor SGs of palate/ nose, etc.
- **Gustatory** / special visceral afferent = to anterior 2/3rd of tongue. (through Chorda Tympanic Nerve)
- General somatic afferent / proprioception from ms = go to mesencephalic nucleus of 5th N.
- Lower facial ms = have unilateral representation through opposite pyramidal tract.
- Upper facial ms = have bilateral representation through both sides pyramidal tract.
- Its sensory root is ka. **nervus intermedius**.
- Motor root lies in a groove on 8th N with sensory root intervening in the internal acoustic meatus.
- The 2 roots fuse at the bottom of meatus and enter the facial canal.
- Comes out of **stylomastoid foramen**.

- Divides behind the neck of condyle in **5 terminal branches** = temporal, zygomatic, buccal, mandibular, cervical.
- Stapedius ms = dampens excessive vibration of the sound.
- **Chorda tympani** = supplies secretomotor fibres to SMG / SLG via lingual n; and carries taste sensation from anterior 2/3rd of tongue.
- Posterior auricular n = supplies to auricularis posterior; occipitalis; intrinsic ms on the back of auricle.
- Temporal br = auricularis superior and anterior ms; intrinsic ms of lateral side of ear; frontalis; orbicularis oculi; corrugator supercilli;
- Cervical br = platysma.
- 2 ganglia = SM ganglion = for p-sympathetic fibres of chorda tympani N; pterygopalatine ganglion for p-sympathetic fibres of greater petrosal n.

TEMPORAL AND INFRATEMPORAL REGION

- **pterion** = where 4 bones, i.e. frontal, parietal, squamous temporal and greater wing of sphenoid bones join; is H –shape (FPTS).
- Masseter, temporalis, lateral pterygoid and medial pterygoid ms are arranged in this order from superficial to deep plane (MTLM).
- Elevators of jaw are = MMT.
- Temporal fascia = splits inferiorly to attach at upper border of zygomatic arch; the gap contains **branch of superficial temporal A, zygomatic temporal N and fat**.
- Superficial surface of temporal fascia = gives origin to **auricularis anterior and superior** ms.
- Deep surface of temporal fascia = gives origin to **temporalis ms**.
- Paralysis of mandibular N = on opening of mouth – the **jaw deviates towards the paralysed side**; which is due to normal lateral pterygoid m of opposite side.
- Maxillary A and buccal br of mandibular N lie = b/w the 2 heads of lateral pterygoid m.

Functions and Nerve supply of masticatory ms

1. Masseter	br of anterior div of mandibular N.
2. Temporalis	2 brs of anterior div of mandibular N.
3. Lateral pterygoid	br of anterior div of mandibular N.
4. Medial pterygoid	br of *main trunk* of mandibular N.
5. Side to side grinding movement = by lateral and medial pterygoids acting alternately.	
6. Depression = mainly by lateral pterygoid; assisted by DG; GH; mylohyoid.	

MAXILLARY A. = is the larger terminal branch of ECA;

It is divided in 3 parts **by lateral pterygoid** m. The pterygopalatine part lies b/w the 2 heads of lateral pterygoid m and PTM fissure. The mandibular part runs along the lower border of the muscle.

TEMPORO-MANDIBULAR JOINT

- Lateral ligament aka TM lig = is the main lig of TMJ.
- Joint cavity is divided in 2 parts by the articular disc.
- Upper compartment = only gliding movement.
- Lower compartment = both rotation and gliding movements.
- **Articular disc** = is **avascular in the center**. It has concavo-convex superior surface and concave inferior surface.
- **Sphenomandibular ligament** = from spine of sphenoid to lingula of mandibular foramen; it is a **remnant of cephalic / dorsal end of Meckel's cartilage**. It is pierced by **mylohyoid Ns and vessels** at its lower end.
- **Stylomandibular lig.** = is thickened part of deep cervical fascia; it separates the parotid gland from the SMG. It runs from the styloid to the angle/posterior border of the ramus.

- Blood supply = by superficial temporal A and br of maxillary A.
- Nerve supply = by auriculotemporal N and masseteric N.

MANDIBULAR N

- Is the **largest** div of 5th n; is the nerve of 1st branchial arch.
- It is **mixed nerve** = large sensory + small motor nerve.
- Comes out through **foramen ovale**.
- Divisions = small anterior + large posterior trunks.

Branches

Main trunk Meningeal br, i.e. nervous spinosus	Anterior div; **mixed** Buccal N / **sensory**	Post div. / **sensory** Inferior alveolar N
Nerve to medial pterygoid, which supplies to medial pterygoid, tensor palatei and tensor tympani ms	**Motor** br, i.e. masseteric; deep temporal; nerve to lateral pterygoid ms,	Auriculo-temporal n Lingual

Nervous spinosus = lies in foramen spinosum with MMA; supplies the dura of middle cranial fossa.

Buccal nerve = is **the only sensory br of anterior trunk**.

Masseteric nerve = passes through the mandibular notch.

Auriculotemporal nerve

1. Arises by 2 roots; encircles the MMA;
2. Ascends on temple behind the superficial temporal vessels;
3. Its auricular part supplies branches to skin of tragus; upper parts of pinna; external auditory meatus and tympanic membrane (the lower parts of these 3 areas are supplied by greater auricular nerve and auricular br of 10th nerve).

4. It is secretomotor and sensory to parotid gland and also supplies to TMJ.

Lingual nerve

1. It is the terminal br; arises 1 cm below skull;
2. It is sensory to anterior 2/3rd of tongue and floor of mouth;
3. Chorda tympani n = a branch of 7th nerve; is secretomotor/p-sympathetic to SMG/SLG; gustatory to anterior 2/3rd of the tongue.
4. Has a direct contact with mandible, medial to 3rd molar; b/w superior constrictor and mylohyoid ms.

Inferior alveolar n

1. Larger terminal br;
2. Its mylohyoid br = **contains all the motor fibres of the posterior div**.; supplies to MH and DGA.
3. Mental n = to skin of chin; skin and mucous membrane of lower lip;

Rx of trigeminal neuralgia = sensory root is divided behind the ganglion; but superomedial ophthalmic fibres should be spared to avoid neuropathic keratitis.

SUBMANDIBULAR REGION

- 4 Suprahyoid ms = DG (5 / 7 th n); SH (7th n); MH (5th n); GH (C 1 n.); derived from 1st / 2nd branchial arches and 1st cervical myotome.
- Structures lying superficial to MH m = DGA; superficial part of SMG, etc.
- Structures lying deep to MH m = hyoglossus m with its superficial relations, i.e. styloglossus, lingual n, SM ganglion; deep part of SMG; SM duct; 12th n; (ie structures lying b/w MH and hyoglossus).
- Structures lying superficial to MH m = i.e. b/w genioglossus and MH = SLG; lingual N,A; SM duct; 12th n.

- Structures passing **deep to posterior bcrder of hyoglossus** m from above downwards are = 9th n; stylohyoid lig; lingual n.

- DG m = 2 heads meet at intermediate tendon which *perforates* the *stylohyoid*. DGA is supplied by mylohyoid br of mandibular n; DGP by br of facial n.

SUBMANDIBULAR GLAND

1. **Mostly serous**; J shaped by mylohyoid ms; fills the digastric triangle; gives 60% of total saliva; **most common site of sialoliths**.
2. Covered by the splitted deep cervical fascia.
3. Superficial part is larger than the deep part. Deep part **lies deep to mylohyoid** m and superficial to hyoglossus and styloglossus ms.
4. Medial surface is related to lingual N, 9th N, 12th N, SM ganglion;
5. SM duct / **Wharton's duct** = runs b/w 12th N and lingual N; opens at the summit of sublingual papillae.
6. **Nerve supply** = secretomotor = chorda tympani through lingual N to SM ganglion. Sensory through lingual N; vasomotor sympathetic N through facial A plexus.
7. This gland is palpable bimanually; but the SM lymph nodes can be felt only outside.
8. SM ganglion = suspended from the lingual N by 2 roots. Functionally related to chorda tympani N (facial N).
9. Motor/p-sympathetic root = is branch of lingual N; posterior root; preganglionic fibres come from the superior salivatory nucleus through facial/chorda-tympani/ lingual n to relay in SMGanglion.
10. Sensory root = is also branch of lingual n.
11. Sympathetic = posterior ganglionic fibres of superior cervical ganglion through facial A plexus.

MAIN BLOOD SUPPLY OF DIFFERENT GLANDS

Gland	Nature	Blood supply
Lacrimal	Serous	Lacrimal A, the branch of ophthalmic A, i.e. of ICA
SLG	Mucus	Lingual A + submental A (of facial A)
SMG	Mixed	Facial A
Parotid	Serous	Transverse facial A (from superficial temporal A/ECA)
Thyroid	Endocrine	Inferior and superior thyroid As
Tonsils	Lymphoid	Facial A
Thymus		Inferior thyroid and internal thoracic As

SUBLINGUAL GLAND

- Is the **smallest** gland; mostly **mucus**;
- Lies **above the mylohyoid m** and below the mucosa of floor of mouth.
- 15 ducts; open at the summit of sublingual folds, as Bartholin's/ Rivinus duct.

DEEP STRUCTURES OF THE NECK

Thyroid gland = lies in the region of C5, 6, 7, and T 1 vertebrae.

- Lobe = from middle of thyroid C to 4 – 5th tracheal ring
- Isthmus = 2nd – 4th tracheal ring.
- False capsule = pretracheal layer of deep cervical fascia; **suspensory ligament of Berry** attached to the cricoid C.
- Its medial surface is related to = external laryngeal and recurrent laryngeal Ns.
- Blood supply = superior and inferior thyroid As.

- *Superior thyroid A* = is a branch of ECA; runs intimately with external laryngeal N. It divides in anterior and posterior branch; anterior branch anastomoses with opposite side branch; the posterior branch anastomoses with ascending branch of inferior thyroid A. It supplies to upper 1/3rd of lobe and upper ½ of isthmus.
- *Inferior thyroid A* = is a branch of thyrocervical trunk of subclavian A, i.e. SCA; its terminal part is intimately related to recurrent laryngeal N; supplies lower 2/3rd of lobe; lower ½ of isthmus and parathyroids.
- Thyroid ima A = branch of brachio-cephalic trunk or arch of aorta.
- Venous drainage = ultimately in IJV through superior, middle, inferior thyroid Vs.
- Lymphatics = mostly in antero-superior and postero-inferior groups of deep cervical LNs.
- Colloid = is drained by Vs and lymphatics both.
- Nerves = Mainly by Middle cervical ganglion; partly by superior and inferior cervical ganglions; are VASOCONSTRICTOR.
- Hormones = **T3 and T4** from follicular cells, it controls BMR; **thyrocalcitonin** from beta-cells/C–cells, it controls Calcium deposition in bones, produces hypocalemia, i.e. **action opposite to that of parathormone**.

Development of thyroid = earliest glandular structure to appear; develops from **median endodermal thyroid diverticulum**; becomes functional during 3rd month of development.

Hyperthyroidism = causes **thyrotoxicosis**; Goitre.

Hypothyroidism = causes **cretinism** in infants; myxoedema in adults.

Parathyroid glands

Superior parathyroids = aka **parathyroid IV** = as they develop from 4th endodermal pouch.

Inferior parathyroids = aka **parathyroid III** = as they develop from 3rd endodermal pouch.

Secrete **PTH** = to control Ca – P metabolism.

Superior parathyroid gland lies dorsal to recurrent laryngeal N; inferior parathyroid gland lies ventral to recurrent laryngeal N.

Blood supply = by mainly inferior thyroid A.

Parathyroid activity is controlled by blood – Ca^{++} levels; low level stimulate the gland; high level inhibit the gland.

Hyperparathyroidism = causes **osteitis fibrosa cystica**; hypercalcemia.

Hypoparathyroidism = causes **tetany**, i.e. hypocalcemia; increases nm irritability; carpopedal spasm; convulsions.

THYMUS GLAND

High rate of lymphopoiesis; develops from **endoderm of the 3rd pouch**.

95 % of lymphocytes / T-cells = are autoallergic; never move out of the thymus; destroyed by phagocytes;

5 % of T-cells = are long lived, i.e. 3 months; move out of thymus; act as uncommitted cells.

Cells from lymph nodes and spleen are committed cells, i.e. react with specific antigens only.

Secrete **lymphopoitin** = stimulates lymphocytes production.

Competence inducing factor = make new lymphocytes competent to react to an antigen.

Normally there are **no germinal centers in thymus**; but appear in autoimmune diseases.

It undergoes involution with age upto puberty.

Thymic hyperplasia/ tumors = cause **myasthenia gravis**.

SUBCLAVIAN A

Principal artery of **upper limb**; on right side it is a branch of brachiocephalic A; on left side it is a branch of arch of aorta.

5 branches = vertebral; internal thoracic; thyrocervical trunk (with its 3 branches, i.e. inferior thyroid; suprascapular; superficial cervical A.); costocervical trunk (it arises from the 2nd part of SCA on right side and from the 1st part of SCA on left side); dorsal scapular A;

Vertebral A = first and the *largest* branch of SCA.

ICA = begins at upper border of thyroid C; opposite the disc b/w C3 and C4.

IJV = is a direct communication of *sigmoid sinus*; begins at jugular foramen; ends by joining subclavian V to form brachio-cephalic V., i.e. IJV + SCV = BCV.

Superior bulb lies in jugular fossa of temporal bone;

Inferior bulb lies beneath the lesser supraclavicular fossa.

Thoracic duct opens in the angle of union of left IJV and SCV.

Right lymphatic duct opens similarly on the right side.

Deep cervical LNs lie on IJV.

Right and left BCVs unite at the lower border of right first costal cartilage to form superior vena cava.

9th Nerve = nerve of the 3rd branchial arch.

- Branchiomotor to *stylopharyngeus* m = branchial efferent. = thro nucleus ambiguus.
- Secretomotor to *parotid* = general visceral efferent = para-sympathetic = through inferior salivatory nucleus.
- Gustatory to *posterior 3rd tongue* = special visceral afferent = gustatory = through nucleus of tractus solitarius.
- Proprioception from stylopharyngeus m.
- **Sensory** to pharynx, *tonsils*, posterior 3rd of tongue.
- In jugular foramen = it is lodged in a deep groove leading to cochlear canaliculus and is separated from the 10, 11 nerves by inferior petrosal sinus.
- Branches = one branch from tympanic plexus is ka *lesser petrosal* nerve; which has preganglionic secretomotor fibres for parotid gland.
- Its carotid branch supplies to *carotid sinus* and *carotid body*.
- Muscular branch supplies to stylopharyngeus m.
- Lingual branch conveys taste and general sensation from posterior 3rd of tongue.

VAGUS NERVE - very vague distribution; is longest cranial nerve.

- Gustatory to epiglottic region, **inhibitor to heart**,
- Leaves cranium thro middle part of jugular foramen.
- Pharyngeal branch contains chiefly fibres of cranial accessory nerve; supply **ms of pharynx, palate (except tensor palati** which is supplied by mandibular N).
- Carotid branch = to carotid body.
- **Superior laryngeal N** = divides in external and internal laryngeal N on middle constrictor m.
- External laryngeal N = pierces inferior constrictor m; supplies cricothyroid ms.
- Internal laryngeal N = pierces *thyrohyoid membrane;* supply sensory fibres to larynx **upto vocal cords**.
- **Recurrent laryngeal** N = enters larynx behind cricothyroid joint; supplies all intrinsic ms of larynx **except cricothyroid** which is supplied by external laryngeal N. It is also sensory to larynx **below the vocal cords**.
- **Clinical testing** of vagus = on affected side, no arching of the palate; and uvula pulled to normal side.
- Stimulation of auricular branch = increases appetite by tickling its cutaneous distribution.

ACCESSORY N

1. Has 2 roots, i.e. cranial and spinal. These 2 roots unite temporarily in jugular foramen and comes out.
2. Cranial root finally fuses with vagus just below inferior ganglion for distribution to palate, pharynx, larynx, heart.
3. Spinal root = is C1 to C5. The nerve enters the cranium thro foramen magnum behind vertebral A. and leaves thro middle of jugular foramen.
4. Spinal root Communicates with C3, C4 nerves and supplies trapezius; i.e. upper half by spinal accessory, lower half by C3 C4 nerves. Also it is the **sole motor supply to SCM m**.

Note = somatic motor nerves are 3, 4, 6, 12 and ventral roots of spinal nerves.

HYPOGLOSSAL N

1. **Supplies to all intrinsic and extrinsic ms of tongue except** palatoglossus which is supplied by pharyngeal plexus, i.e. cranial accessory thro vagus.
2. Also supplies thyrohyoid m and geniohyoid m through descendens hypoglossi or upper root of ansa cervicalis (12th N with C1 N.)
3. **Clinical testing** = protruded tongue deviates to paralysed side.

Trachea = 4 – 66" long; begins at lower border of cricoid C, opposite the lower border of C6 vertebra.

Oesophagus = 10" long; begins at lower border of cricoid C, opposite the lower border of body of C6 vertebra Same level as trachea).

Pharynx – oesophageal junction is narrowest part of GIT except appendix.

Lymph nodes of head and neck = finally in deep cervical nodes, which lie along IJV.

Jugulo-digastric lymph nodes = lies below DGP m; b/w angle of mandible and anterior border of SCM. It is the **main lymph node of tonsil**.

Jugulo-omohyoid LNs = lies above the tendon of omohyoid m. It is the **main lymph node of tongue**.

Efferents of deep cervical LNs = in Jugular lymph trunk;

Left Jugular trunk opens in thoracic duct.

Right Jugular trunk opens in right lymphatic duct or in angle of junction b/w IJV and SCV.

Peripheral LNs = 2 circles, i.e. superficial and deep.

Superficial LNs = submental; submandibular; buccal and mandibular/facial; preauricular/parotid; posterior auricular/mastoid; occipital; anterior cervical; superficial cervical.

Deep/inner circle LNs = prelaryngeal; pretracheal; paratracheal; retropharyngeal.

Lymph nodes	Drain area	End in
Buccal; **on buccinator**; on anteroinferior angle of buccinator ms	Part of cheek and **lower eyelid**	Antero-superior group of deep cervical LN
Post-auricular/ Mastoid nodes	Strip of scalp just above and behind the auricle; posterior wall of external acoustic meatus	Posterior-superior group of deep cervical LN
Occipital	Occipital region of scalp	Supraclavicular
Anterior cervical	Skin of anterior part of neck below hyoid	Deep CLNs
Superficial Cervical LN; lie along EJV superficial to SCm	Lobule of auricle; floor of meatus; skin of lower parotid region; angle of mandible.	Upper and lower deep CLNs
Submental; +nt b/w anterior bellies of DG m	Drain superficial tissue of chin; adj gum; central part of lower lip; anterior part of floor of mouth; tip of tongue.	
Submandibular; lie below deep fascia of surface of SMG	Centre of forehead; nose; frontal, maxillary, ethmoidal sinus; inner canthus of eye; upper lip and anterior part of cheek with underlying gum/teeth; outer part of lower lip with lower gum and teeth excluding incisors; anterior 2/3 of tongue	

Lymph nodes	Drain area	End in
	excluding tip; floor of mouth; submental LNs.	
Parotid; lie over parotid gland	Temple; side of scalp; lateral surface of auricle; external auditory meatus; middle ear; parotid gland; upper part of cheek; parts of eyelid; orbit;	Upper deep cervical LNs

Lymph drainage of tongue = from submental to submandibular to JO nodes.

1. Tip = bilaterally to submental LNs.
2. Each half of the anterior 2/3 rd = unilaterally to SM LNs.
3. Posterior 1/3 = bilaterally to jugulo-omohyoid LNs; so carcinoma is more dangerous.
4. **Jugulo-omohyoid** LNs = is ka **LN of the tongue**.

1. **Thoracic duct is the largest lymph trunk** of body. It begins at cisterna chyli. Ends in angle b/w left IJV and left SCV. It drains most of the body except for the right upper limb, right halves of head, neck, thorax and superior surface of liver.
2. Jugular trunk = drains half of the head and neck.
3. Subclavian trunk = drains upper limb.
4. On right side = subclavian trunk + jugular trunk = form right lymph trunk which ends in thoracic duct.

MOUTH AND PHARYNX

- Parotid duct opens opposite the crown of upper 2nd molar.
- Central part of lower lip drains in = submental LNs. Rest of the lip in submandibular LNs.

- Junction of cheek and lip is ka = nasolabial sulcus.
- Lymphatics of cheek = mainly in submandibular LNs and preauricular LNs. Partly in buccal and mandibular LNs.
- Isthmus of fauces is bound on each side by = palatoglossal arches.

Lymphatics of different areas are

Anterior part of floor of mouth	Submental LNs
Hard / soft palate	Retropharyngeal (partly) and upper deep cervical LNs (mainly).
Gums and rest of floor of mouth	Submandibular
Upper gums	Submandibular
Anterior part of lower gum	Submental
Posterior part of lower gum	Submandibular

- PDL acts as a periosteum to both the cementum and socket.

Nerve supply

Posterior superior alveolar	Upper molars
Middle superior alveolar	MB root of upper first molar and upper premolars
Anterior superior alveolar	Upper incisors and canine
Inferior alveolar nerve (IAN)	Mand. premolars and molars
Incisive branch of IAN	Mand. incisors and canine

Soft palate

- *Main bulk* of soft palate is by large volume of numerous *mucous glands* on its anterior oral surface.

- **Palatoglossal arch** = anterior pillar of fauces. Also forms the lateral boundaries of oropharyngeal isthmus.
- **Palatopharyngeus fold** = posterior pillar of fauces. And posterior boundary of tonsillar fossa.
- Palatine aponeurosis = flat tendon of tensor palati m; encloses the musculus uvulae in median plane.
- Palatoglossus m = attached on inferior surface of aponeurosis.
- Palatopharyngeus m and levator palati = attached on superior surface of aponeurosis.
- All ms of soft palate are supplied by **pharyngeal plexus** except the **tensor palati** m which is supplied by mandibular N.
- Gustatory is through = lesser palatine N, derived from nucleus of tractus solitarius through *greater petrosal* N.
- **Passavant ridge** = is upper part of *palato-pharyngeus* m which has not come down with other fibres during the descent of the inlet of larynx. It lies at the *level of hard palate*. It is aka palatopharyngeus *sphincter of Whillis*. It is best developed in CLP cases compensatory.

PHARYNX

- 5" long; continues with oesophagus at C 6 / lower border of cricoid C.
- 3 parts = naso-, oro-, laryngo-.

Nasopharynx

- Its m.m. is supplied by 5th N (pharyngeal branch of pterygopalatine ganglion).
- Rest of the pharynx is supplied by 9th, 10th Ns.
- Opening of the auditory tube is at the level of inferior nasal concha.
- *Pharyngeal tonsils* = opposite the basi-occiput. Are the **adenoids**.
- **Pouch of Luschka** = *endodermal* pit drawn out by cranial end of notochord.

Oropharynx

- Tonsillar fossa is bound by palatoglossal and palatopharyngeus arches.

- **Waldeyer's** lymphatic ring = ring has 4 main masses = 2 palatine + 1 pharyngeal + 1 lingual.
- Capsule of tonsil is the extension of pharyngobasilar fascia.
- Intratonsillar cleft = is the *largest crypt* in tonsil. It is the internal opening of 2nd pharyngeal pouch; quinsy starts here.
- Tonsil is the **only lymphoid tissue of** the body which is lined by squamous epithelium with mucous glands in submucosa; it has no afferent lymphatics. Its main blood supply is from **facial A**.

Laryngopharynx

- Extends from the upper border of epiglottis to lower border of cricoid C.
- **Vocal cords** = at upper border of cricoid C.
- *Internal laryngeal* N lies below the mucosa of piriform fossa; can get damaged by foreign body removal here.

Wall of pharynx

- Mucosa = lined by sq. epithelium. Except nasopharynx which is columnar ciliated.
- Pharyngobasilar fascia = fills the gap b/w upper border of superior constrictor and base of the skull (i.e. sinus of morgagni)
- Nerve supply = by *pharyngeal plexus* which lies chiefly on middle constrictor m. It is formed by :

Motor = pharyngeal br of 10th n., i.e. cranial 11th n;

Sensory = pharyngeal br of 9th n;

Sympathctic and vasomotor = pharyngeal br of superior cervical ganglion.

- **All ms of pharynx are supplied by pharyngeal plexus except stylopharyngeus m which is supplied by 9th n.**
- Inferior constrictor m is **thickest** m of the 3 constrictors; it is also supplied by external and recurrent laryngeal Ns, which supply cricopharyngeus part of inferior constrictor.
- Lower part of thyropharyngeus m (part of inferior constrictor m) = is the **weak part** and lies below the level of vocal folds / upper

border of cricoid; it is ka KILLIAN'S DEHISCENCE. Thyropharyngeus part is supplied by pharyngeal plexus.

- **Pharyngeal plexus** supplies all ms of **soft palate except tensor palati** which is supplied by mandibular n.

STRUCTURES RELATED IN THIS AREA

1. **Sinus of Morgagni** = is the gap b/w skull base and superior constrictor m. It is closed by strongest pharyngobasilar fascia. Structures passing through this area are auditory tube; levator palati m.; ascending palatine A.
2. Structures passing b/w superior and middle constrictor ms = stylopharyngeus m; 9th N.
3. Structures passing b/w middle and inferior constrictor ms = internal laryngeal N and superior laryngeal vessels pierce thyrohyoid membrane.
4. Structures passing b/w inferior constrictor ms and oesophagus = recurrent laryngeal N and inferior laryngeal vessels.

Auditory tube

- Bony part = lies in petrous temporal; opens in anterior wall of middle ear cavity.
- Cartilagenous part = lies in sulcus tubae;
- Tubal tonsils = lymphoid tissue at its pharyngeal opening.
- Nerve supply = by br of 5th and 9th Ns.
- Lymph = drains in retropharyngeal LNs.

NOSE AND PARANASAL SINUSES

1. Olfactory mucosa / receptors = in upper $1/3^{rd}$ of nasal cavity and roof and walls of superior concha; olfactory cells are BIPOLAR.
2. Beneath the epithelium = serous glands ka BOWMAN'S GLANDS are present.
3. Septum = formed by vomer and perpendicular plate of ethmoid bone; lower margin of septum is ka **columella**.

4. **Vomeronasal organ of Jacobson** = lies immediately above the incisive canal; lined by olfactory epithelium; better seen in fetal life.
5. Antero-inferior part of septum = is ka LITTLE'S AREA / KIESSELBACH'S AREA. It is the anastomosis b/w superior labial and sphenopalatine A.
6. Lymph goes to = Submandibular LNs from anterior half and to retropharyngeal and deep cervical LNs from posterior half.

LATERAL WALL OF NOSE

1. Nasal conchae = are 3; extend down and medially; help in increasing the surface area.
2. Inferior concha = is an *independent bone.*
3. Middle concha = from ethmoid labyrinth.
4. Superior concha = *smallest;* from ethmoid labyrinth.
5. Inferior meatus = *largest*, nasolacrimal duct opens at Hansen's valve at the junction of anterior $1/3^{rd}$ and posterior $2/3^{rd}$.
6. **Middle meatus**

> Structures seen are ethmoidal bullae as round elevation of middle ethmoidal sinus; *hiatus semilunaris*; infundibulum at the anterior end of hiatus.
>
> Opening of frontal sinus = in anterior part of hiatus.
>
> Opening of maxillary sinus = in posterior part of hiatus.
>
> Opening of anterior ethmoidal sinus = in middle part of hiatus.
>
> Opening of middle ethmoidal sinus = at the upper margin of bulla.

7. Opening of posterior ethmoidal sinus = in *superior meatus*.
8. Sphenoethmoidal recess = just above the superior concha; opening of sphenoid sinus.
9. **Olfactory region** = area below the cribriform plate to superior concha.
10. Blood supply = br of ophthalmic A / br of ICA (anterosuperior part); rest by br of maxillary A / br of ECA.

11. Nerve supply = antero-superior part by branch of ophthalmic N (branch of 5th N); rest by branch of maxillary N / 5th N.
12. Special sensory supply = by branch of olfactory N.

Quadrant	Artery	Nerve
Antero-superior	ICA	Ophthalmic, br of 5th n.
PS/ AI/ PI	ECA	Maxillary, br of 5th n.

PARANASAL SINUSES: 4 in no.; lined by respiratory m.m.

- Maxillary sinus is the **largest** of all; aka **antrum of Highmore**; first to develop in the body at the 4th mo. I.U age. Opens in the middle meatus near the roof rather than the floor so the drainage is difficult.
- Sinuses enlarge rapidly at 6 – 7 yrs age and then after the puberty.
- **Functions of sinuses** = to lighten the skull; to warm up the inspired air; to add **resonance** to the voice.

Sinus	Artery	Nerve	Veins	Lymph	Opening
Frontal	Supraorbital	Supraorbital	Anastomose b/w supra orbital and superior ophthalmic v	SM	Middle meatus/ anterior end
Maxillary	Facial; infraorbital; greater palatine	IO n; anterior/ middle/ posterior superior alveolar Ns.	Facial v; pterygoid plexus	SM	Middle meatus in lower part
Sphenoidal	Post. ethmoidal A; ICA	Post. eth. N, a br of ophthalmic N; pterygoplatine gang		Retropharyngeal	Sphenoethmoidal recess

Sinus	Artery	Nerve	Veins	Lymph	Opening
Ant. Ethmoidal, 11 in no.	Ant. Ethm. A	Ant. Ethm. V	Ant. Ethm. N	SM	Anterior part of hiatus
Middle ethmoidal, 3 in no.	Ant. Ethm. A	Ant. Ethm. V	Ant. Ethm. N	SM	Upper part of bulla
Post eth, 7 in no.	Post eth	Post eth, orbital br of pterygopalatine gang	Post eth	Retropharyngeal	Superior meatus

Contents of pterygopalatine fossa

1. 3rd part of Maxillary A.
2. maxillary N with zygomatic and posterior alveolar branch= maxillary n continues as the infraorbital N.
3. Pterygopalatine ganglion/ sphenopalatine ganglion.

PTERYGOPALATINE GANGLION

1. *Largest* peripheral parasympathetic ganglion. Topographically it is associated with maxillary N; functionally to 7th n./ greater petrosal N.
2. Preganglionic fibres come from the *superior salivatory nucleus* and posterior ganglionic fibres are secretomotor to lacrimal gland and mucous glands of nose/ PNS/ palate, etc.
3. Motor / p-sympathetic root = from the nerve of pterygoid canal.
4. Sympathetic root = from the nerve of the pterygoid canal.
5. Sensory root = from maxillary n.

LARYNX

- Extends from C3 – C6 in males; but at higher level in females and children.

- Has 9 cartilages = 3 unpaired, i.e. thyroid (hyaline); cricoid (hyaline); epiglottic (elastic) and 3 paired, i.e. arytenoid (hyaline except apex which is elastic); corniculate and cunieform (elastic).
- Thyroid lamina = has more obtuse angle in females than males;
- Arytenoid C = its base forms the **vocal process**.
- **Thyrohyoid membrane** = pierced by internal laryngeal N and superior laryngeal vessels.
- Fibroelastic membrane of larynx = its cricovocal part, i.e. conus elasticus forms cricothyroid lig and its upper free border forms the **vocal cords**.
- Cavity of larynx = extends from inlet of larynx to lower border of cricoid C; lower fold of m.memb forms the **vocal fold**. Space b/w them is ka **rima glottidis**.
- Rima glottidis = is the *narrowest part* of larynx.

Intrinsic ms of larynx

1. Cricothyroid = only muscle outside the larynx.
2. All intrinsic ms of larynx are supplied by recurrent laryngeal n **except cricothyroid** which is by external laryngeal N.
3. Ms which **open the glottis** = posterior cricoarytenoid m
4. Ms which **close the glottis** = lateral cricoarytenoid and transverse arytenoid.
5. Ms which **tense the vocal cords** = cricothyroid
6. Ms which **relax the vocal cords** = thyroarytenoid and vocalis
7. Ms which **close the inlet of larynx** = oblique arytenoid and aryepiglottics
8. Ms which **open the inlet of larynx** = thyroepiglottic.
9. At rest = intermembrane part of rima is triangular and intercartilagenous part is quadrangular.
10. During phonation = rima is like a chink by ADDUCTION of vocal cords.
11. Damage to both recurrent laryngeal Ns = vocal cords lie in cadaveric position and phonation is completely lost.

12. **Damage to external laryngeal N** = weakness of phonation due to loss of cricothyroid m force.

	Upto vocal cords	**Below vocal cords**
Artery	Superior laryngeal	Inferior laryngeal / br of inferior thyroid A
Veins	Superior laryngeal V drains in superior thyroid A	Inferior laryngeal V drains in inferior thyroid A
Sensory N Lymph drainage	Internal laryngeal N Anterosuperior group of deep cervical LNs	Recurrent laryngeal N Posteroinferior group of deep cervical LNs

TONGUE

- Sulcus terminalis = separates the anterior 2/3rd and posterior 1/3rd parts; is V shaped; its median pit is foramen cecum; and the 2 limbs reach upto the palatoglossal arches.
- Foramen cecum represents the = upper part of thyroid diverticulum.
- Epithelial lining develops from the *endoderm* of 1st branchial arch; thro 2 lingual swellings and a median tuberculum impar.
- Pharyngeal / lymphoid part of tongue = has no papillae but plenty of lingual tonsils; it develops from the 3rd branchial arch / anterior ½ of the hypobranchial eminence. Its m.m forms the median and lateral glossoepiglottic folds.

Papillae of tongue = develop from the m.m /corium.

Papilla	**Size**	**No.**	**Dev.**	**Taste buds**	**Site**
Vallate	**Largest**; 1 – 2 mm dia	8 – 12	11 wk IU	Yes	In front of sulcus terminalis
Fungiform	< vallate; > filiform	Numerous	11 wk IU	Yes	Tip; margins dorsum of tongue

Papillae of tongue = develop from the m.m /corium. (*Contd.*)

Papilla	Size	No.	Dev.	Taste buds	Site
Filiform/ conical	**Smallest**	**Most numerous**	11 wk IU	**No**	Presulcal area; velvetty appearance
Foliate		4 –5	11 wk IU	Yes	In front of **palato-glossal** arches

- **Muscles of the tongue** = each half contains 4 intrinsic and 4 extrinsic ms (genio-, hyo-, palato-, styloglossi).
- Intrinsic ms alter the shape of the tongue.
- Genioglossus m =forms the **main bulk of tongue**; upper fibers retract the tip; middle fibers depress the tongue; lower fibers protrude the tongue.
- **Main artery** = lingual A, a branch of ECA. Root is also supplied by tonsillar and ascending pharyngeal A.
- Main vein = deep lingual V;
- **Lymph drainage** = from submental to submandibular to JO nodes.
- Tip = bilaterally to submental LNs.
- Each half of the anterior 2/3 rd = unilaterally to SM LNs.
- Posterior 1/3 = bilaterally to jugulo-omohyoid LNs; so carcinoma is more dangerous.
- **Jugulo-omohyoid** LNs = is ka **LN of the tongue**.

Nerve supply

1. Motor = all intrinsic and extrinsic ms of the tongue are supplied by 12th N **except palatoglossus** which is supplied by cranial 11th through pharyngeal plexus.
2. Sensory N = lingual n is general sensory; **chorda tympani** is special sensory/gustatory to anterior 2/3rd; 9th N is both general and special sensory to posterior 3rd; internal laryngeal / 10th n is to posterior most part of the tongue.

3. Mucous glands are abundant in pharyngeal part; **serous glands** are near taste buds which **open in the sulci of vallate papillae.** Seromucous glands are on inferior surface of tongue near the apex.

Taste buds

- Most numerous on the sides of vallate papillae;
- Plenty over foliate papillae; posterior 1/3rd of tongue.
- More in infants than in adults.
- None in mid-dorsal region of oral part of tongue.
- Filiform papilla do not have any taste bud.

DEVELOPMENT

- Anterior 2/3 rd = from 2 lingual swellings and tuberculum impar, i.e. first branchial arch. The posterior – trematic nerve is lingual N from 5th n; and pretrematic N is chorda tympani N from the 7th N.
- Posterior 1/3rd = from the cranial ½ of hypobranchial eminence, i.e. 3rd arch; supplied by 9th N.
- Posterior most part = from the 4th arch; by 10th N.
- Muscles = from occipital myotomes; from 12th N.
- Connective tissue = from local mesenchyme.

EAR

- Inner ear lies in the petrous temporal bone.
- Root of auricle is supplied by = auricular branch of 10th N.
- Motor supply of auricular ms = 7th N.
- External meatus = its greater diameter is vertical at its lateral end; and AP at the medial end.
- Its Bony part is formed by tympanic plate; is C-shaped = its posterosuperior gap is filled by squamous temporal bone.

- Ceruminous / wax glands are present in the cartilagenous part = are the modified sweat glands.
- **Ear cough** = due to irritation of auricular branch of 10th N. It may lead to death due to sudden cardiac inhibition;
- **Tympanic membrane** = is tensed by tensor tympani m attached at the upper end of handle of malleus, i.e. pars tensa.
- **Umbo** = point of **maximum convexity;** at the tip of the handle.
- **Pars flaccida** = aka SHARPNELL'S MEMBRANE; is a small triangular area above the malleolar fold; is crossed by chorda tympani N; more *liable to rupture.*
- Bones of the middle ear = malleus is largest; stapes is smallest; incus resembles lower molar tooth; stepes is fixed in — window?
- **Joints** = incudo-malleolar joint is saddle joint; incudo- stapedial joint is ball and socket type of the joint.
- Tensor tympani m = from 1st branchial arch; for malleus; supplied by mandibular N; dampens the sound waves.
- Stapedius m = from 2nd branchial arch; for stapes; supplied by facial N; **opposes the action** of tensor tympani m.

Internal ear = lies in petrous temporal bone; 2 parts

1. Bony labyrinth = cochlea + vestibule + semicircular canals; contains the perilymph.
2. **Membranous labyrinth** = spiral ducts of cochlea (the organs of hearing); utricles and saccule (organs of **static balance** present in the vestibule); semicircular ducts (organs of **kinetic balance**). It contains the endolymph. Its is specialised in 3 parts as : receptors of sound (the organs of corti); static balance (macula); kinetic balance (crista).
3. **Semicircular canals** open into the posterior wall of the vestibule; these canals are at right angle to each other, each describes 2/3 of a circle; open in the vestibule by 5 openings.
4. The peripheral processes of ganglion cells pass to the organ of corti and the **central processes form the cochlear nerve**.
5. Maculae are static balance receptors which are sensitive to gravitational stimuli = the impulses pass through VESTIBULAR N.

6. Medial wall of each ampulla of all ducts forms a transverse crest ka **cristae** = which **responds to pressure changes** in endolymph caused by the movements, i.e. kinetic balance.
7. **8th nerve** = its **vestibular part**, i.e. **nerve of balance** and **cochlear part is nerve of hearing** are special somatic afferent nerves.
8. Cochlear impulses pass through 3 neuron pathways and vestibular impulses pass through 2 neuron pathways.
9. Vestibular receptors are in saccule and utricle (static balance) and in cristae of ampullae of semicircular ducts (kinetic balance).
10. Aerial conduction of sound is better than the bony conduction.

EYEBALL

Ciliary body = suspends the lens and helps in accommodation for near vision.

Ciliary ms = supplied by p-sympathetic N, i.e. 3rd N.

Iris = has sphincter pupillae ms; supplied by p-sympathetic 3rd N. and the dilator pupillae m by sympathetic N.

Sclera is **avascular**. Sclero-corneal junction is ka **limbus**. Cornea is also avascular.

Retina = optic part is sensitive to the light upto ora-serrata.

Blind spot = has *no rods and cones*; insenstive to light;

Fovea centralis = only **cones** present; *thinnest part* of retina; maximum acuity of vision.

Rods = contain the visual purple; sensitive to dim light / **scotopic vision**; periphery of retina contains only rods but fovea has no rods; has low threshold.

Cones = have a high threshold, i.e. **photopic vision**; sensitive to **color vision**; fovea has only cones.

Suspensory lig. / zonula of ZINN of lens = attached to the lens; its tension keeps the anterior surface of lens flattened; it is **relaxed by contraction of ciliary ms**.

Aqueous humor = secreted in the posterior chamber; drained in the anterior ciliary Vs through the spaces of FONTANNA and canals of Schlemm.

CONTENTS OF THE FORAMINA

Foramen	Contents
Carotid canal	ICA; and its venous and sympathetic plexus
F. lacerum	Meningeal branch of ascending pharyngeal A; emissary V from cavernous sinus; upper part is traversed by ICA and its plexus; in upper part = greater petrosal N unites with deep petrosal N to form nerve of pterygoid canal/ *vidian* N.
F. Magnum	♦ Thro wide posterior part = lower part of medulla/ tonsils of cerebellum/ meninges. ♦ Thro subarachnoid space = spinal accessory N/ vertebral A/ sympathetic plexus of vertebral A/ anterior and posterior spinal As. ♦ Thro anterior narrow part = apical lig. of dens; membrana tectoria.
F. Ovale (Male)	Mandibular N; lesser petrosal N; accessory meningeal A; emissary V which connects cavernous sinus with pterygoid plexus of Vs.
F. spinosum (3M)	MMA; meningeal br of mandibular N, i.e. nervous spinosus; posterior trunk of MMV.
Gap b/w zygomatic arch and side of skull	Tendon of temporalis m and deep temporal N and vessels.
Greater palatine	Greater palatine vessels and anterior palatine N
Incisive	Terminal parts of greater palatine vessels from palate to nose and of nasopalatine nerve from nose to palate.
Mastoid	Emissary V and meningeal br of occipital A.
Mental	Mental N and vessels; directed U and B.
Palatovaginal canal	Opens in the posterior wall of pterygopalatine fossa; has pharyngeal br from pterygoplatine ganglion; a small pharyngeal br. of Maxillary A.

CONTENTS OF THE FORAMINA (*Contd.*)

Foramen	Contents
Parietal	Emissary V from the superior sagittal sinus.
Petrotympanic fissure	Chorda tympani N and anterior tympanic A.
Supra-/ infra -orbital	N and vessels of same names.
Cribriform plate	♦ anterior ethmoidal vessels and nerves pass to nasal cavity; olfactory Ns.
F. rotundum	♦ maxillary N; opens in the pterygo-palatine fossa.
F. caecum	♦ a vein from upper nose to superior saggital sinus.
F. of Vesalius	♦ lies in front and medial of F. ovale in greater wing of sphenoid; sphenoid emissary V.
F ovale	♦ opens in the infratemporal fossa.
F spinosusm	♦ opens in the infratemporal fossa.
Hypoglossal canal	12th N; meningeal br of 12th N; meningeal br of ascending pharyngeal A; emissary v connecting sigmoid sinus with IJV.
Inferior orbital fissure	♦ maxillary N; zygomatic N; orbital br of pterygo-palatine ganglion; infraorbital vessels; and a communication b/w inferior ophthalmic V and pterygoid venous plexus.
Jugular F	♦ Anterior part = inferior petrosal sinus; meningeal br of ascending pharyngeal A ♦ mid part = 9, 10, 11 th nerves ♦ posterior part = IJV; meningeal br of occipital A.
Jugular fossa	♦ superior bulb of IJV lies.
Mandibular F	♦ inferior alveolar N and vessels; lies at the level of occlusal plane.

CONTENTS OF THE FORAMINA (*Contd.*)

Foramen	Contents
Mandibular notch	♦ masseteric N and vessels
Optic canal	♦ optic N; meningeal sheath of optic n; ophthalmic A
Stylomastoid	♦ facial N and stylomastoid br of postauricular A
Superior orbital fissure	♦ lateral part = LFT Ns; superior ophthalmic V; meningeal br of lacrimal A; anastomotic br of MMA with recurrent br of lacrimal A. ♦ middle part = U/L div of 3rd n; nasociliary N in b/w 2 div of 3rd N; 6th N ♦ medial part = inferior ophthalmic V; symp N from the plexus around ICA

OSTEOLOGY

- Skull has 22 bones; 8 in calvaria (2 are paired and 4 unpaired); 14 in face + mandible (6 paired + vomer + mandible).
- **Fusion in cranial sutures** begins at 30–40 yrs of age on inner surface and 40–50 yrs on outer surface.

- **Coronal suture** = b/w frontal and 2 parietal bones.
- **Sagittal suture** = b/w 2 parietal bones.
- **Lambdoid suture** = b/w 2 parietal bones and the occipital bone.
- **Metopic suture** = b/w the 2 halves of the frontal bone.

- **Vertex** is the highest point on the sagittal suture.

- **Bregma** = meeting point b/w coronal and sagittal sutures (i.e. anterior fontanelle which closes at 1½ yrs of age).
- **Lambda** = meeting point b/w sagittal and lambdoid suture. It is the site of posterior fontanelle which closes at 2–3 mos age.

- **Inion** = most prominent point on external occipital protuberance. Upper part of EOP gives rise to trapezius.
- **Obelion** = point on sagittal suture b/w 2 parietal foramen; site of pineal / 3rd eye.
- **Glabella** = median elevation connecting 2 superciliary arches.
- **Nasion** = median point where internasal suture meets with frontonasal.
- **Rhinion** = lower part of internasal suture.
- **Occipital point** = median point a little above inion which is farthest from glabella.

- Parietal tuber/ eminence = common site of fracture of skull; area of maximum convexity.
- Superior temporal line = attachment of epicranial aponeurosis.
- Infraorbital margin = formed by zygomatic bone and maxilla.
- Lateral orbital margin = by frontal process of zygoma and zygomatic process of frontal bone.
- Medial orbital margin = by frontal bone above and lacrimal crest of frontal process of maxilla.
- In fetal skull = the facial skeleton is 1/8th of calvarium; there are no diploe; the tables appear later by 4th year of age; internal ear / tympanic cavity/tympanic antrum/ and ear ossicles are almost the adult size.

- 2 halves of frontal bones = at metopic suture.
- 4 parts of occipital bone = 1 squamous + 2 condylar + 1 basilar.
- 4 parts of temporal bone = tympanic; squamous; petrous; styloid.
- 6 fontanelles at the angles of parietal bones; help in easy passage of fetus through the birth canal.

- **Closure of anterior fontanelles** at 18 mos of age; of **posterior fontanelles** at 2 – 3 mos; of **sphenoidal fontanelles** at 2 – 3 mos; and of **mastoid fontanelles** at 12 mos of age occurs (MAPS).
- Mastoid process appears during the later part of 2nd yr of age and mastoid air cells during the 6th year.

- In adult skull = facial skeleton is ½ of the calvarium
- Growth of vault = rapid during the 1st yr; slows upto 7th yr when it is almost of adult size.
- Growth of orbit and ethmoid is complete by 7th yr of life.
- Obliteration of suture of vault = on inner surface at 30 – 40 yrs of age; on outer surface in 40 – 50 yrs of age; first in lower part of coronal suture and then in posterior part of sagittal suture; then in lambdoid suture.
- Capacity of skull in males is > females; by 10 %.
- Forehead of males is sloping; of females is vertical.
- Frontal and parietal tubera are more prominent in females than males.
- **Wormian / sutural bones** = found in region of the fontanelles; common in hydrocephalic skulls.
- Sutural bones are most common at lambda and asterion; common at pterion epipteric bone and rare at bregma and at occipital fontanelle.
- **Cephalic index** = breadth x 100 / length ; if < 75 = dolichocephalic; if 75 – 80 then meso-; if > 80 then brachy.
- Facial skeleton / **splanchnocranium** and calvaria / **neuro-cranium** are inversely proportional to each other.
- **Oxycephaly** = tower skull = premature closure of suture b/w presphenoid and postsphenoid, and coronal suture; s.t. very short AP dimensions but height increases very much.
- **Scaphocephaly** / boat skull = premature closure of sagittal suture, so the skull is v. narrow but greatly elongated.
- **Mandible is the largest and strongest bone of the face**.
- Sphenomandibular lig attached at lingula. Remnant of cephalic end of Meckel's cartilage.
- Mandible is the 2nd bone (next to clavicle) to ossify in the body. Parts which ossify in cartilage are incisive part below incisors/ coronoid and condyloid process/ upper ½ of the ramus above the level of mandibular foramen.
- Each half of the mandible ossifies from only one centre at 6th wk i.u. near the future mental foramen.

- Ventral end of **Meckel's cartilage** ossifies at 10th wk to form incisive part below incisors.
- Parts ossifying intramembranous = except the lower incisive part/ lower half of the ramus upto the mandibular foramen.
- Secondary / accessory cartilages develop in condyle / coronoid / symphysis and ossify from the parent center.
- Condyle and coronoid cartilages ossify a little later than 10th wk i.u.
- Cartilage of symphysis menti ossify at 7th month = to form the mental ossicles. Ossicles unite with the body during 1st yr of life.
- At **symphysis menti** = bony union begins from below upwards and during 1st yr of life and complete at beginning of the 2nd yr.
- **Zygomatic arch** = anterior 1/3rd (temporal process of zygomatic bone) + posterior 2/3rd (zygomatic process of temporal bone)
- Articular tubercle lies on zygoma lower border at the junction of anterior and posterior roots; lateral lig of TMJ is attached to it.
- **Macewen's triangle** = suprameatal triangle; forms lateral wall of mastoid antrum.
- Mastoid process appears during the 2nd yr of life.

- **Jugal point** = anterior end of upper border of zygomatic arch
- **Asterion** = point where parietomastoid and occipitomastoid sutures and lambdoid sutures meet = is the site of mastoid fontanelles.
- **Entomion** = point near anterior part of parietomastoid suture where a process of parietal bone is received into parietal notch of mastoid.
- **Pterion** = where frontal / parietal/ sphenoid/ and temporal bones meet. It lies 4 cm above the midpoint of zygomatic arch, 1 inch behind the frontozygomatic suture. Deep to it lies MMV, anterior div of MMA, sylvian point of brain.

- Deep temporal A,V, N lie beneath the temporalis m.
- Pterygoid process is a part of sphenoid bone and tympanic plate is a part of temporal bone. Styloid and mastoid processes are part of temporal bone.

- **Pterygoid fossa** = contains the deep head of medial pterygoid m and tensor palati m.
- Long axis of occipital condyle is = forward and medially.
- Bones covered by ms are thinner than those covered by scalp.
- Skull bones derive their main blood supply by meningeal artery from inside.
- **Diploe** = is the spoongy bone filled with red bone marrow. Blood from diploe is drained by 4 diploe vs and MMVs.
- **Posterior boundary** of anterior cranial fossa = is formed by lesser wing of sphenoid bone.
- **Fracture** of anterior cranial fossa causes discharge and bleeding thro nose and the black eye.
- Fracture of middle cranial fossa causes discharge and bleeding thro ear. Thro nose also if sphenoid is involved. **Fracture of middle cranial fossa are most common fracture.**
- Fracture of posterior cranial fossa causes bruising over the mastoid region extending down the SCM m. (**Battle's sign**).
- Cerebellum, pons, medulla are infratentorial structures.
- **Clivus** is related to basilar plexus of Vs; supports the pons and medulla.
- Petro-occipital fissure is continuous behind with the jugular foramen.
- Superior sagittal sinus is continuous with right transverse sinus.
- **Sigmoid sinus continues as IJV**.

ORBIT

- Medial walls are parallel and lateral walls are perpendicular to each other. Lateral wall of orbit is strongest/ thickest.
- Optic canal lies in / bounded by lesser wing of sphenoid.
- **Trochlear fossa** = attachment of fibrous pully of superior oblique m.

- Medial wall is formed by 4 bones, i.e. the frontal process of Maxilla/Lacrimal bone/orbital plate of Ethmoid/body of Sphenoid bones (i.e. MALES).
- **Whitnall's tubercle** = attachment to lateral cheek ligament.

Summary

NERVOUS SYSTEM

Sympathetic outflow	Thoraco-lumbar, i.e. all thoracic and L 1,2 (anterolateral cell column of grey substance).
Para-Sympathetic outflow	Craniosacral, i.e. 3,7,9,10 cranial nerves and S 2,3,4 spinal nerves.

Cell bodies of sympathetic preganglionic neurons are in thoracolumbar segment of s. cord.

Pyramidal tract = for fine voluntary movements

Extrapyramidal tract = for involuntary movements

Vagus is predominant over sympathetic nerves = as on the effect on the basal heart rate.

Pulp has no p-sympathetic fibres and proprioceptors.

Ventral column of s. cord = is motor.

Dorsal column of s. cord = is sensory

Visual area lies in occipital lobe of brain.

Auditory area lies in temporal lobe of brain.

Sensory area is posterior – central gyrus.

Motor area is pre– central gyrus.

Vomiting centre = is chemoreceptor trigger zone, i.e. CTZ

SPINAL CORD

Lower limit is = L1 vertebra in adults; L3 in children

Duramater ends at S2 vertebra level

Filum terminale ends at = first piece of coccyx.

NERVE SUPPLY; SUMMARY

- TMJ is supplied by auriculo-temporal and masseteric N
- Buccinator m. by facial N
- Ms of mastication by mandibular N.
- Tongue anterior 2/3rd sensory by lingual N
- Tongue anterior 2/3rd Special sensory = by facial n; chorda tympani
- Tongue anterior 2/3rd Motor = hypoglossal N
- Posterior 1/3 rd sensory = glossopharyngeal
- Posterior 1/3 rd special = 9th
- Posterior 1/3 rd motor = hypoglossal
- Posterior most part vagus; through internal laryngeal
- Ms of tongue by 12th n except palatoglossus (by cranial part of accessory N)
- Circumvallate papillae by 9th N.

ANSA CERVICALIS / ANSA HYPGLOSSI

- Supplies infrahyoid ms

Superior root	**Inferior root**
Continuation of descending branch of 12th N	C2, C3
From C1	
Supply superior belly of omohyoid	Sternohyoid; sternothyroid; inferior belly of omohyoid

Thyrohyoid and geniohyoid are supplied by separate branches from C1 through 12th N.

Suprathyroid ms

Stylohyoid is supplied by facial N

Mylohyoid by mylohyoid br of 5th N

Anterior belly of digastric by mylohyoid br of 5th N.

Posterior belly of digstric by facial N

Submandibular gland by facial N

Sublingual gland by facial N

Parotid gland

Parasympathetic Route	**Sympathetic**	**Sensory**
Inferior salivary nucleus/preganglionic fibres	From plexus around external carotid A	Auriculotemporal N
9th N		
Tympanic br		
Tympanic plexus		
Lesser petrosal N		
Otic gang/posterior ganglionic fibres		
Auriculotemporal N		
Parotid gland		

Parotid fascia = by sensory fibres of greater auricular N.

Nucleus ambiguus is related to 9, 10, 11 N

Cranial N = attached to

1. 1,2 crerebrum
2. 3,4 midbrain
3. 5,6,7,8 pons
4. 9,10,11,12 medulla

Auricle / pinna is supplied by

Part	**Lateral surface**	**Medial surface**
Upper 2/3	Auriculotemporal	Lesser petrosal
Lower 1/3	Greater auricular	Greater auricular

Root of auricle = by auricular br of vagus N

Auricular ms = by facial N

Sternocleidomastoid by spinal accessory n for motor supply; branches from ventral rami of C2, C3 are sensory.

The **smallest cranial n** = is trochlear n; but **it has longest intracranial canal course**.

Superior oblique	by 4th N
Lateral rectus	by 6th N
Rest of ocular ms	by 3rd N
Levator palpebrae superioris	by 3rd N
Ptosis is	paralysis of 3rd N
Medial squint is	paralysis of 6th N
Lateral squint is	paralysis of 3rd N
Crow eye / strabismus is due to	paralysis of 6th. N
Bell's palsy	due to 7th N
Trigeminal N is	largest cranial n.

Skin at the angle of mandible is supplied by greater auricular N; also supplies parotid fascia and lower 1/3 rd of pinna.

Nasal septum

- general sensory = from trigeminal N;
- anterosuperior part of septum = anterior ethmoid Ns
- postero-inferior part = nasopalatine N
- special sensory n = olfactory N. upto olfactory area.

Lateral wall of nose = general sensory n from 5th N.

- anterosuperior part — anterior ethmoidal n
- anteroinferior part — anterior superior alveolar n

- posterosuperior part — posterior superior lateral nasal n
- posteroinferior part — anterior palatine n
- abducent / 6th n lacks parasympathetic fibres.
- Stapedius m is supplied by facial n.
- Pure motor nerve contains 40% of sensory fibres.
- Vestibule of nose is supplied by superior labial artery.
- Palatine tonsil is supplied by 9th n.
- N. to pterygoid canal is aka **vidian n**.
- Nerve involved in **Saturday night palsy** is = radial n.
- Impulses of taste are carried to brain through = 7, 9, 10 Ns.
- Pure sensory cranial nerves = 1,2,8
- Pure motor = 3, 4, 6, 12
- Mixed = 5, 7, 9, 10, 11
- **Palatine tonsil** is supplied by **9th and lesser palatine** n.
- **Thyroid gland** = middle cervical ganglion; partly from superior and inferior cervical ganglia.
- **Parathyroid gland** = middle and superior cervical ganglia
- **Thymus** = stellate ganglia.
- Hard palate = greater palatine and nasopalatine Ns.

Soft palate

1. Motor n = all ms of soft palate are supplied by pharyngeal plexus from cranial part of accessory n. *except tensor palati* which is supplied by mandibular N.
2. General sensory = lesser palatine n; 9th n
3. Special sensory = lesser palatine
4. Secretomotor = lesser palatine

- Carotid body = by vagus n
- Phrenic n = formed by C3,C4,C5
- Primary motor area of speech = frontal area
- Sylvian fissure of cerebrum separates temporal and frontal lobes.

LARYNX

- Muscles = all intrinsic ms of larynx are supplied by recurrent laryngeal n *except cricothyroid* which is supplied by external laryngeal n.
- Sensory n = the internal laryngeal n supplies mucous membrane above the level of vocal cords. And recurrent laryngeal n below the level of vocal cords.
- After exertion, an athlete is puffing. **Posterior crico-arytenoid** pair of ms helps to maintain a wide airway thro the larynx.

SINUSES

1. Frontal = supraorbital n.
2. Maxillary = infraorbital and anterior, middle, posterior superior alveolar Ns.
3. Sphenoidal = posterior ethmoid n.

AUDITORY TUBE

1. At ostium = pharyngeal br of pterygopalatine ganglion / maxillary n.
2. Cartilagenous part = nervous spinosus / mandibular n
3. Bony part = tympanic plexus / 9th n.

NERVE SUPPLY OF FACE

Motor supply	Facial n = temporal; zygomatic; buccal; mandibular; cervical	
Sensory	Trigeminal	
Ophthalmic div of 5th N	Supratrochlear; supraorbital; lacrimal; infratrochlear; external nasal.	Scalp upto vertex, forehead, upper eyelid, conjunctive, root – dorsum – tip of nose.

NERVE SUPPLY OF FACE (*Contd.*)

Maxillary	Infraorbital; zygomatico-facial; zygomatico-temporal.	
Mandibular	Auriculotemporal; buccal; mental.	

Cervical plexus = auricular div of greater auricular N / C2, C3 and upper div of transverse cervial Ns / C2, C3.

NERVE SUPPLY OF PHARYNX = by pharyngeal plexus of nerves which lies on middle constrictor ms.

- Motor = by cranial accessory n. through vagus; they supply ms of pharynx *except stylopharyngeus* which is supplied by 9th n.
- Inferior constrictor also receives additional supply from external and recurrent laryngeal n.
- Sensory = 9th, 10th Ns.
- Taste = from vallecula and epiglottic by internal laryngeal branch of 10th n.
- Parasympathetic = greater petrosal n.

Quick revision Important points

- Largest organ of the body = skin
- Largest gland = liver
- Largest ganglion of neck = superior cervical ganglion
- First artery to appear in the embryo = right and left primitive aorta
- First bone to ossify in body = clavicle
- Second bone to ossify = mandible
- Most sensitive part of bone = periosteum.
- Nerve supply to the tip of nose = mandibular n
- Nerve supply of skin over the angle of mandible = great auricular n
- Embryonic disc develops during = 3rd wk

- **P**terion = **s**phenoid meets **p**arietal bone; (PSP)
- **B**regma = **s**agittal suture meets **c**oronal; (BSC)
- **L**ambda = **s**agittal suture meets **l**ambdoid suture; (LSL); it lies at the location of posterior fontanelles.
- Sagittal suture = forms where parietal bones meet.
- **C**oronal suture = **f**rontal and **p**arietal bones meet; (CFP)
- **L**ambdoid suture = **p**arietal and **o**ccipital bones meet; (LPO)
- SCM m is innervated by = spinal accessory n and C2, C3 spinal Ns
- Trapezius = by spinal accessory n and C3, C4 spinal Ns
- Cranial n having longest intra-cranial course = 6th / abducent n
- Cranial n most commonly involved in intra-cranial aneurysm = 3rd / occulomotor.
- First endocrine gland to appear in fetus = thyroid gland
- Clinically, most imp layer of scalp = 4th; loose areolar tissues.
- Flexion and extension at neck occurs at = atlanto-occipital joint / AO = YES
- Rotational movement at neck occurs at = atlanto-axial joint / AA = NO
- Lateral flexion at the neck occurs at = b/w 2nd to 7th cervical vertebrae
- Nucleus pulposus is the remnant of = notochord
- Common carotid artery divides into ECA and ICA at = upper border of thyroid C / C4 level.
- Lateral geniculate body is concerned with = light reflex
- Medial geniculate body is concerned with = auditory reflex
- Arch of aorta develops from = artery of 4th branchial arch of left side.
- Pulmonary artery develops from = artery of 6th branchial arch.
- Artery of 1st branchial arch = maxillary A
- Artery of 2nd branchial arch = stapedial A
- No. of primary centres of ossification of clavicle = 2
- Musician's nerve = ulnar

- Labourer's nerve = median
- Nerve of deltoid m = axillary
- Blood supply of S. A. node of heart is from = right coronary A
- Apex of heart is present at = left 5th intercostal space
- Tricuspid orifice of heart is located at = right 5th intercostal space.
- Chief muscle of inspiration = is diaphragm; supplied by phrenic n. / C3,4,5
- Thinnest wall of all the 4 chambers of heart is of = right atrium
- Bundle of His is supplied by = right coronary A
- Action of vagus nerve on heart = inhibitory
- Action of vagus on gut = facilitatory
- **Angle of Louis** / sternal angle is present at = articulation of 2nd rib anteriorly
- Pharyngo-tympanic tube is supplied by = 9th N
- Ligamenum arteriosum is present b/w = left pulmonary A and arch of aorta
- Trachea bifurcates at the level of = lower border of T4 vertebra.
- IVC enters right atrium at the level of = 6th chondro-sternal joint.
- Arch of aorta begins at = T 4 vertebra.
- Oesophagus passes through the diaphragm at = T 10 level
- Length of oesophagus = 25 cm.
- IVC pierces the diaphragm at = T 8 level
- Left umblical V ends into = left branch of portal V
- Content of free margin of lesser omentum = common bile duct ; hepatic artery; portal V (BHP).
- **Space of Disse** = is the space b/w hepatocytes and hepatic sinusoids
- Eustachian tube connects = middle ear to nasopharynx.
- **Signet ring** cartilage is = cricoid cartilage
- Safety m of tongue = genioglossus
- Length of filum terminale = 25 cms
- Spinal cord extends upto = lower border of first lumbar vertebra in adults; L1 level.

- **Transverse facial A** is branch of = superficial temporal A
- Trigeminal ganglion is lodged in = **Meckel's cave**
- Thyroid gland is attached to cartilages of larynx by = pretracheal fascia
- Middle meningeal A / MMA is the branch of = maxillary A
- **MMA overlies** the = motor cortex
- Olfactory epithelium is = pseudostratified
- Lacrimation occurs when facial N gets injured at the level of = geniculate ganglion.
- **Vein of Galen** is formed by = fusion of superior sagittal sinus and straight sinus, i.e. it drains into straight sinus.
- Lymphatics are absent in = brain; spinal cord; eye, cornea; internal ear; nail, hair, epidermis; cartilage; splenic pulp.
- **Maximum representation in brain** is of = thumb
- Tympanic plexus is found in = petrous part of the temporal bone; it is formed by the tympanic br of 9th n.
- **Nerve of pterygoid canal** is formed by the = lesser petrosal N and sympathetic Ns.
- Great superficial petrosal N is the br of = 7th N
- **Apoptosis** = is the normal process of replacement of epithelial cells by the new cells
- A depressor of mandible is = lateral pterygoid m.
- Ms which elevates and retracts the mandible = temporalis
- Right upper motor neuron lesion of 7th n cause = paralysis of lower facial ms of the left side.
- Cartilage which calcify most frequently are = hyaline
- Structures passing through sinus of Morgagni, i.e. b/w the base of skull and superior constrictor ms = levator palati ms and cartilagenous part of eustachian tubes.
- Submandibular ganglion supplies sensory fibres to = sublingual salivary gland
- Middle constrictor ms of pharynx takes origin from the = stylohyoid ligament
- In cavernous sinus, a direct content is = the 6th / abducent nerve.

Functions of cell organelles

Organella	Functions
Endoplasmic reticulum	Contains membrane system for protein synthesis; esp rough ER
Golgi apparatus	Modifies proteins and their secretion
Lysozyme	Causes degradation of macromolecules; contains hydrolytic enzymes
Mitochondria	Contains enzymes for metabolism; respiratory enz; helps in energy production aka **power house** of the cell.
Nucleolus	Helps in RNA and ribosomes production.
Nucleus	Contains chromosomal material for cell multiplication esp DNA.
Ribosomes	Catalyses peptide bond formation during protein synthesis.

EPITHELIUM LININGS OF DIFFERENT ORGANS

Organ	Epithelium Lining
Larynx	Ciliated columnar
Maxillary sinus	Pseudostratified ciliated columnar aka **Schnederian membrane;** it is bluish in colour.
Nose, trachea	Stratified ciliated columnar
Oesophagus	Stratified squamous/nonkeratinizing
Oral cavity	Stratified squamous/nonkeratinized
Respiratory tract	Ciliated columnar
Tonsil	Nonkeratinised stratified squamous
Urethra	Transitional
Vocal cords	Stratified squamous

SITES OF IMPORTANT RECEPTORS

Receptors	Sites
Arterial blood pressure	Stretch receptors in carotid sinus and aortic arch
Arterial PO_2 and PCO_2	Glomus cells of aortic and carotid bodies
Blood glucose difference/ glucostat	Hypothalamus
Blood temperature in head/thermostat	Hypothalamus
Central venous pressure (CVP)	Stretch receptors in walls of great veins and atria; esp right IJV
Hearing	Hair cells in Organ of corti
Linear acceleration	Hair cells in utricle and saccules
pH of CSF	Receptors at ventral part of medulla
Rotational acceleration	Hair cells on semicircular canals

MULTIPLE CHOICE QUESTIONS in Anatomy

1. **The function of which cells is most affected in scurvy**
   A. Eosinophils
   B. Fibroblasts
   C. Osteoclasts
   D. Plasma Cells

2. **Scurvy results due to a defect in**
   A. Collagen cross-linking
   B. Elastin biosynthesis
   C. Fibronectin binding
   D. Tropocollagen biosynthesis

3. **The fundamental lesion involved in the etiology of scurvy is:**
   A. Deficient synthesis of collagen alpha chains
   B. Increased collagen turnover
   C. Increased hydrolysis of tropocollagen telopeptides
   D. Leakage of capillaries

4. **The most powerful flexor muscle of the thigh is**
   A. Adductor longus
   B. Iliopsoas
   C. Rectus femoris
   D. Sartorius

5. **A chief abductor muscle of the thigh is**
   A. Gluteus maximus
   B. Gluteus medius
   C. Piriformis
   D. Quadratus femoris

6. **Which costal cartilage articulates with the sternum at the level of the sternal angle:**
   A. 1st rib
   B. 2nd rib
   C. 3rd rib
   D. 4th rib

7. Which costal cartilage is the lowest costal cartilage contributing to the costal margin of the rib cage ?

A. 9th
B. 10th
C. 11th
D. 12th

8. For central venous pressure (CVP), the best barometer is which jugular vein?

A. Right external jugular vein
B. Right internal jugular vein
C. Left external jugular vein
D. Left internal jugular vein

9. When the head – neck – trunk of a supine adult are elevated 30–45 degrees from the horizontal, then the pulsatile activity in the jugular veins will be observed at what normal vertical distance above the level of the sternal angle:

A. 0–1 cm
B. 2–3 cm
C. 4–5 cm
D. 6–7 cm

10. The right border of the heart lies to the right of the right border of the sternum in a normal healthy adult by

A. 0–1 cm
B. 2–3 cm
C. 4–5 cm
D. 6–7 cm

11. All of the following viscera are retroperitoneal except:

A. Abdominal aorta
B. Inferior vena cava
C. Right kidney
D. Spleen

12. All of the following viscera are secondarily retroperitoneal EXCEPT:

A. Body of the pancreas
B. Descending colon

C. Head of the pancreas
D. Tail of the pancreas

13. Following segments of the small and large intestines are intraperitoneal EXCEPT:
A. 2nd, 3rd and 4th parts of the duodenum
B. Jejunum
C. Ileum
D. Transverse colon

14. The normal range for the height of the liver along the right mid-clavicular line in an adult on percussion, is
A. 3–6 cm
B. 6–9 cm
C. 9–12 cm
D. 6–12 cm

15. Pain from an inflamed appendix is most often referred to the
A. Epigastric and/or umbilical regions
B. Hypogastric region
C. Right lumbar region
D. Right inguinal region

16. Vagus nerves supplies preganglionic parasympathetic fibres to the large intestine as far distally as
A. Near the border between the cecum and ascending colon
B. Near the border between the descending colon and sigmoid colon
C. Near the splenic flexure
D. Near the border between the sigmoid colon and rectum

17. The height of an adult kidney averages ____ times the thickness of the body of the 2nd lumbar vertebra.
A. 1.5
B. 2.6
C. 3.7
D. 4.8

18. The fibers of the olfactory nerve pass through which part of the ethmoid bone from the nasal cavity to the cranial cavity
A. Cribriform plate

B. Crista galli
C. Perpendicular plate
D. Superior concha

19. The ethmoid bone contributes to all of the following parts EXCEPT

A. Floor of the nasal cavity
B. Medial wall of the orbital cavity
C. Nasal septum
D. Roof of the nasal cavity

20. All of the following nerves except one passes through the superior fissure:

A. Abducent nerve
B. Oculomotor nerve
C. Ophthalmic division of the trigeminal nerve
D. Optic nerve
E. Trochlear nerve

21. Injury to the nerves that pass through the superior orbital fissure can lead to all EXCEPT

A. The ability to move the eyeball from the primary position to a position in which the cornea faces directly medially could be weakened or lost.
B. The ability to forcibly close the eyelids could be weakened or lost.
C. The ability to raise the upper eyelid could be weakened or lost
D. The ability to decrease the size of the pupil could be weakened or lost

22. All of the following pass through the interior of the cavernous sinus or its lateral wall EXCEPT:

A. Postganglionic sympathetic fibers that innervate dilator pupillae
B. Internal carotid artery
C. Trochlear nerve
D. Mandibular division of the trigeminal nerve

23. Following statements concerning the cavernous sinus are correct EXCEPT:

A. The cavernous sinus lies immediately lateral the pituitary gland

B. The cavernous sinus lies immediate medial to the frontal lobe of the cerebrum.

C. The cavernous sinus can drain blood from the facial vein.

D. The superior ophthalmic vein is a tributary of the cavernous sinus.

E. The internal jugular vein can drain blood from the cavernous sinus.

24. Tapping a patient's lower jaw causes a reflexive raising of the lower jaw due to jaw jerk / deep tendon reflex. It tests sensory fibers of the

A. Facial nerve

B. Hypoglossal nerve

C. Mandibular division of the trigeminal nerve

D. Vagus nerve and cranial root of the accessory nerve

25. The jaw jerk tests motor fibers of the

A. Mandibular division of the trigeminal nerve

B. Facial nerve

C. Glossopharyngeal nerve

D. Hypoglossal nerve

26. On palpating masseter muscle as the patient is asked to clench the teeth to test motor fibers of the

A. Mandibular division of the trigeminal nerve

B. Facial nerve

C. Glossopharyngeal nerve

D. Vagus nerve and root of the accessory nerve

27. During laryngoscopy, the right vocal fold is not abducted when the patient says "e-e-e" in a high pitched voice, it indicates paralysis of muscles innervated by the

A. Facial nerve

B. Glossopharyngeal nerve

C. Vagus and cranial root of the accessory nerve

D. Hypoglossal nerve

28. Disease or injury to the motor fibers in which of the nerve leads to the left deviation of a tongue in protrusion

A. Mandibular division of the trigeminal nerve
B. Right vagus nerve cranial root of the right accessory nerve
C. Left hypoglossal nerve
D. Right hypoglossal nerve

29. On saying "AH", a left deviation of the uvula is a result of injury to motor fibers in one or more nerves in the

A. Left vagus nerve and cranial root of the left accessory nerve
B. Right vagus nerve cranial root of the right accessory nerve
C. Left hypoglossal nerve
D. Right hypoglossal nerve

30. If left corner of mouth does not move upwards on smiling, it indicates injury to the motor fibres of

A. Mandibular div of left 5th n.
B. Left facial n
C. Left 9th n
D. Left hypoglossal n.

31. A reflexive decrease in the rate of heart beat on massaging neck in the region of carotid pulse is mediated by pregang-lionic p – sympathetic fibres of the:

A. Facial nerve
B. 9th n
C. 10th n
D. Cranial root of 11th n

32. The taste fibers for sugar on the tip of tongue lie in:

A. Mandibular div of 5th n
B. Facial n
C. Vagus n and cranial root of the 11th n
D. 12th n

33. Nerve giving the sensation of light touch on the tip of the tongue is :

A. Mandibular div of 5th n
B. Facial n
C. Vagus n and cranial root of the 11th n
D. 12th n

34. Muscle responsible for protrusion of the tongue is

A. Genioglossus
B. Hyoglossus
C. Intrinsic ms of tongue
D. Styloglossus

35. The branch of ICA giving blood supply to the lateral aspect of the frontal and parietal lobes is

A. Anterior cerebral
B. Middle cerebral
C. Posterior cerebral
D. Superior cerebral

36. The blood supply to the visual cortex is severely compromised by the occlusion of

A. Basilar
B. Internal carotid
C. Middle cerebral
D. Posterior cerebral

37. The oculomotor nerve may be affected by an aneurysm of which of these arteries as it passes between them at the base of the brain

A. Middle cerebral-anterior cerebral
B. Anterior cerebral-anterior communicating
C. Posterior cerebral-superior cerebellar
D. Basilar-vertebral

38. The skeletal muscle which raises the eyelid is supplied by:

A. III
B. IV
C. V
D. VII

39. Axons controlling pupillary constriction with light stimulation and during accommodation originate in the

A. Lateral geniculate nucleus
B. Superior colliculus
C. Nucleus solitarius
D. Edinger-Westphal nucleus

40. Preganglionic parasympathetic nerve fibers carried by the oculomotor nerve synapse in the

A. Ciliary ganglion
B. Otic ganglion
C. Pterygopalatine ganglion
D. Superior cervical ganglion

41. Vein of Galen drains its contents into:

A. Cavernous sinsus
B. Superior sagittal sinus
C. Inferior sagittal sinus
D. Straight sinus

42. Ansa cervicalis supplies to which muscle:

A. Cricohyoid
B. Thyroyhyoid
C. Posterior transverses
D. Vocalis

43. Nerve supply to the Lateral rectus muscle of eye is:

A. II
B. III
C. IV
D. VI

44. One of the following is not draining in the cavernous sinus:

A. Superficial middle cerebral vein
B. Ophthalmic vein
C. Sphenoparietal sinus
D. Great vein of Galen

45. PDA(Patent Ductus Arteriosus) is the embryonic remnant of:

A. 2nd arch
B. 4th arch
C. 6th arch
D. 8th arch

46. True about the sphenoid air sinus is that it :

A. Opens into the middle meatus
B. Is lined by stratified squamous epithelium
C. Is present at birth
D. Occupies the greater wing of sphenoid

47. The deep cerebellar nuclei:
A. Lie in the roof of 4th ventricle
B. Are related to lateral recess of 4th ventricle
C. Receives a connecting branch from trigeminal nerve
D. Joins the sphenopalatine ganglion

48. The lesser petrosal nerve is characterised by that it:
A. Contains the secretomotor fibres to parotid gland
B. Passes through the foramen rotundum
C. Receives a connecting branch from trigeminal nerve
D. Joins the sphenopalatine ganglion, etc.

49. The structure passing through sinus of Morgagni, i.e. between superior constrictor muscle and base of skull is:
A. Tensor tympani
B. Tensor palati + Auditory tube
C. Tensor palati
D. Only auditory tube

50. Ultrastructure of β - cells of pancreas represent as :
A. Rectangular and crystalline shaped vesicles
B. Spherical shaped vesicles
C. Numerous mitochondria
D. Increased vesicles in active state.

51. The location of Ductus arteriosus is between:
A. Left and right pulmonary arteries
B. Aortic arch and left pulmonary artery
C. Aortic arch and right pulmonary artery
D. Aortic arch and right subclavian artery

52. Commonest part of aorta which gets ruptured during trauma is:
A. Ascending
B. Descending
C. Abdominal
D. Junction of thoracic and abdominal aorta

53. All are the branches of internal carotid artery except:
A. Middle cerebral
B. Posterior communicating

C. Anterior communicating
D. Posterior cerebral.

54. Source of bleeding in Duodenal ulcer is from:
A. Gastroduodenal artery
B. Left gastroepiploic artery
C. Right gastroepipolic artery
D. Superior pancreatic duodenal artery.

55. The location of the Brunner's glands is in the mucosa of:
A. Stomach
B. Duodenum
C. Oesophagus
D. Colon

56. All are draining in cavernous sinus except:
A Basilar sinus
B. Inferior petrosal sinus
C. Inferior sagittal sinus
D. Superior sagittal sinus

57. The following ms are the depressors of mandible except:
A. Hyoglossus
B. Mylohyoid
C. Geniohyoid
D. Digastric

58. Nerve supply of the Meninges is by all except:
A. Anterior ethmoidal nerve
B. Posterior ethmoidal nerve
C. Frontal nerve
D. Nervous spinosus

59. Broca's area is in (it is related with speech):
A. Superior temporal gyrus
B. Inferior temporal gyrus
C. Angular gyrus
D. Inferior frontal gyrus

60. The opening of the Duct of Wirsung is at (i.e. Wharton's duct of submandibular gland):
A. Minor papilla
B. Major papilla
C. Opposite upper 2nd molar
D. Side of frenulum of tongue

61. Structures passing through Foramen Magnum include all except:
A. Ascending cervical A
B. Jacobson's nerve
C. Vertebral venous plexus
D. Spinal cord

62. The taste sensation to the anterior 2/3 of the tongue is through:
A. Chorda tympani nerve
B. Jacobson's nerve
C. Glossopharyngeal nerve
D. Trigeminal nerve

63. The blood to the inner ear is supplied by:
A. Middle
B. Posterior inferior cerebellar A
C. Superior cerebellar A
D. Anterior inferior cerebellar A

64. The gland derived from Foramen caecum is:
A. Pituitary
B. Thyroid
C. Thymus
D. Parathyroid

65. Sensory nerve supply to the Tip of nose is:
A. Facial nerve.
B. Mandibular nerve of V nerve
C. Maxillary nerve of V nerve
D. Ophthalmic nerve of V nerve

66. Pulmonary vasculature is different because:

A. Mean pressure difference of arteries is low
B. Absent sympathetic vasoconstrictor tone
C. Can accommodate large amount of blood volume
D. All of the above.

67. Distance between upper incisors and gastroesophageal junction is:

A. 15 cm
B. 25 cm
C. 40 cm
D. 60 cm

68. Purkinje cells found in cerebellum are:

A. Input cell
B. Output cell
C. Interneuron cell
D. Glial component

69. The structure which disappears in umbilical cord is:

A. Right Artery
B. Left Artery
C. Right Vein
D. Left Vein

70. The most common site for Lung sequestration is in which lobe:

A. Left posterior basal
B. Right lateral basal
C. Apical
D. Left posterosuperior

71. The most important characteristic of protective epithelium is:

A. Microvilli
B. Pinocytic vesicles
C. Infolding of membrane
D. Thinness

72. H_2O_2 is produced and destroyed in which component of the cell:

A. Lysosome
B. Ribosome
C. Peroxisome
D. Golgi bodies

73. The structures dividing the liver in two lobes is by all except:

A. Portal vein
B. Hepatic artery
C. Common bile duct
D. Right hepatic vein

74. Untrue about ectodermal cleft is:

A. Dorsal part of first cleft forms lining of external cartilage,
B. Cervical sinus is found between 2nd to 6th arches
C. Ventral part of cleft is obliterated
D. None of the above

75. The structure common to Oesophagus and duodenum is :

A. Mucous cells
B. Submucosal glands
C. Pseudostratified column epithelium
D. All of the above.

76. Portal vein is related to all except:

A. IVC
B. CBD
C. Pancreas
D. Gallbladder

77. Organ having skeletal muscles, str. squamus epithelium, serous and mucus glands is :

A. Tongue
B. Gastric cells in antrum
C. Mucus cells in cardia
D. Mucus cells in antrum

78. Shape and size of the cell is determined by:

A. Nuclear growth
B. ER
C. Cell wall
D. Golgi bodies

79. The muscle not supplied by Ansa cervicalis is:

A. Inferior Belly of omohyoid
B. Sternothyroid
C. Sternohyoid
D. Thyrohyoid

80. Pulsation in the neck felt inferiorly at medial border of sternocleidomastoid muscle is of:

A. Subclavian
B. Vertebral
C. CCA
D. Brachial

81. Structure found at the midpoint of Anterior Superior Iliac spine and pubic symphysis is:

A. Femoral A
B. Femoral V
C. Femoral Nerve
D. Saphenous opening

82. The level at which the trachea bifurcates is:

A. T_{3-4}
B. T_{4-5}
C. T_{5-6}
D. T_{6-7}

83. Mandibular nerve lesion at its origin involves all of the following except:

A. Buccinator
B. Masseter
C. Tensor Palati
D. Tensor Tympani

84. Lymphatics are found in:
A. Brain
B. Internal ear
C. Dermis
D. Eye

Answer Key to MCQs in Anatomy

1	B	2	A	3	B	4	B
5	B	6	B	7	B	8	B
9	B	10	A	11	D	12	D
13	A	14	D	15	A	16	C
17	C	18	A	19	A	20	D
21	B	22	D	23	B	24	C
25	A	26	A	27	C	28	C
29	B	30	B	31	C	32	B
33	A	34	A	35	B	36	D
37	C	38	A	39	D	40	A
41	D	42	B	43	D	44	D
45	C	46	C	47	A	48	A
49	D	50	B	51	B	52	D
53	D	54	A	55	B	56	D
57	A	58	C	59	D	60	D
61	A	62	A	63	D	64	B
65	D	66	D	67	C	68	B
69	C	70	A	71	C	72	C
73	D	74	D	75	B	76	D
77	A	78	C	79	D	80	A
81	A	82	B	83	A	84	C

2

Embryology

GENERAL POINTS

⇒ Cells of theca interna secrete a hormone known as OESTROGEN. Ovum which is shed from ovary is known as SECONDARY OOCYTE.

⇒ Corpus luteum secretes PROGESTERONE.

⇒ It contains YELLOW PIGMENT known as LUTEIN and that is why it is known as corpus luteum, i.e. yellow body.

⇒ If ovum is not fertilised, CL persists for 14 days and secretes progesterone and changes into CORPUS ALBICANS (white body).

⇒ If ovum is fertilised, CL persist for 3–4 month. It secretes progesterone for maintenance of pregnancy. After 4th month, the placenta starts secreting progesterone.

⇒ During the first meiosis, 2 chromosomes of a pair separate at ANAPHASE.

⇒ Turner syndrome 44 X

⇒ Klinefelter syndrome 44 X X Y

⇒ Triploidy 46 + 23 = 69 chromosomes

⇒ Trisomy 46 + 1 = 47

⇒ Isochromosomes: When the centromere splits transversely, producing 2 dissimilar chromosomes.

⇒ Just before the start of next menstrual cycle, there is a decrease of both progesterone and estrogen levels and it is believed that this withdrawal leads to the onset of menstrual bleeding.

⇒ Ovulation occurs 14 days before the next menstrual bleeding.

⇒ After ovulation, ovum is viable for 2 days and sperms die within 4 days.

⇒ FSH stimulates
- Formation of follicle
- Secretion of estrogen

⇒ LH stimulates
- Secretion of progesterone
- Conversion of ovarian follicle into CL.

GERM LAYERS

⇒ **3 germ layers**

i. ENDODERM, which is the first germ layer to be formed.

ii. Remaining cells of inner cell mass become COLUMNAR and form ECTODERM.

⇒ Amniotic cavity develops between ectoderm and trophoblasts.

⇒ Primary yolk sac is lined by ENDODERM.

⇒ Extraembryonic mesoderm (primary mesoderm) does not give rise to any tissues of the embryo itself.

Prochordal plate is formed by endoderm.

⇒ Cells from primitive streak migrate between ecto - and endoderm to form MESODERM (Intraembryonic) which is the 3rd germ layer.

⇒ prochordal plate forms later bucco-pharyngeal membrane.

Bulk of tissues of body is formed by mesoderm.

⇒ Henson's node is the thickened cranial end of primitive streak.

⇒ Notochord forms the central axis of the body. It lies in midline, in the position to be later occupied by the vertebral column. Remnants of it persist at nucleus pulposus.

⇒ Neural tube

* gives rise to brain and spinal cord.
* formed from ECTODERM.

⇒ Mesoderm separates ecto- and endoderm in all parts except:

i. Prochordal plate

ii. Cloacal membrane

iii. In midline caudal to prochordal plate,

⇒ In human placenta, known as Hemochoreal

* Maternal tissue - Blood
* Fetal tissue - Chorion

⇒ Progesterone secreted by the placenta is essential for maintenance of pregnancy after degeneration of corpus luteum.

⇒ Endoderm forms the epithelium of whole GIT (except the parts of mouth and anal canal lined by ectoderm).

BONE

⇒ Smallest unit of bone = LAMELLAE
(It contains collagen fibres + matrix + Ca^{++} salts).

⇒ Spongy bone = has trabeculae and numerous bone marrow spaces.

⇒ Compact bone = Very small spaces, lamellae are arranged as OSTEONE (or HAVERSIAN SYSTEM).

* Bone marrow is present in Haversian canals only.
* Concentrically arranged lamellae.

⇒ <u>All bone is of MESODERMAL ORIGIN</u>.

⇒ Diaphysis = shaft of bone, formed by extension of primary centre of ossification.

⇒ Cartilagenous ends = secondary centres of endochondral ossification appear. <u>Part of bone formed from one secondary centre is known as EPIPHYSIS</u>.

⇒ Bone of diaphysis and of epiphysis are separated by EPIPHYSEAL PLATE.

⇒ Metaphysis = part of diaphysis adjacent to epiphyseal plate.

* It is the region of active bone formation, is highly vascular, no marrow cavity.
* Calcium turnover function of bone is most active here and acts as a store house of Ca^{++}.

MUSCLES

i. Sclerotome = gives rise to vertebral column and ribs.
ii. Myotome = gives rise to striated muscles.
iii. Dermatome = gives rise to dermis and subcutaneous tissues.

⇒ Occipital somites = supplied by Hypoglossal N

⇒ Preoccipital (Pre-otic) somites by 3, 4, 6 N.

⇒ In human - myotomes give origin only to the muscles of trunk.

⇒ Occipital myotomes - form tongue ms.

⇒ Preoccipital myotomes - Extrinsic ms of eyeball (supplied by 3, 4 and 6 N)

⇒ Myotome of neck and trunk divide in:

i. Dorsal part - ms supplied by dorsal primary ramus of spinal ns.
ii. Ventral part - ms supplied by ventral ramus of spinal N.

⇒ Smooth ms - almost all are formed from MESENCHYME

⇒ Smooth muscles of walls of viscera and cardiac ms. by splanchnopleuric mesoderm.

⇒ Myoepithelial cells of sweat glands = Ectodermal

GLANDS

⇒ Develop as diverticula from epithelial surfaces.

⇒ Derived from one diverticulum = Parotid gland

⇒ Derived from several diverticula = Lacrimal, prostate

⇒ Ectodermal origin = Sebaceous glands, sweat glands, mammary glands

⇒ Endodermal origin = Pancreas, liver

⇒ Mesodermal origin = Adrenal cortex.

⇒ Mixed = Prostate

⇒ Adrenal medulla = ectodermal origin. Adr. medulla has some embryonic origin as symp. ganglion.

⇒ Hypophysis cerebri (Pituitary gland)

* Ant part develop from = ectoderm (Rathke's pouch)
* Post part develop from = diencephalon (as downgrowth)

BLOOD

⇒ Blood formation occurs in Red bone marrow in post natal life.

⇒ In prenatal life - blood formation is first seen i.r.t. wall of the yolk sac and i. r. t. the allantoic diverticulum.

⇒ In 2nd mo. IU - Liver is formed, becomes imp. site of blood formation.

⇒ In 3rd mo. IU - Bone marrow begins to be formed and blood formation starts here and is completely taken over by the marrow by 6th month.

⇒ Precursor of blood forming cells are MESENCHYMAL ORIGIN. Head starts taking shape in 3rd /4th week IU.

SKIN

⇒ Epidermis - from surface ectoderm

⇒ Melanoblasts (or dendritic cells) = from neural crest.

⇒ Dermis from mesenchyme underlying the surface ectoderm.

NAIL

⇒ Derived from ectoderm

⇒ Nail substance corresponds to stratum lucidum of skin.

HAIR

⇒ Derived from surface ectoderm.

PHARYNGEAL ARCHES

⇒ are mesodermal thickenings in the wall of cranial most part of foregut—six bars which run dorsoventrally in the side wall of the foregut.

⇒ 5th arch disappears soon after its formation.

⇒ 1st arch is known as mandibular arch.

⇒ 2nd arch is known as hyoid arch.

In mesoderm of each arch - following structures are found:

i. A skeletal element.

ii. Striated muscle = supplied by the nerve of the arch.

iii. An arterial arch.

⇒ A double innervation is seen only in first arch in human.

Derivatives of pharyngeal arches

1. First arch - cartilage is Meckel's cartilage.
   * Incus from dorsal end.
   * Malleus from dorsal end.
   * Ventral part forms frame-work for mandible.
   * Anterior ligamentum of malleus and sphenomandibular ligament from perichondrium.

2. 2nd Arch: (5 S) – Its cartilage is ka Reichter's cartilage.
   * Stapes
   * Styloid process
   * Stylohyoid ligaments (from sheath)
   * Smaller (lesser) cornu of hyoid.
   * Superior part of body of hyoid.

3. 3rd arch:
   * Greater cornu of hyoid
   * Lower part of body of hyoid.

4. 4th and 6th - cartilages of larynx, thyroid C are formed.

Arch	**Artery**	**Nerve**	**Pouch, derivatives**	**Ms. of arch**
I. Mandibular	Maxillary	Trigeminal, Mandibular	Eustachian tube middle ear	Tensor tympani, tensor palati, DG (Anterior) mylohyoid, (masseter, temporalis, medial and lateral pterygoids) (8 ms.)
II. Hyoid	Stapedial	Facial	Palatine tonsils	Stapedius, stylohyoid, DG post auricular ms, platysma, occipitofrontalis, facial ms.
III. Glossopharyngeal	CCA, part of ICA	Glossopharyngeal	Thymus, inferior parathyroid	Stylopharyngeus
IV. and	Aorta	Vagus, Sup. laryngeal	Superior parathyroid	Ms of soft palate, pharynx and larynx.
VI.		Recurrent laryngeal		

⇒ <u>Only mandibular arch has a double nerve supply</u> - mandibular N = post trematic; and chorda tympani = Pre trematic (Br of 7th N)

This double innervation is reflected in the anterior 2/3rd tongue, which is derived from ventral part of the first arch.

Ectodermal clefts	**Endodermal pouches**
I * Epithelium lining of external auditory meatus from dorsal part. * Pinna is formed from a series of swellings which arise on Ist and 2nd arches * Ventral part is obliterated.	I. Ventral part is obliterated by formation of TONGUE. Dorsal part of 1st and 2nd arch forms tubotympanic gives rise to auditory tube recess = Its proximal part (pharyngotympanic tube) and distal part forms Middle ear cavity and tympanic antrum.
II Cervical sinus is the space between overhanging 2nd arch and 3, 4, 6 arches. * If cervical sinus is not obliterated, then branchial cyst remains, which lie along anterior border of SCM ms.	II. Epithelium of ventral part forms **Tonsil** Dorsal part contributes to tubotympanic recess. III. Inf. parathyroid and thymus. IV. Sup. parathyroid and contribution to thyroid. V. Known as ultimobranchial pouch: which forms: Para-follicular cells of thyroid. - Sup. parathyroid with 4th pouch) - Many times - 4, 5th pouch fuse.to form CAUDAL - PHARYNGEAL COMPLEX.

THYROID GLAND

⇒ Epithelium of floor of pharynx form a thickening which is depressed below as diverticulum known as thyroglossal duct (at foramen cecum).

⇒ Bifurcated ends of diverticulum - form 2 lobes of thyroid gland (so it develops from thyroglossal duct).

SKULL

⇒ Develop from mesenchyme

⇒ Otic capsule and nasal capsules are mesenchymal.

⇒ Mandibular and maxillary process from Ist branchial arch-mesoderm of these processes form some bones of skull.

A. Intramembranous bones:

i. Frontal, parietal - from mesenchyme covering the brain

ii. Maxilla, zygomatic, palatine (excluding Pre-mx) from mesenchyme of maxillary process.

iii. Nasal, lacrimal, vomer from membrane covering the nasal capsule.

B. Endochondral bones:

- Ethmoid, Inf. nasal concha - from cartilage of nasal capsule.
- Septal and alar C. are parts of capsule which do not ossify.

C. Bones which partly form in cartilage and partly in membrane:

* Occipital - Interparietal part is Membranous.
  - Rest is Endochondral
* Sphenoid - Lateral part of greater wing and pterygoid lamina is membranous.
  - Rest is Endochondral
* Temporal - Squamous and tympanic part is membranous
  - Petrous and mastoid part - Endochondral from cartilage of otic capsule.
  - Styloid from cartilage of second arch.
* Mandible - Most is membranous in mandibular process
  - Ventral part of Meckel's cartilage is embedded in bone.

- Condylar and coronoid process ossify from secondary cartilage which appear in these situations.
- Clavical is a membranous bone.

Developmental disturbances

* Anencephaly - greater part of skull - vault is missing
* Scaphocephaly - Premature <u>sagittal suture</u> closure forms <u>boat-shaped skull</u>.
* Acrocephaly - Premature <u>coronal suture</u> closure forms <u>pointed - skull</u>.
* Plagiocephaly - Asymmetrical union of sutures results in a <u>twisted skull</u>.
* Syndactyly - Fused digits
* Synphalangia - Fused phalanges of a digit.
* Macrodactyly - Longer digit
* Brachydactyly - Abnormally small digit
* Arachnodactyly - Fingers are long and thin.
* Polydactyly - More fingers

Summary of origin of Different parts of mouth and face

Stomodeum	- Rathke's pouch -	Anterior Pituitary
		- Lips / teeth
		- Hard palate
		- Anterior part of soft palate.
MNP	- Premaxilla - 2 central incisors.	
	Nasal septum	
	Philtrum (?)	
	Frenum of upper lip	
LNP	- Cribriform plate and lateral mass of ethmoid	
	Inferior nasal concha	
	Upper part of body of maxilla and frontal process.	

Summary of origin of different parts of mouth and face ***(Contd.)***

	Lacrimal and other nasal bones.
	Lat. cartilage of nose and part of alar cartilage of nasal septum.
Maxillary process	- Part of body of maxilla.
	- Upper alveolar process
	- Lateral part of premaxilla
	Hard palate except premaxillary part
	zygomatic bones, zygomatic process of temporal bone.
	Upper lip except philtrum.
Mandibular process	- Body of mandible.
	- Lower alveolar process.
	- Lower lip.
	- Part of cheek.

Corner of mouth is formed by the fusion of maxillary and mandibular processes

Bifid uvula is due to incomplete fusion of palatine shelves

EMBRYOLOGY (FACE / PALATE)

⇒ Mesoderm covering the forebrain proliferates to form-Frontonasal process.

⇒ Floor of stomodeum – by buccopharyngeal membrane (ecto + endoderm)

Stomodeum gives rise to mouth.

⇒ Face is derived from :

- FNP and Mandibular arch (Maxilla Process and Mandibular Process)

⇒ Nasal placodes - are Ectodermal thickenings

⇒ Lips are derived from = Maxillary + Mandibular + MNP.

Lower lip	Mandibular process
Lower jaw	Mandibular process
Mouth	Stomodeum
Upper lip	Mesodermal base of lateral part = by Maxillary Process Its overlying skin = Ectoderm of Maxillary Process Mesodermal basis of median part, i.e. philtrum by FNP. Overlying skin = Ectoderm of Maxillary Process So skin of entire upper lip - by Maxillary Process (Maxillary Nerve) Muscles of face and lips - Mesoderm of 2nd arch (7th N).
Anterior nares	MNP + LNP (Maxillary Process fuses with MNP also)
Nasal septum	Deep part of FNP.
Prominence of nose	Mesoderm becomes heaped up in median plane so nares now open downwards.
Cheeks	Maxillary and mandibular processes
Nasolacrimal sulcus	Maxilla Process + LNP
Nasolacrimal duct	By ectoderm which gets buried along this furrow.
Lens placodes	Ectodermal thickening Lie lateral and cranial to nasal placode Lie in the angles between maxillary process and LNP.

Eye lids	Folds of ectoderm - formed above and below the eyes : - by mesoderm - within the folds.
External ear	- On dorsal part of first ectodermal cleft. - Mesodermal thickenings appear on Ist, IInd arches which fuse to form PINNA.
Primitive palate	FNP
Lateral nasal wall	LNP
Olfactory epithelium	From olfactory placodes

ANOMALIES OF FACE

How it develops: due to non-fusion of:

CLP	FNP + Maxillary Process
Cleft Lip	MNP + Maxillary Process
Midline cleft of Upper lip	FNP (lowest part)
Midline cleft of Lower lip	Mandibular Process + Mandibular Process (Do not fuse) of other side
Oblique facial cleft	Maxillary Process + LNP (do not fuse)
Nasolacrimal duct not formed	Maxillary Process + LNP (do not fuse)
Macrostomia	Maxillary + Mandibular Process
Lateral facial cleft	Unilateral non-fusion of Maxillary + Mandibular Process
Microstomia	Too much fusion of Maxillary + Mandibular Process
Cyclops	Fusion of 2 eyes.
Mandibulofacial dysostosis	Underdevelopment of entire Ist arch on one or both sides.

PALATE

⇒ Palatal process - from Maxillary Process

3 processes which form palate are:

i. 2 palatal process fusion starts anteriorly and goes posteriorly.

ii. FNP—forms Primitive palate (premaxilla).

⇒ Palatal process fuse with free lower edge of nasal septum.

⇒ Mesoderm in palate by intramembranous ossification forms hard palate.

MOUTH

⇒ Partly from stomatodeum and foregut.

⇒ Epithelial linings is - partly ectodermal

- partly endodermal

⇒ Epithelium of lips, cheek, palate, teeth, gum are **Ectodermal**.

⇒ Epithelium of tongue - **Endodermal.**

⇒ Mandibular process forms - 3 structures:

* L. lip and lower part of cheeks.
* L. jaw and tongue

TOOTH

Dental lamina	- from epithelium overlying the alv. process
Enamel organ	- cells of dental lamina **(ectodermal)**
Dental papilla	- **Mesenchymal**
Tooth germ	- Dental papilla + enamel organ
Ameloblasts	- from enamel organ, i.e. **ectodermal**
Odontoblasts	- **Mesodermal** cells of dental papillae.
Pulp	- from dental papilla.

TONGUE

Pharyngeal arches are MESODERMAL THICKENINGS in lateral wall of foregut.

⇒ Two **Lingual swellings** - from medial most part of mandibular arches.

⇒ One **Tuberculum impar** - also from mandibular arch in midline.

⇒ Behind tuberculum impar- epithelium proliferates to form **Thyroglossal duct** - which forms Thyroid gland at F. caecum.

⇒ One **hypobranchial eminence** - i.r.t. medial ends of 2, 3, 4th arches.

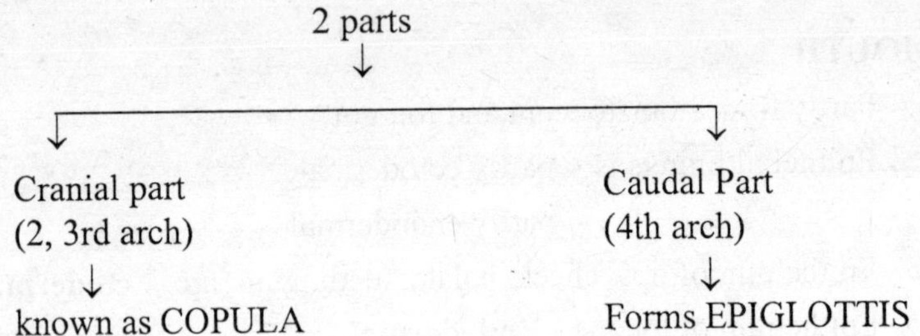

Anterior 2/3rd tongue is formed by :

* Tuberculum impar, i.e. from **Mandibular arch.**
* 2 lingual swellings, i.e. from **Mandibular arch.**

Posterior 1/3 - from COPULA, and 3rd arch mesoderm.

* 2nd arch mesoderm gets buried below the surface
* 3rd arch mesoderm overgrows 2nd to join 1st.

Posterior most part - from 4th arch.

Nerve Supply

1	Anterior 2/3	=	Lingual br. of mandibular N (5th) Chorda tympani N of 7th N (Pretrematic)
2	Posterior 1/3	=	Glossopharyngeal N (9th)
3	Posterior most	=	Superior laryngeal N (10th)
4	Ms. of tongue	=	Hypoglossal N (12th); (derived from occipital myotomes)

SALIVARY GLANDS

⇒ Outgrowth for parotid gland arises i.r.t. the line of fusion of Maxillary Process and Mandibular Process. It is **ectodermal**.

⇒ Submandibular and sublingual glands arise i.r.t. linguogingival sulcus - **endodermal**

TONSILS (Palatine)

⇒ Develop i.r.t. 2nd pharyngeal pouch.

⇒ Similarly epithelial proliferations and aggregation of lymphoid tissue give rise to: tubal, lingual and pharyngeal (adenoid) tonsils,

⇒ Pharynx develop from uppermost part of foregut.

⇒ Respiratory system develop from floor of foregut.

ARTERIES

⇒ First arteries to appear in the embryo are R and L primitive aortae.

⇒ Greater part of Ist and 2nd, 5th arch arteries disappear.

⇒ In adult life ; **first arch artery = Maxillary A.**

But = 2nd arch artery persists for some part of fetal life as STAPEDIAL and it may contribute to the formation of ECA.

⇒ Aortic sac is connected with arteries of 3, 4 and 6th arches.

Ventral part of aortic sac = 3, 4th A; receives blood from ascending aorta. Dorsal part of aortic sac = 6th arch A, receives blood from pulmonary trunk.

⇒ 3rd arch A. gives off a bud to form CCA, ICA and ECA.

⇒ 6th arch A. gives artery to LUNG BUD.

⇒ Truncus arteriosus = forms Asc. aorta and pulmonary trunk.

⇒ Ventral part of aortic sac, its left horn and left 4th arch A arise from Arch of aorta.

FETAL CIRCULATION

⇒ Source of oxygenated blood = PLACENTA through UMBILICAL V. greater part of blood passes direct to the inferior vena cava through DUCTUS VENOSUS.

⇒ From R ventricle - Deoxygenated blood enters pulmonary trunk - greater part of blood is short- circuited to AORTA via DUCTUS ARTERIOSUS.

⇒ Umbilical A. carry deoxygenated blood to placenta for OXYGENATION, which is then returned to heart.

	Artery	**Vein**
Umbilical	Carry impure blood	Carry pure blood
Pulmonary	Carry impure blood	Carry impure blood
Ductus	Carry impure blood	Carry pure blood

CHANGES IN CIRCULATION AFTER BIRTH

⇒ Ductus arteriosus gets occluded such that all blood from R. ventricle goes to lungs.

⇒ Pressure in Left Atrium now is greater than Right atrium, which causes closure of valves of F. ovale.

Remnants of

Umbilical A.	Medial umbilical ligament.
Left Umbilical V	Ligamentum teres of liver (LUV = LTL)
Ductus venosus	Ligamentum Venosum
Ductus arteriosus	Ligamentum Arteriosum

3

Histology

MORPHOLOGY OF CELL

BASIC MEMBRANE: 2 layered - Formed by phospholipid molecules

Polar end/head end (has PO_4 part), soluble in water, hydrophilic.

Nonpolar/tail end, non-soluble in water, hydrophobic

CELL MEMBRANE: Large molecules enter the cell by PINOCYTOSIS.

CONTACT BETWEEN ADJACENT CELLS

Desmosome: Most common type; thick areas are joined together by fibrils.

Zonula Adherens (ZA): Seen at apices of epithelial cells, it is in the form of a continuous band around the apical part of epithelial cells and the gap between 2 cells is not traversed by fibrils.

Zonula Occludens (ZO): Known as tight junctions, near apices of epithelial cells, two plasma membranes are in actual contact,

Junctional Complex (JC): when **ZO, ZA, MA** are arranged in that order near the apices of epithelial cells, it is known as J.C.

Gap junction: Membranes lie very close to each other, the gap being 3 nm, also known as MACULAE COMMUNICANTES.

CELL ORGANELLES

Rough (granular) endoplasmic reticulum (RER) = have ribosome (RNA particles), here proteins are synthesised.

Smooth (agranular) ER (SER) - associated with various biochemical processes like carbohydrate metabolism.

RIBOSOMES: Help in protein synthesis.

MITOCHONDRIA: Greatest in number in cells with high metabolic activity. ATP and GTP are formed in it to provide energy.

GOLGI COMPLEX: Carbohydrate synthesis.

Phagosomes - ingest solid material.

Pinocytotic vesicles - ingest fluid material

Exocytic vesicles - Expel the material from inside the cell to outside the cell.

Lysosomes - destroy unwanted material present within a cell.

Peroxisomes contain CATALASE to destroy H_2O_2.

CENTRIOLES: It contains 9 groups of microtubules arranged in a circle, each group has 3 tubules **(9+3)**, Help in forming Mitotic spindles,

Cilia and flagella, tail of sperm, have **9+2** configuration of tubules.

Proteins of microtubules are TUBULIN

Proteins of microfilaments are ACTIN.

Some cilia like structures, which perform sensory functions:

Olfactory cilia	-	Smell
Kinocilia	-	Internal ear
Stereocilia	-	are large microvilli.

NUCLEUS

Cytoplasmic DNA = associated with mitochondria

Heterochromatin - Where chromatin is in the form of irregular dark masses, chromatin fibres are tightly coiled.

Euchromatin = where chromatin is loose and stains lightly, coiling is not so marked.

Nucleoli - have high RNA content. rRNA is synthesised in nucleoli.

Structure of DNA: PO_4 of one nucleotide is linked to sugar of other nucleotide. Base may be A, G, T, C — A = T, G = C

Structural Gene / Cistron - that part of DNA molecule which bears the code for a complete polypeptide chain.

⇒ DNA $\xrightarrow{\text{transcription}}$ mRA $\xrightarrow{\text{translation}}$ Protein

Types of chromosomes

Acrocentric - when centromere is not in the centre of chromatids, 2 arms are of unequal lengths.

Metacentric - when 2 arm are of equal length.

Telocentric - when centromere lies at one end.

CELL DIVISION: MITOSIS

Period between 2 mitoses = **Interphase**

1. Greater part of interphase is **G1 stage**
2. Approx. 12 hours before mitosis, DNA synthesis occurs and is completed in 7 hours—This period is known as **S-Stage**.
3. Last 5 hours before mitosis are used for protein synthesis required for cell division = known as **G2-Stage**.

⇒ Stages - 4 - PROPHASE
⇒ - META PHASE
⇒ - ANA PHASE
⇒ - TELO PHASE

DNA duplicated = S-stage of interphase

Chromosomes become recognisable and distinct in **prophase**.

Each chromosome becomes attached to the microtubules of spindle = in **METAPHASE.**

Centromere of each chromosome splits and cell has 46 pairs (46 × 2) chromosomes = **ANAPHASE**.

2 daughter nuclei are formed by appearance of nuclear membrane. = **TELOPHASE**

Centrioles duplicate = **Early interphase**

Colcemide: is the drug which can arrest cell division, is used during karyotyping.

COLCHICIN: can arrest mitosis at metaphase and helps in chromosomal study.

MEIOSIS: 2 stages—I, II

1st Meiotic:

1. Leptotene: **Chromosomes become visible.**

Chromatids not distinct.

2. **Zygotene**: 2 homozygous chromosomes come to lie side by side forming a bivalent known as **synapsis / conjugation.**
3. **Pachytene**: Chromatids become distinct (bivalent has 4 chromatids known as **TETRAD)**

   Crossing over of central chromatid occurs = crossing points are known as CHIASMATA.
4. **Diplotene:** 2 chromosomes of a bivalent try to move apart, exchange of genetic material takes place.

2. **Metaphase**: 46 Chromosomes become attached to spindle at the equator.
3. **Anaphase**: No splitting of centromeres takes place (as compared to in mitosis)
   - 23 chromosomes in each pair move.
4. **Telophase**: Same as mitosis.

IInd MEIOSIS: is like mitosis.

1. **Short interphase** - but no DNA duplication.

Determination of chromosomal sex:

- Other inactive X- chromosome of female forms a mass of HETEROCHROMATIN known as SEX CHROMATIN/BARR BODY/ nucleolar satellite in neurons or drum-stick in WBCs.

Active X-Chromosomes = is of EUCHROMATIN

Epithelia are devoid of blood vessels = get nutrition by DIFFUSION.

MUCOUS MEMBRANE: Layer of epithelium along with its lamina propria is known as MUCOUS MEMBRANE.

GLANDS

Simple gland: When all secretory cells discharge into one duct.

Compound gland: When group of secretory cells discharge in their own ducts, which then unite to form a common duct to discharge on epithelial surface.

MUCOUS GLANDS: Secretions have mucopolysaccharides, e.g. **Goblet cells** in intestine.

Serous glands: secretions are PROTEIN.

ECCRINE: (merocrine, epicrine), secretions occur by exocytosis and cell remains intact.

APOCRINE: Apical part of cells are shed off to discharge their secretion, e.g. atypical sweat glands, mammary gland.

HOLOCRINE: Entire cell disintegrates, e.g. sebaceous gland.

SALIVARY GLANDS: All salivary glands are "compound racemose" glands

Parotid, SMG = Primarily **Serous**

Sublingual, Minor glands = **Mucous**

Parotid gland = Largest, **Stenson's duct** -opens against maxillary second molar.

SMG gland = 2nd largest, Wharton's duct

SLG = Smallest, **ducts of Rivinus** are multiple ducts, some may join to form **Bartholin's duct** which then opens in submandibular duct.

Myoepithelial cells are present in respect to alveoli and intercalated ducts - which are contractile to squeeze out secretions.

CONNECTIVE TISSUES

Fibres: Collagen (most numerous), Reticular, Elastic.

Collagen fibril shows cross striations after every 64 nm, made of protein COLLAGEN which is made of small units known as TROPOCOLLAGEN - 280 nm size.

Tropocollagen is rich in Glycine, hydroxyproline and hydroxylysine (GHH)

Reticular fibres: also known as ARGENTOPHILE FIBRES, Periodicity at 64 nm. Are essentral component of all basement membranes.

ELASTIC FIBRES: run singly (not in bundles), branch and anastomose.

Protein is ELASTIN, made of TROPO-ELASTINS, Digested by enzyme ELASTASE

Elastin contains high quantity of VALINE, also rich in glycine and proline.

FIBROBLASTS: Most numerous cells of CT.

Produce collagen and reticular fibres.

Macrophage Cells: also HISTIOCYTES / CLASMATOCYTES, Can eat ORGANIC material (bacteria) and inorganic material.

MAST CELLS: Granules contain polysaccharides

Mast cells release following :

Heparin (prevents blood clotting)

Histamine and serotonin are associated with allergic reactions.

Eosinophils are found in CT; Increase in number in allergies.

Lymphocytes - Increase during inflammation.

T-Lymphocytes= destroy foreign tissues, grafts, etc.

T-lymphocytes = in thymus - lymphoid tissues

B-lymphocytes = in blood - lymphoid tissues

(B= from Bursa of fabricius in birds)

Abs are produced by B-lymphocytes.

T-Cells = Cell mediated response

Rejection of graft = by T-cells.

Ground substance contains PPS complexes mainly chondroitin sulfate and hyaluronic acid.

Fat cells or lipoblasts arise from undifferentiated mesenchymal cells.

Macrophage system: also known as RE system or mononuclear phagocyte system. Most of the cells arise in BONE MARROW and pass in blood as circulating monocyte.

Neutrophils = Collect at sites of INFECTION, cause phagocytosis, lysis of bacteria.

Eosinophils = Immune response, increase in ALLERGY.

Basophils =Contain Heparin, histamine, serotonin (like mast cells).

In **Liver** = They also known as KUPFFER CELLS.

In **Lungs' alveoli** = They also known as DUST cells.

NUCLEI

In Lymphocytes = Spherical, may be indented.

In Monocytes = Ovoid, may be indented, eccentric.

In Basophils = S-shaped

In Eosinophils = 2–3 lobed

In Neutrophils = Several lobed (also known as PMN cells or polymorphs).

CARTILAGE

Hyaline and elastic C. are covered by PERICHONDRIUM but fibrocartilage is not.

Elastic and fibrocartilage C do not undergo calcification.

Hyaline C. especially costal C. and C. of larynx can undergo calcification.

Cartilage is AVASCULAR - nutrition is by DIFFUSION.

COMPACT BONE: Made of lamellae,

Lamellae are arranged in concentric rings which surround a narrow **HAVERSIAN CANAL** which contains - blood vessel + nerve + cells.

Haversian system **(OSTEON)** One H canal + lamellae around it—run along the length of the bone. Average number of lamellae in each osteon = Six

H. canals communicate with marrow cavity and external surface through = **CANALS of VOLKMANN** (for nutrition).

OSTEOBLASTS = Bone forming, Lay down organic matrix of bone + collagen., Rich in ALKALINE PHOSPHATASE, Osteoblasts move inwards while laying down lamellae, so the first lamella (peripheral) is OLDEST.

OSTEOCLASTS: Bone removing cells, Contains more than 20 nuclei /cell. Rich in ACID PHOSPHATASE,

Primary centre of ossification = forms **diaphysis.**

Secondary center of ossification = part of bone formed by one secondary centre of ossification is known as **EPIPHYSIS**.

Metaphysis: Part of diaphysis adjacent to epithyseal plate is known as Metaphysis.

- Region of active bone formation, highly vascular, no marrow cavity
- Ca^{2+} turnover function is most active here even after bone growth has ceased. It acts store house of Ca^{2+}.

NASAL CAVITIES: Olfactory mucosa - present on superior nasal concha and adjacent part of nasal septum

Trachea bifurcates in R and L primary bronchi at the level of STERNAL ANGLE, i.e. T4.

H/E feature which most readily distinguishes AORTA is presence of a TUNICA MEDIA composed primarily of elastic membrane.

Amount of muscle in the bronchial wall increases as the bronchi become smaller.

In tongue, the Taste buds: are present i.r.t. circumvallate, fungiform papilla, and folia - linguae on posterolateral part of tongue. Filiform papillae have no taste buds.

GASTROINTESTINAL TRACT

Gastric glands: present all over the stomach except in PYLORIC REGION and a small area near cardiac end.

1. Most numerous cells are **chief cells / peptic cells / zymogen cells,** esp in basal part of glands, secrete PEPSIN which is formed from pepsinogen.
2. **Oxyntic / Parietal cells**: Produce **HCl** and intrinsic factor which combines with Vit. B_{12} (extrinsic factors) = complex is necessary for formation of RBCs.

Mucus neck cells: Near the neck (upper end) of the gland - secrete mucous.

Argentaffin cells - near the basal part of gastric glands,

- Secrete **GASTRIN** and contain serotonin (5-HT)

CARDIAC GLANDS: are mucous secreting.

PYLORIC GLANDS : occupy lower 1/3rd of mucosa, secrete mucous

Epithelial lining:

1. **Goblet cells** - secrete mucous,
2. **Undifferentiated cells** - in the wall of crypts, active mitosis
3. **Zymogen / Paneth cells** - produced digestive enzymes.
4. **Argentaffin cells** (Endocrine cells of gut)
   i. **T-Cells having 5 HT (serotonin)** - known as Entero-chromaffin cells.
   ii. **Argyrophile cells** - produce amines which have endocrine functions (neurotransmitters).

Lymphoid tissue (Peyer's patches) maximum in terminal ileum.

LIVER: It is an exocrine gland.

Along the periphery of lobule, the angular intervals known as PORTAL CANALS, contains: branch of hepatic A, a branch of portal V, and an interlobular bile duct which form **a portal triad.**

True functional unit of liver - PORTAL LOBULE

PANCREAS

Partly exocrine + partly endocrine - main bulk of gland by its exocrine part.

Both derived from endodermal lining of gut

EXOCRINE PART

1. 2 types of secretions:
   a. Watery: it neutralises ACID contents, production is influenced by SECRETIN,
   b. Thicker: has enzymes, e.g. trypsinogen, chymotrypsinogen, amylase, lipase, etc., which is stimulated by PAN-CREOZYMIN, by VAGAL stimulation.
2. ENDOCRINE PART- as **Islets of LANGERHANS**

- 3 types of cells-

A-Cells (α)	Glucagon (A-2)		20%
B-Cells (β)	Insulin		≃ 80%
D-Cells (δ)	Gastrin and somatostatin	Somatostatin inhibits secretion of glucagon and insulin.	

KIDNEYS

When first formed, the glomerular filtrate (GF) is **isotonic** with blood.

With reabsorption of ions, it becomes Hypotonic.

Considerable amount of Na, Cl are reabsorbed from DC Tubule.

The GF entering the collecting ducts is HYPOTONIC.

Urine entering the renal pelvis = HYPERTONIC (1.5 litres / day).

REPRODUCTIVE ORGANS

Sertoli cells (Sustentacular cells) are supportive / nutritive.

Interstitial cells of Leydig secrete male sex hormones (Testicular androgens).

ENDOCRINE GLANDS

(Ductless glands)

A. PITUITARY GLAND / HYPOPHYSIS CEREBRI

a. PARS ANTERIOR:

- Chromophil cells - have granules — Acidophils (α-cells)
  Basophils (β-cells)
- Chromophobe cells - no granules

B. PARS INTERMEDIA: some cells produce MSH (melanocyte SH) which increases skin pigmentation.

C. PARS POSTERIOR: 2 hormones:

VASOPRESSIN / ADH: controls water reabsorption by kidney tubules.

OXYTOCIN: controls **smooth m. contraction of uterus** and mammary gland. (Produced in para-ventricular nuclei and secreted here.)

Posterior lobe of hypophysis has = <u>Unmyelinated nerve fibres</u>

Cells	**Produced**	**Influence**
Somatotrophs	Somatotropin/GH	Growth
Mammotrophs	Mammotropin/ Prolactin	Mammary gland
Corticotrophs	ACTH	Adrenal cortex hormones secretion
Thyrotrophs	Thyrotropin	Thyroid gland
Gonadotrophs	FSH	Growth of ovarian follicle Secretion of oestrogen from ovaries Spermatogenesis in males
	LH	Maturation of corpus luteum and progesterone secretion in females Production of androgens by interstitial cells in males

THYROID GLAND

Folliclular cells secrete 2 hormones which **influence rate of metabolism**, e.g. T3 (triiodothyronine), T4 (thyroxine). It is influenced by TSH (thyrotropine).

Parafollicular cells, also known as C-cells, clear cells or light cells, secrete **thyrocalcitonin**, which has an action **opposite to PTH** on Ca^{2+} metabolism. This hormones comes into play when serum - Ca^{2+} level is high. It decreases Ca^{2+} level by suppressing Ca^{2+} release from bone.

PARATHYROID GLAND

Two types of cells:

1. **Chief or principal cells** - produce **PTH** - which increases serum Ca^{2+} level by bone resorption, Ca^{2+} resorption from renal tubules, and increasing Ca^{2+} resorption from GUT.

2. **Oxyphil/ eosinophil cells** - granules of oxyphil cells are MITOCHONDRIA.

ADRENAL GLANDS

Four **S**'s — **S**alt, **S**ugar, **S**ex, **S**urvival

Layers of cortex : 3 layers

1. **Zona glomerulosa** produce **mineralocorticoids** (Aldosterone, deoxycorticosterone) which influence electrolyte and water balance of body.

2. **Zona fasciculata** produce **glucocorticoids,** (cortisone, cortisol, i.e. dihydroxycortisone), which affect carbohydrate and protein metabolism, decrease Antibody-responses, have antiinflammatory effects.

3. **Zona reticularis** produce some glucocorticoids and sex hormones - both estrogens and androgens.

Secretion of **aldosterone is influenced by RENIN** secreted by JG cells of kidney. Secretion of hormones of ZG (mineralocorticoids) is independent of pituitary.

Adrenal medulla

PARAGANGLIA: Cells similar to Adr. medulla, found in close relation to AUTONOMIC GANGLIA.

Serve as alternative site for production of **catecholamines** in fetus and early postnatal life.

MUSCLE TISSUE

Skeletal muscle: made up of single, multinucleated cell.

Striations: with H and E stain, alternate light and dark bands are seen in myofibril.

A-bands	=	Dark
I-bands	=	Light
Z-bands	=	in the middle of each I-band.
H-zone	=	in the middle of each A-band
M-bands	=	in the middle of each H-band

I-band = **only ACTIN** fibres.

A-band = **Myosin + actin**, myosin filaments are **confined to A-band only**

H-Band (Hensen's line) = Central part of A-band into which actin filaments do not extend, i.e. **only myosin**. Seen only when muscle is in relaxed state.

I. band = only **actin, H-band** = only **myosin**

Z-band = **Actin** filaments of adjacent sarcomeres, i.e. in the **centre of I-band**.

M-band = Fine interconnection between adjacent myosin filaments (in the **centre of H-zone**).

H-band gets **obliterated** in a contracted fibril, by **sliding of actin** filament between myosin filaments.

Myosin **(i.e. thick filament) are present in** A-band **only.**

Sarcomere: Part of a myofibril **between two consecutive Z-bands** (1/2 I band + A band + ½ I-band)

Sarcolemma = Each muscle fibre covered by a plasma membrane.

Endomysium = Surrounds individual muscle fibres.

Perimysiun = Surrounds fasciuli

epimysium = Surrounds entire muscle.

Gamma (g)- efferents supply to special fibres, present only within sensory receptors (called **muscle-spindles**); these special muscle fibres are known as **INTRAFUSAL FIBRES.**

Skeletal M = is a True anatomical syncytium.

Junction between adjacent myosites = known as intercalated discs and lie **opposite to I-bands and are characteristics of cardiac muscle.**

NERVOUS TISSUE

Functional unit of nervous system = NEURONS

No lymphatic vessels in nervous tissue.

Schwann Cells - Provides myelin sheath to the axons lying outside the CNS.

Oligodendrocytes - Provides sheath to the axons lying within the CNS.

Most common type of Neuron - MULTIPOLAR.

PERIPHERAL NERVES

Each nerve fibre surrounded by ENDONEURIUM.

Each fasciculus surrounded by PERINEURIUM.

Each nerve surrounded by EPINEURIUM.

1. **Efferent /Motor fibres** : Carry impulses from S. cord or brain to peripheral structure. They are axons of neurons located in grey matter of spinal cord or brainstem.
2. **Afferent / Sensory fibres**: Carry impulses from peripheral organs to brain or spinal cord. They are the processes of neurons located in SENSORY GANGLI. Neurons in it are PSEUDOUNIPOLAR.

In case of vestibulo- cochlear nerve, they are BIPOLAR neurons.

In spinal nerve = Ganglia are located in DORSAL NERVE ROOTS.

In Cranial nerves = ganglia located on the nerve concerned.

This description does not apply for 1, 2 nerves.

CLASSIFICATION OF FIBRES

Type A = **fastest** conduction, (15–100 meter / sec.)

Type B = 3–15 m/sec., **slow,** 3 mm dia.

- Pre-ganglionic autonomic efferent fibres.

Type A and B are myelinated.

Type C = Unmyelinated, 0.3–1.6 m/sec. (Vel.), 0.2–1.5 m (Dia)

SYNAPSE = Junction between neurons.

<u>Most common</u> = **Axo-Dendritic Synapse.**

BOUTON - If axon may terminate in a single, bulb-like end.

RECEPTORS

1 **Cutaneous / exteroceptive** for (TTPP) Temperature, Touch, Pain, Pressure.

2 **Proprioceptive:** Provide informations about the state of muscle contraction, joint position and movement, required for <u>precise control of movement</u> and maintenance of body posture; these activities occur due to reflex - action.

3 **Interoceptive**: These are in thoracic and abdominal viscera, blood vessels, carotid sheath and bodies.

4 **Special sense receptors** of vision, hearing, smell, taste.

Exteroceptive receptors

1. **Free nerve endings**: Numerous i.r.t. hair follicle, hair are touch receptor, also respond to pain.
2. **Tactile corpuscles (Meissner)**: i.r.t. dermal papillae on hand, foot; are **touch** receptors, for tactile touch.

3. **Pacinian corpuscles (Lamellated):** on subcutaneous tissue of palm, sole, digits, for pressure sensation.
4. **Krause corpuscles (Bulbous)**: for COLD.
5. **Tactile disc (of Merkel):** seen i.r.t. enlarged epithelium cells in Stratum spinosum of epidermis, for touch.

6. Ruffinil's end organs: for heat.

PROPRIOCEPTORS

1. **Golgi-tendon organs:** Located at the junction of muscles and tendon.

   Stimulated by pull upon the tendon during active contraction of the muscle.
2. **Muscle-spindles:** Located within STRIATED muscle.

Sensory endings — 2 types:

- Primary : wind spirally around the nuclear region of intrafusal fibres and also known as ANNULOSPIRAL ENDINGS.
- Secondary : known as Flower Spray Ending.

Function: Spindles provide information to the brain about the extent and rate of stretching of muscle.

Neuromuscular junction: Preganglionic of both SNS/PNS are cholinergic (Ach.).

In SNS = N Adr - Postganglionic

PNS = Ach

GANGLIA: Aggregation of cell bodies of neurons present outside the brain and S. cord : 2 types—Sensory and autonomic

A. Sensory ganglia

i. Present on the dorsal nerve roots of spinal nerves (known as Dorsal nerve root ganglia) and

ii. On 5, 7, 8, 9, 10 cranial nerves

Regeneration of several Axons does not occur in CNS – due to absence of Neurilemma.

Neurons in these ganglia are pseudounipolar except vestibulo-cochlear nerve (where bipolar neuron).

B. Autonomic ganglia - Supply smooth muscles or glands by 2 neurons.

Preganglionic = Cell bodies are located in the spinal cord / brain stem.

Post ganglionic - Cell bodies in autonomic ganglia. These neurons are MULTIPOLAR.

In sympathetic ganglia - **catecholamines** (Adr, N. Adr) are synthesised.

In p-symp. ganglia - **Ach.** is synthesised.

DIFFERENT CELLS: **in Nervous System are :**

1. Neuroglial - found in grey and white matter of brain and S. cord.
2. Ependymal - Line the ventricular system.
3. Schwann - form sheaths for axons of peripheral nerve.
4. Capsular / satellite -Surround neurons in peripheral ganglia.
5. Supporting cells: i.r.t. motor and sensory terminals of nerve fibres.

ARTERIES

Smallest arteries = known as Arterioles

In proceeding distally along the artery, there is a gradual reduction in elastic fibers and increase in smooth muscle content of media.

Diff. between V. and A. - V. has more prominent tunica adventitia, but lesser smooth ms. in Tunica media.

Muscular arteries do not have an **internal elastic lamina.**

VEINS: wall of vein is thinner than A.

T. media has much larger quantity of collagen than artery. Amount of elastic tissue and muscle is less.

In As, TM is thicker than TA.

In Vs, TA is thicker than TM.

VENULES: Smallest veins, into which capillaries drain are known as venules. 20–30μ dia.

Lymphocytes and other **cells pass out** / in blood at venules only.

Capillaries

Exchange between blood and tissue occurs through the walls of capillary plexus.

Wall = made of endothelial cells, PERICYTES and no muscles in the wall.

SINUSOIDS: As compared to capillaries- Wall may be incomplete at places.

Wall may be lined by phagocytic RE cells instead of endothelial cells.

Diff. between capillaries and sinusoids is that capillaries have constant lumen and a complete endothelial lining, whereas sinusoids are irregular , tortuous tubes.

Arterioles have maximum % age of smooth muscle and so are the main resistance vessels.

VASA-VASORUM - Supply to the walls of large and medium sized vessels, i.e. to adventitia and outer part of media.

Lymphatics

Smallest lymph vessel= Lymphatic capillaries.

Peyer's patches: present in small intestine esp ilium in mucosa/ submucosa.

Chyle - lymph rich in fat - globules

B- lymphocytes - matures to **plasma cells** and form **antibodies**.

Thymus is the primary lymphoid organ.

Lymph nodes, spleen are known as secondary lymph organs.

SPLEEN: Largest lymphoid organ of body.

Lymphatic nodules of white pulp has B-cells, while rest of the white pulp is made of T-cells .

Red pulp has **sinusoids,** space between sinusoids is filled with B, T-cells, macrophages and blood cells arranged as cords known as **splenic cords of BILLROTH.**

Lymphoid tissue of spleen has the function of filtering **Blood only**

- Kupfer cells = RE (macrophages) cells of liver.
- Microglial cells = Macrophages in CNS.

In GIT—Largest aggregations are - R/L palatine tonsils

Peyer's patches = always lie along the ante-mesenteric border of intestine, **most numerous in terminal ileum.**

In adenoids - pharyngeal tonsils are involved.

SKIN

Epidermis + dermis

Epidermis - Stratified squamous epithelium. 5 layers (BSGLC)

1. Basal layer: also known as germinal or Malpighian layer.
2. Str. spinosum : also known as Prickle cells. Get keratinized - so also known as Keratocytes.

Germinative zone of epidermis = Str. basale + Str. spinosum.

3. Str. granulosum - Granules contain Keratohyaline.
4. Str. lucidum - cytoplasm has a derivative of keratohyaline known as ELEIDIN.
5. Str. corneum - Contain keratin (from ELEIDIN)

1. Str. germinativum = Str. basale + Str. spinosum
2. Zone of Keratinisation = Str. granulosum + Str. lucidum + Str. corneum
3. Seen well on non-hairy skin are:
   - Str. granulosum = contains keratohyaline
   - Str. lucidum = contains eleidine
4. Thickest in palm and sole :

   Str. corneum = contains keratin

5. Str. lucidum is absent in very thin skin.

   Stratum germinativum forms epithelial root sheath of the hair follicles.

Basal cells and adjacent cells of S. spinosum = contain **melanin** (from melanoblasts which is also known as dendritic cells.

Tyrosine → DOPA → Melanin

Blood vessels do not penetrate into the EPIDERMIS, which get nutrition by DIFFUSION.

HAIR

Hair root is a modified part of Str. corneum, has keratin, [cortex (outer) + medulla (inner)]

- Sebaceous glands are HOLOCRINE
- Meibomian (Tarsal) glands of eyelids are modified sebaceous glands.

Typical sweat glands: are eccrine (mesocrine) type

NAILS: It is modified part of zone of keratinisation of epidermis, a thickened continuation of **stratum lucidum**.

4

MCQs in Anatomy, Histology and Embryology

1. The Golgi apparatus functions to

A. Give form to the cell and control passage of materials in and out of the cell

B. Serve as a matrix substance in which chemical reactions occur

C. Synthesize complex carbohydrate molecules which combine with protein produced by rough endoplasmic reticulum to form secretory products such as lipoproteins

D. Release energy from food molecules and transform energy into usable **ATP**

2. All of the following statements concerning the sphenoid bone are true except:

A. The greater wing of the sphenoid bone forms the lateral wall of the orbit and the roof of the infratemporal fossa

B. The lesser wing of the sphenoid bone contains the optic canal (optic foramen) and helps from the superior orbital fissure and roof of the orbit

C. The medial pterygoid plates of the sphenoid bone provide attachment sites fcr two muscles of mastication

D. Foramina within the greater wing of the sphenoid bone provide access to both the pterygopalatine and infratemporal fossa

E. The body of the sphenoid bone contains the sella turcica and the sphenoid sinus

3. **The os coxa or hipbone is formed by the fusion of the three structures listed below except?**
   A. Ilium
   B. Ischium
   C. Acetabulum
   D. Pubis

4. **Which part of the face listed below is the first to form in the embryo?**
   A. The maxilla
   B. The mandible
   C. Both of the above
   D. None of the above

5. **All of the following are functions of the skeletal system, except:**
   A. Support
   B. Protection
   C. Body movement
   D. Hemopoiesis
   E. Fat storage
   F. Mineral storage

6. **The auxiliary vein begins at the border of the teres major muscle as the continuation of the basilic vein. As it ascends to the inferior margin of the first rib it becomes which vein listed below?**
   A. Brachial vein
   B. Brachiocephalic vein
   C. Cephalic vein
   D. Subclavian vein

7. **Mitosis results in:**
   A. One daughter cell
   B. Two daughter cells
   C. Three daughter cells
   D. Four daughter cells

8. **Which type of tissue listed below supports or binds other tissues and provides metabolic needs to all body organs?**
   A. Epithelial tissue
   B. Connective tissue

C. Muscle tissue
D. Nervous tissue

9. All of the following structures empty into the cavernous sinus, excepts the
A. Superior ophthalmic vein
B. Inferior ophthalmic vein
C. Maxillary artery
D. The cerebral veins
E. Sphenoparietal sinus
F. Central vein of the retina

10. The greater petrosal nerve originates from which ganglion listed below?
A. Otic ganglion
B. Pterygopalatine ganglion
C. Geniculate ganglion
D. Celiac ganglion

11. Which structures listed below form the root of the lung?
A. Bronchi
B. Pulmonary artery
C. Pulmonary vein
D. Lymph vessels
E. Bronchial vessels
F. Nerves
G. All of the above

12. Which cranial nerve provides preganglionic parasympathetic fibers through the otic ganglion to the parotid gland?
A. Trigeminal nerve (CN V)
B. Facial nerve (CN VII)
C. Glossopharyngeal nerve (CN IX)
D. Vagus nerve (CN X)

13. Which of the following has the most extensive distribution of all the cranial nerves?
A. Facial nerve (CN VII)
B. Trigeminal nerve (CN V)
C. Hypoglossal nerve (CN XII)
D. Vagus nerve (CN X)

14. Which nerve listed below is the largest of the 12 cranial nerves and is the principal general sensory nerve to the head, particularly the face?
A. Vagus (CN X)
B. Glossopharyngeal (CN IX)
C. Facial (CN VII)
D. Trigeminal (CN V)

15. Which organ listed below extends from the pyloric opening to the ileocecal junction and is that where digestion and food absorption mainly takes place?
A. Stomach
B. Liver
C. Small intestine
D. Large intestine

16. The thymus gland produces which hormone listed below?
A. Glucagon
B. Thymopoietin
C. Calcitonin
D. Insulin

17. In relationship to the occlusal plane of the mandibular molars, the mandibular foramen is:
A. Below the occlusal plane and posterior to the molars
B. Above the occlusal plane and posterior to the molars
C. Above the occlusal plane and anterior to the molars
D. Below the occlusal plane and anterior to the molars

18. All of the following statements concerning neurons are true except:
A. They are unipolar, bipolar, or multipolar in shape
B. They are specialized for the reception, integration, and transmission of information
C. They are the basic structural and functional component of the nervous system
D. Their axons carry impulses toward the cell body
E. They consist of cell bodies, axons and dendrites

19. Wharton's duct is associated with which salivary grand listed below?

A. Parotid gland
B. Submandibular gland
C. Sublingual gland
D. von Ebner's glands

20. Specialized structures, which are found periodically along lymph vessels, are

A. Thrombocytes
B. Lacteals
C. Lymph nodes
D. Gap junctions

21. Which of the following is the hardest substance in the body?

A. Enamel
B. Dentin
C. Cementum
D. Bone

22. All of the following structures are found in the superior mediastinum, except:

A. The arch of the aorta
B. The branchio-cephalic veins
C. Trachea
D. Lungs
E. Thymus gland

23. In which type of muscle fiber listed below, would you expect to find fusiform cells?

A. Skeletal muscle fibers
B. Smooth muscle fibers
C. Cardiac muscle fibres
D. Neither of the above

24. Which type of epithelium listed below would be found lining the stomach?

A. Simple squamous epithelium
B. Simple columnar epithelium
C. Stratified cuboidal epithelium
D. Pseudostratified columnar epithelium

25. All muscles listed below are considered to be the circular muscles of the pharynx except?
A. Superior constrictor
B. Middle constrictor
C. Inferior constrictor
D. Stylopharyngeus

26. Which group of gingival fibers listed below connects all teeth and maintains the integrity of the dental arches?
A. Alveolo-gingival fibers
B. Transseptal fibers
C. Dentoperiosteal fibers
D. Dentogingival fibers

27. Muscle fiber contraction results from the interaction of contractile proteins in which the length of the sarcomeres is reduced. Which two proteins listed below are responsible for this muscle contraction?
A. Elastin
B. Myosin
C. Collagen
D. Actin

28. The exchange of nutrients and wastes between blood and tissue takes place across the walls of:
A. Veins
B. Arteries
C. Capillaries
D. Venules
E. Arterioles

29. Thrombosis in the coronary sinus might cause dilation of all of the following veins except:
A. Small cardiac veins
B. Great cardiac vein
C. Middle cardiac vein
D. Anterior cardiac veins

30. Which structure listed below gives rise to cementoblasts?
A. Dental papilla
B. Enamel organ

C. Dental sac
D. Inner enamel epithelium

31. Which of the following are the two terminal branches of the internal thoracic artery?
A. Superior epigastric and musculophrenic arteries
B. Anterior and posterior intercostal arteries
C. Subclavian and inferior epigastric arteries
D. None of the above

32. Compared to companion arteries, veins show all of the following except:
A. Less muscles
B. Lower blood pressure within them
C. Less elastic tissues
D. Same general tissues
E. Smaller diameter

33. Which two structures listed below join to form Hertwig's epithelial root sheath?
A. Stratum intermedium
B. Inner enamel epithelium
C. Stellate reticulum
D. Outer enamel epithelium

34. All of the following statements concerning the nasal cavity are true, except
A. The roof is formed by the nasal, frontal, sphenoid (the body) and ethmoid (the cribriform plate of bones)
B. The floor is formed by the palatine process of the maxilla and the horizontal plate of the palatine bone.
C. The lateral walls are formed by the superior, middle, and inferior conchae.
D. The medial wall or nasal septum is formed entirely by the vomer bone
E. The bridge of the nose is formed by the two nasal bones

35. The middle ear cavity and the sphenoid sinus are separated by a thin layer of bone from which part of the cranial fossa listed below?
A. Anterior cranial fossa

B. Middle cranial fossa
C. Posterior cranial fossa
D. None of the above

36. The common carotid artery divides into its external and internal branches at the level of the superior border of the:
A. Jugular notch
B. First cervical vertebra
C. Cricoid cartilage
D. Thyroid cartilage
E. Hyoid bone

37. Which of the following is the principal artery to the nasal cavity, supplying the conchae, meatus, and paranasal sinuses?
A. Anterior tympanic artery
B. Sphenopalatine artery
C. Middle meningeal artery
D. Lingual artery

38. Which cell listed below is considered to be a phagocytic cell and is concerned with defense against bacterial invasion?
A. Plasma cell
B. Mast cell
C. Macrophage
D. Schwann cell

39. The cell cycle consists of all of the following except:
A. Growth
B. Synthesis
C. Fusion
D. Mitosis

40. Which of the following is the best way to palpate the posterior aspect of the mandibular condyle?
A. Intraorally
B. Through the external auditory meatus
C. Lateral to the external auditory meatus
D. Any of the above

41. Which structure listed below is a band or cord of dense, regular fibrous connective tissue that attaches muscle to bone?

A. Ligament
B. Tendon
C. Joint
D. Disc

42. The external laryngeal branch of the superior laryngeal nerve innervates which muscle listed below?

A. Thyrohyoid muscle
B. Middle pharyngeal constrictor muscle
C. Cricothyroid muscle
D. Superior pharyngeal constrictor muscle

43. Anatomically the dental pulp is divided into two portions, the coronal and radicular pulp. Which portion is located in the pulp chamber and pulp horns?

A. Coronal pulp
B. Radicular pulp
C. Both of the above
D. None of the above

44. Which nerve listed below innervates the facial muscles with motor fibers, the lacrimal gland and salivary glands with parasympathetic fibers, and the anterior tongue with sensory fibers?

A. Trigeminal
B. Vagus
C. Facial
D. Glossopharyngeal

45. Which of the following is the main function of cementum?

A. Compensation for tooth wear
B. Reparative
C. To attach the principle fibers of the periodontal ligament to the tooth
D. Protection

46. The splanchnic nerves (greater, lesser and least) arise from which region of the sympathetic trunks listed below?

A. Cervical region
B. Thoracic region
C. Lumbar region
D. Sacral region

47. Which nerve listed below carries general sensation from the anterior two-thirds of the tongue?

A. Hypoglossal nerve
B. Chorda tympani
C. Lingual nerve
D. Recurrent laryngeal nerve
E. Glossopharyngeal nerve

48. Non-neuronal tissue of the CNS that performs supportive and other ancillary functions is called:

A. Dermatome
B. Neuroglia
C. Bursa
D. Synapse

49. All structures listed below make up the brainstem except?

A. Diencephalon
B. Pons
C. Medulla oblongata
D. Mesencephalon

50. Which part of the adrenal gland listed below behaves more like neural tissue as opposed to a typical endocrine gland?

A. Adrenal cortex
B. Adrenal medulla
C. None of the above
D. Both of the above

51. Which salivary gland listed below is the smallest and contains both serous and mucous acini?

A. Submandibular gland
B. Parotid gland
C. Sublingual gland
D. None of the above

52. Which pharyngeal pouch listed below gives rise to the inferior parathyroid gland and the thymus gland?
A. First
B. Second
C. Third
D. Fourth
E. Fifth

53. Which endocrine gland listed below plays a vital role in the regulation of calcium and phosphorus metabolism?
A. Adrenal gland
B. Parathyroid gland
C. Pancreas
D. Pineal gland

54. The soft palate ends posteriorly in the midline as a conical projection called the:
A. Palatine aponeuroses
B. Uvula
C. Piriform fossa
D. Pharyngeal isthmus

55. Which longitudinal muscle of the pharynx listed below is innervated by the glossopharyngeal nerve?
A. Stylopharyngeus
B. Palatopharyngeus
C. Salpingopharyngeus
D. None of the above

56. Most of the joints of the body are:
A. Fibrous joints
B. Cartilaginous joints
C. Synovial joints
D. Fibrocartilaginous joints

57. Bruner's glands are found in which area listed below?
A. Submucosa of the stomach
B. Submucosa of the duodenum
C. Submucosa of the jejunum
D. Submucosa of the ileum

58. Which type of oral mucosa listed below covers the dorsum of the tongue and the taste buds?

A. Masticatory mucosa
B. Lining or reflective mucosa
C. Specialized mucosa
D. None of the above

59. All of the following statements concerning the periodontal ligament are true except:

A. It is a specialized connective tissue that is soft, fibrous, cellular and vascular
B. Its average width is 2.0 mm
C. Its principal function is to support the tooth, in its socket
D. It occupies the space between the cementum and the alveolar bone

60. Which muscle of the soft palate listed below draws the soft palate down to the tongue closing the oropharyngeal isthmus

A. Tensor veli palatini
B. Levator veli palatini
C. Palatoglossus
D. Palatophyaryngeus
E. Muscularis uvulae

61. Which muscle of the larynx listed below is the only one innervated by the external laryngeal branch of the vagus nerve?

A. Cricothyroid
B. Posterior cricoarytenoid
C. Lateral cricoarytenoid
D. Oblique arytenoid
E. Thyroarytenoid

62. The arterial blood supply of the heart is provided by

A. The right and left pulmonary arteries
B. The right and left coronary arteries
C. The right and left subclavian arteries
D. The right and left innominate arteries

63. Which heart valve listed below guards the opening between the right atrium and right ventricle?
A. Mitral (bicuspid) valve
B. Tricuspid valve
C. Pulmonary semilunar valve
D. Aortic semilunar valve

64. Which branch of the external carotid artery listed below supplies the submandibular gland?
A. Posterior auricular artery
B. Ascending pharyngeal artery
C. Maxillary artery
D. Facial artery

65. The maxillary artery divides into three parts. Which one of the following is not one of those parts?
A. Pterygopalatine part
B. Pterygoid part
C. Infratemporal part
D. Mandibular part

66. Histologically, the dentin of the root is distinguished readily from the dentin of the crown by the presence of which structure listed below?
A. Incremental lines of Retzius
B. Rete pegs
C. Tomes granular layer
D. Sharpey's fibers

67. Epithelia with two or more layers of cells, with only the deepest layer in contact with the basal lamina, are classified as:
A. Simple epithelia
B. Stratified epithelia
C. Pseudostratified epithelia
D. Columnar epithelium

68. The oral epithelium is covered by a layer of
A. Stratified cuboidal epithelium
B. Stratified squamous epithelium
C. Stratified columnar epithelium
D. Pseudostratified columnar epithelium

69. The pterygoid processes are part of which bone listed below?

A. Palatine bone
B. Temporal bone
C. Sphenoid bone
D. Occipital bone

70. The portal vein is formed by the union of splenic vein and:

A. Superior mesenteric vein
B. Inferior phrenic vein
C. Paraumbilical vein
D. None of the above

71. Under the microscope, erythrocytes (red blood cells) appear as:

A. Oval discs with multilobed nuclei
B. Circular discs with centrally located nuclei
C. Biconcave discs without nuclei
D. Circular discs with several nuclei

72. Which fossa listed below is an irregular-shaped space lying posterior to the maxilla, between the pharynx and the ramus of the mandible?

A. Pterygopalatine fossa
B. Mandibular fossa
C. Infratemporal fossa
D. Coronoid fossa

73. Which cell listed below is considered to be the most versatile in the body?

A. Macrophage
B. Hepatocyte
C. Kupffer cell
D. Erythrocyte

74. Platelets are best described as

A. Giant multinucleated cells
B. Cytoplasmic fragments of cells
C. Immature leukocytes
D. Lymphoid cells

75. The articular surfaces of the TMJ are covered by:

A. Elastic cartilage
B. Hyaline cartilage

C. Fibrocartilage
D. Periosteum

76. The basophils in the circulating blood are similar to which cell listed below?
A. Platelets
B. Mast cell
C. Macrophage
D. Kupffer cell

77. Which cranial nerve listed below supplies motor function to the trapezius and sternocleidomastoid muscles?
A. Vagus nerve
B. Glossopharyngeal nerve
C. Accessory nerve
D. Hypoglossal nerve

78. Which of the following ligaments normally is found in the inguinal canal of the female?
A. Ovarian ligament
B. Broad ligament
C. Round ligament of the uterus
D. Suspensory ligament of the ovary

79. Apical abscesses of which teeth listed below have a marked tendency to produce cervical spread of infection most rapidly?
A. Mandibular central and lateral incisors
B. Mandibular canine and first premolar
C. Maxillary first and second molars
D. Mandibular second and third molars

80. Which of the following statements concerning urine are true?
A. Adults pass about a quart and a half of urine each day depending on the fluids and foods consumed.
B. The volume of urine formed at night is about half that formed in the daytime.
C. Normal urine is sterile. It contains fluids, salts and waste products but is free of bacteria, viruses and fungi.

D. The tissues of the bladder are isolated from urine and toxic substance by a coating that discourages bacteria from attaching and growing on the bladder wall.
E. All of the above statements concerning urine are true.

81. Most skull joints found between the flat bones of the skull are

A. Fibrous joints
B. Cartilaginous joints
C. Synovial joints
D. Ligamentous joints

82. All of the following statements concerning the temporalis muscle are true, except:

A. It is fan-shaped and originates from the bony floor of the temporal fossa and from the deep surface of the temporal fascia.
B. The anterior and superior fibers elevate the mandible; the posterior fibers retract the mandible.
C. It inserts on the coronoid process of the mandible and the posterior fibers retract the mandible.
D. It is innervated by the maxillary division of the trigeminal nerve (V-2).
E. It is considered to be one of the muscles of mastication.

83. Which of the following can classify exocrine glands?

A. Type of secretion
B. Mode of secretion
C. Structure of duct system
D. Shape of secretory unit
E. All of the above

84. Metabolically active follicular colloid in the usual thyroid follicle stains

A. Acidophilic
B. Basophilic
C. Mixed
D. None of the above

85. Which of the following is the function of hyaline cartilage during endochondral ossification in a long bone of an extremity?

A. Provides a region where a long bone can grow in length.
B. Provides a region where a long bone can grow in width.
C. Hyaline cartilage has no function during endochondral ossification in a long bone.
D. All of the above

86. The cardiac notch is a deep indentation on the

A. Superior lobe of the left lung.
B. Inferior lobe of the left lung
C. Inferior lobe of the right lung
D. Middle lobe of the right lung
E. Superior lobe of the right lung

87. Which space listed below is entered when performing a spinal tap?

A. Arachnoid space
B. Central canal
C. Subarachnoid space.
D. Conus medullaris

88. Which division of the trigeminal nerve listed below passes through the foramen ovale and supplies motor innervation to the tensor veli palatini, tensor tympani, muscles of mastication (Temporalis, masseter and lateral and medial pterygoid and the anterior belly of digastric and mylohyoid muscles?

A. Ophthalmic division
B. Maxillary division
C. Mandibular division
D. None of the above

89. Resting lines as seen in a histologic section of cortical bone of the mandible are the result of which of the following?

A. Growth of the mandible by the interstitial growth
B. Growth of the mandibular by appositional growth.
C. Growth of the mandible by both interstitial and appositional growth
D. None of the above

90. Which of the following statements concerning the breast and mammary gland are true?

A. The mammary glands lie in the superficial fascia

B. The mammary gland is actually a modified sweat gland.

C. The breast receives arterial blood through branches of the lateral thoracic (branch of the axillary artery) and internal thoracic arteries

D. Fibrous Copper's ligaments support the breasts

E. All of the above statements are true.

91. Which of the following characteristics are true concerning veins?

A. Thin tunica media with few muscle fibers

B. Thick tunica adventitia with little elastic tissue

C. Larger lumen and thinner walls than the arteries they accompany

D. Some contain valves and vasa vasorum

E. They receive blood from the venules and carry it from the body (except the lungs) to the right atrium of the heart.

F. All of the above are true.

92. Which cell listed below is the most common type found in the epidermis of the skin?

A. Melanocytes

B. Keratinocytes

C. Langerhans cells

D. None of the above

93. The primary purpose of cilia in mammalian cells is to

A. Move solids over their surfaces

B. Move fluid, mucous, or cells over their surfaces

C. Absorb fluid, mucous of cells over their surfaces

D. Absorb solids and liquids over their surfaces

94. Which of the following is the distinctive array of microtubules in the core of cilia and flagella composed of a central pair surrounded by a sheath of nine doublet microtubules (Characteristic ("9+2" pattern)?

A. Tubulin

B. Centriole

C. Axoneme
D. Malleolus

95. The mandibular fossa is a part of which bone listed below:?
A. Ethmoid bone
B. Sphenoid bone
C. Temporal bone
D. Parietal bone

96. Which method of bone development or formation involves a cartilaginous model being laid around it?
A. Intramembranous ossification
B. Endochondral ossification
C. Both of the above
D. None of the above

97. Which structure below gives the first indication of tongue development in the embryo?
A. The stomodeum
B. The tuberculum impar
C. The copula
D. The hypobranchial eminence

98. Calcitonin and thyroxine are produced and stored in which gland listed below?
A. Parathyroid glands
B. Adrenal glands
C. Thyroid gland
D. Thymus

99. The veins of the brain are direct tributaries of the
A. Internal jugular vein
B. Dural sinuses
C. Diploic veins
D. Emissary veins
E. Pterygoid venous plexus

100. The ductus venosus present in the fetus becomes what in the newborn?
A. Ligamentum arteriosum
B. Ligamentum teres

C. Fossa ovalis
D. Ligament venosum

101. Which type of epithelium listed below lines the mucous membranes of the nasopharynx?
A. Simple squamous epithelium
B. Stratified squamous epithelium
C. Pseudostratified ciliated columnar epithelium
D. Transitional epithelium

102. Which of the following cells form cementum?
A. Cementoblasts
B. Odontoblasts
C. Cementoblasts
D. Ameloblasts

103. Which area of the oral cavity has mucosa that is lined with keratinized epithelium?
A. Soft palate
B. Gingiva
C. Sublingual regions
D. Buccal regions

104. Which of the following is the region where the optic nerve exits the eye?
A. Lens
B. Iris
C. Cornea
D. Optic disc.

105. The two optic nerves unite in the floor of the diencephalon to form which of the following?
A. Optic tract
B. Lateral geniculate body
C. Optic chiasma.
D. Lateral geniculate nuclei

106. Which parasympathetic ganglion listed below lies in the infratemporal fossa just below the foramen ovale between the mandibular nerve and the tensor veli palatini muscle?
A. Ciliary ganglion

B. Pterygopalatine ganglion
C. Submandibular ganglion
D. Otic ganglion.

107. Which of the following nerves innervate the TMJ?
A. Auriculotemporal nerve
B. Masseteric nerve
C. Deep temporal nerve
D. All of these

108. A lesion occurring in the jugular foramen may damage all of the following structures except:
A. Spinal accessory nerve
B. Vagus nerve
C. Glossopharyngal nerve
D. Internal jugular vein
E. Facial nerve

109. Which of the following is a pear-shaped muscular sac lying on the undersurface of the liver
A. Pancreas
B. Gallbladder
C. Stomach
D. Esophagus

110. Which gland listed below is the major gland of immune system?
A. Thyroid gland
B. Adrenal gland
C. Thymus glands
D. Pineal gland

111. Which of the following contains mucous- secreting cells?
A. Submandibular gland
B. Sublingual gland
C. Buccal glands
D. Glands of the esophagus
E. Mucosa of the trachea
F. All of the above

112. The nervous system can be divided into which two main parts listed below?

A. Central nervous system (CNS)
B. Somatic nervous system (SNS)
C. Peripheral nervous system (PNS)
D. Autonomic nervous system (ANS)

113. Myelin is the fat-like substance forming a sheath around certain nerve fibers in the PNS (peripheral nervous system) which type of cell listed below form myelin?

A. Oligodendrocytes
B. Schwann cells
C. Astrocytes
D. Microglia

114. The middle ear (tympanic cavity) communicates anteriorly with the nasopharynx via the

A. Acoustic apparatus
B. Vestibular apparatus
C. Eustachian (auditory) tube
D. External acoustic (auditory meatus)

115. Which of the following statements concerning the thoracic duct are true?

A. Begins below in the abdomen as a dilated sac, the cisterna chyli
B. Ascends through the aortic opening in the right side of the descending aorta
C. Empties into the junction of the left internal jugular vein and the left subclavian vein (which is the beginning of the left brachiocephalic vein)
D. Contains valves and ascend between the aorta and azygos vein in the thorax
E. Conveys to the blood all lymph from the lower limbs, pelvic cavity, abdominal cavity, left side of the thorax and left side of the head and left arm
F. All of the statements concerning the thoracic duct are true

116. Which of the following explains how the epidermis of the skin obtains nourishment?

A. By diffusion of tissue fluid from capillary beds in the hypodermis
B. By diffusion of tissue fluid from capillary beds in the dermis
C. By diffusion of tissue fluid from capillary beds in the subcutaneous tissue
D. By diffusion of tissue fluid from capillary beds in the stratum corneum

117. Which of the following is the fundamental morphologic unit of enamel?

A. Enamel tuft
B. Enamel spindle
C. Enamel rod
D. Enamel lamellae

118. The epithelium of the oral mucous membrane may be

A. Keratinized
B. Parakeratinized
C. Nonkeratinized
D. All of the above

119. Which of the following refers to the sarcoplasmic reticulum present in skeletal muscle?

A. Releases and stores phosphate ions during muscle contraction and relaxation
B. Releases and stores glucose during muscle contraction and relaxation
C. Releases and stores calcium ions during muscle contraction and relaxation
D. None of the above

120. Which muscle listed below can flex the thigh and extend the leg?

A. Biceps femoris
B. Sartorius
C. Rectus femoris
D. Semimembranosus

121. All of the following statements concerning skeletal muscles are true, except:

A. Are considered voluntary in that they may be consciously contracted

B. Are usually long and narrow, span a joint, and are attached at either end by a tendon

C. Their origin is the more movable attachment and their insertion is the more stationary attachment

D. They may be classified according to their fiber arrangement as parallel, convergent, circular or pinnate

E. Each individual muscle fiber is innervated by a motor neuron terminal at a motor end plate

F. They are enclosed by epimysium, perimysium, and endomysium

G. They comprise approximately 40% of a person's body weight

122. All of the following statements concerning cardiac muscle are true, except:

A. It makes up the muscular component of the heart known as the myocardium

B. Cardiac muscle cells are faintly striated, branching cells which connect by means of intercalated disks to form a functional network

C. It contracts voluntarily

D. Its fibers are separate cellular units which (unlike other striated muscle fibers) don't contain many nuclei

E. It responds to increased demands by increasing the size of its tissue; this is known as compensatory hypertrophy

123. The fossa ovalis and the anulis ovalis lie on the:

A. SA node

B. Atrial (interatrial) septum

C. Interventricular (ventricular) septum

D. AV node

124. The liver is one of the organs, along with lungs to receive a dual blood supply. Which two structures listed below are responsible for that dual blood supply to the liver?

A. Common carotid artery

B. Hepatic artery
C. Splanchnic vein
D. Hepatic portal vein

125. Which of the following is the first layer of dentin formed?
A. Mantle dentin
B. Peritubular dentin
C. Intertubular dentin
D. Interglobular dentin

126. Which muscle listed below has fibers that insert into neck of the mandibular condyle and into the capsule and articular disc of the TMJ?
A. Temporalis muscle
B. Buccinator muscle
C. Medial pterygoid muscle
D. Lateral pterygoid muscle

127. Which of the following is the main function of the dental pulp?
A. Nutritive
B. Sensory
C. Protective
D. Formative

128. All of the following statements concerning the left vagus nerve are true except?
A. It can be cut on the lower part of the esophagus to reduce gastric secretion (termed as vagotomy)
B. It forms the anterior vagal trunk at the lower part of the oesophagus.
C. It passes in front of the left subclavian artery as it enters the thorax
D. It contains parasympathetic postganglionic fibers
E. It contributes to the anterior esophageal plexus

129. All of the following are the four distinct layers of the enamel organ except?
A. Outer enamel epithelium
B. Inner enamel epithelium
C. Stratum granulosum

D. Stratum intermedium
E. Stellate reticulum

130. Listed below are the usual events in the histogenesis of a tooth. Place them in their correct sequence (from what happens first to what happens last)

1. Deposition of the first layer of dentin
2. Differentiation of odontoblasts
3. Deposition of the first layer of enamel
4. Elongation of inner enamel epithelial cells

A. 4,2,1,3
B. 1,2,3,4
C. 2,3,4,1
D. 3,2,1,4

131. The first sign of human tooth development is seen during the:

A. First week
B. Third week
C. Sixth week
D. Ninth week

132. The ground substance of hyaline cartilage is basophilic because it contains which substance listed below?

A. Muramic acid
B. Glycogen granules
C. Sulfated proteoglycans
D. Polysaccharides

133. Which organelle listed below contains centrioles which are short cylinders adjacent to the nucleus that take part in cell division?

A. Mitochondria
B. Peroxisomes
C. Ribosomes
D. Centrosomes

134. What is the collective name given to lifeless substances, such as yolk, fat and starch - that may be stored in various parts of the cytoplasm?

A. Ectoplasm

B. Metaplasm
C. Protoplasm
D. Nucleoplasm

135. Which artery listed below gives rise to the right subclavian and the right common carotid arteries?
A. Maxillary artery
B. Coronary artery
C. External iliac artery
D. Brachiocephalic artery

136. Which one of the meninges that cover the spinal cord and brain is a dense, strong fibrous sheet?
A. Dura mater
B. Arachnoid mater
C. Pia mater
D. All of the above

137. Which cranial nerve listed below sends motor fibers to levator palpebrae superioris and all extrinsic eye muscles except superior oblique and lateral rectus?
A. Trochlear nerve
B. Abducens nerve
C. Oculomotor nerve
D. Optic nerve

138. Which structures listed below makes up the forebrain?
A. Cerebrum
B. Pons
C. Medulla oblongata
D. Diencephalon

139. Which hormones listed below are released from the posterior pituitary?
A. Prolactin
B. Growth hormone (GH)
C. Antidiuretic hormone (ADH)
D. Luteinizing hormone (LH)
E. Oxytocin

140. Which of the following determines whether gigantism or acromegaly will occur when there is over-secretion of growth hormone by the pituitary gland?

A. Whether or not the epiphyses of the short bone have fused with the shaft

B. Whether or not there is enough calcium present to cause fusion of the epiphyses

C. Whether or not the epiphyses of the long bones have fused with the shaft

D. None of the above

141. Which structure listed below divides the anterior body cavity into an upper thoracic cavity and a lower abdomino-pelvic cavity?

A. Liver

B. Diaphragm

C. Stomach

D. Lungs

142. During the fourth week of embryonic development, the first branchial arch divides to form

A. The two lateral nasal processes

B. The mandibular and maxillary process

C. The two medial nasal processes

D. The lateral and medial nasal process

143. All of the following comparisons between the large intestine and small intestine are true, except:

A. The large intestine is about one-fourth the size of the small intestine

B. The lumen of the large intestine is of a greater diameter than that of the small intestine

C. The smooth muscle coat of the large intestine consists of three bands called teniae coli that cause the colon to form pouches (called Haustra). The small intestine lacks this characteristic.

D. The walls (or tunics) of the large intestine have more villi than the small intestine.

E. The external surface of the large intestine has small areas of fat-filled peritoneum called epiploic appendages. The small intestine lacks this characteristic.

144. Which two muscles listed below form a sling around the angle of the mandible?

A. Buccinator muscle
B. Masseter muscle
C. Medial pterygoid muscle
D. Lateral pterygoid muscle

145. Gingival fibers are found

A. In the free gingiva
B. At the DEJ
C. In the attached gingiva
D. At the muco-gingval junction

146. The point of exit from the stomach, where the stomach joins with the small intestine is guarded by a:

A. Greater omentum
B. Pyloric sphincter
C. Lesser omentum
D. Cardiac orifice

147. Which type of smooth muscle listed below has numerous gap junctions?

A. Single-unit smooth muscle
B. Multiunit smooth muscle
C. Both of the above
D. None of the above

148. The periodontal ligament is composed primarily of:

A. Elastic fibers
B. Reticulin fibers
C. Collagen fibers
D. Spindle fibers

149. Which heart valve is best heard over the apex of the heart?

A. Tricuspid valve
B. Mitral valve
C. Pulmonary valve
D. Aortic valve

150. Which muscle of the neck listed below separates the anterior and posterior triangles of the neck?
A. Digastric
B. Mylohyoid
C. Sternocleidomastoid
D. Omohyoid

151. Which artery listed below supplies the tongue?
A. Palatine artery
B. Inferior alveolar artery
C. Lingual artery
D. Vertebral artery

152. The thick middle muscular layer of the heart wall is called the:
A. Epicardium
B. Myocardium
C. Endocardium
D. Pericardium

153. Which chamber of the heart listed below is associated with the apex of the heart?
A. Right atrium
B. Left atrium
C. Right ventricle
D. Left ventricle

154. Of the following blood vessels, which one plays a significant role in peripheral vascular resistance and in the regulation of pressure?
A. Capillaries
B. Arterioles
C. Veins
D. Venules

155. Which one of the five layers of epidermis listed below contains the pigment producing melanocytes?
A. Stratum basale (basal layer)
B. Stratum spinosum (spiny layer)
C. Stratum granulosum (grainy layer)

D. Stratum lucidum (clear layer)
E. Stratum corneum (horny layer)

156. Which structure listed below is considered to be remnants of Hertwig's epithelial root sheath?
A. Accessory root canals
B. The epithelial rests of Malassez
C. Dentino-enamel junction (DEJ)
D. Cemento-enamel junction (CEJ)

157. Which vein listed below drains venous blood from structures of the posterior abdominal and thoracic body wall
A. External jugular vein
B. Internal jugular vein
C. Azygos vein
D. Femoral vein

158. Which type of tissue below can be classified according to the shape of the cell and the number and arrangement of cell layers?
A. Nervous tissue
B. Muscle tissue
C. Connective tissue
D. Epithelial tissue

159. Which of the following is the basic structural unit of adult compact bone?
A. Lamellae
B. The osteon
C. Volkmann's canals
D. Osteocytes

160. Which of the following is known as the sex chromatin body?
A. Golgi body
B. Barr body
C. Pineal body
D. Lateral body

161. Which of the following is a bone-forming cell that is derived from mesenchyme?
A. Osteoclast

B. Osteoblast
C. Osteoid
D. Osteocyte

162. Which structure listed below is a sieve-like bone at the base of the skull, behind the root of the nose that runs through the mid-sagittal plane and aids to connect the cranial skeleton to the facial skeleton?
A. Temporal bone
B. Maxilla
C. Ethmoid bone
D. Vomer bone

163. Mitosis includes all of the following stages except:
A. Prophase
B. Metaphase
C. Hypophase
D. Anaphase
E. Telophase

164. Which of the following is the cartilaginous bar of the first branchial arch?
A. Meckel's cartilage
B. Reichert's cartilage
C. John's cartilage
D. Smith's cartilage

165. At each intervertebral foramen the spinal nerves are formed by the union of which of the following?
A. Fibers originating in the cranial nerves
B. Anterior and posterior roots
C. Fibers originating in the cervical plexus
D. Mediolateral roots

166. Which veins listed below unite in the superior mediastinum to form the superior vena cava?
A. Right and left external jugular veins
B. Right and left subclavian veins
C. Right and left brachiocephalic veins
D. Right and left gastric veins

167. The gonads are the:

A. The uterus in females and the epididymis in males
B. The vagina in females and the ductus deferens in males
C. The ovaries in females and the testis in males
D. The uterine tubes in females and the ejaculatory ducts in males

168. Which of the following is formed very rapidly in response to irritants

A. Primary dentin
B. Secondary dentin
C. Reparative dentin
D. Sclerotic dentin

169. Which of the following are the last bronchioles of the bronchial tree?

A. Terminal bronchioles
B. Respiratory bronchioles
C. Primary bronchioles
D. Tertiary bronchioles

170. Which form of connective tissue listed below can be described as cells and fibers embedded in a gel-like matrix (amorphous ground substance)?

A. Bone
B. Cartilage
C. Adipose tissue
D. Vascular tissue

171. Which types of nerves listed below are the principal types found in the dental pulp?

A. Parasympathetic and efferent fibers
B. Sympathetic and afferent fibers
C. Parasympathetic and afferent fibers
D. Sympathetic and efferent fibers

172. Which nerve listed below innervates the posterior belly of the digastric muscle?

A. Oculomotor nerve
B. Facial nerve
C. Abducens nerve
D. Trochlear (CN IV)

173. Which ganglia listed below is located at the level of the cricoid cartilage?

A. The superior cervical ganglia
B. The middle cervical ganglia
C. The inferior cervical ganglia
D. All of the above

174. Which of the following causes the folding of the embryo during the fourth week of development?

A. Growth of the epithelial tissues
B. Growth of the connective tissues
C. Growth of the muscle tissues
D. Growth of the neural tissues

175. The internal acoustic meatus transmits which two of the following structures?

A. Vestibulocochlear nerve
B. Trigeminal nerve
C. Facial nerve
D. Vagus nerve

176. All of the following nerves pass through the superior orbital fissure, except:

A. Ophthalmic nerve
B. Abducens nerve
C. Optic nerve
D. Oculomotor nerve
E. Trochlear nerve

177. Which duct listed below is the main excretory duct of the pancreas?

A. Wharton's duct
B. Duct of Wirsung
C. Bartholin duct
D. Wolffian duct

178. Which gland listed below is both an exocrine and endocrine gland?

A. Thyroid gland
B. Thymus

C. Pancreas
D. Parathyroid glands

179. Which spinal cord tracts listed below convey impulses concerned with touch and pressure?
A. Anterior spinothalamic tracts
B. Lateral spinothalamic tracts
C. Lateral corticospinal tracts
D. Anterior corticospinal tracts

180. Which lobe of the cerebrum listed below is responsible for hearing?
A. Temporal lobe
B. Occipital lobe
C. Frontal lobe
D. Parietal lobe

181. In the head and neck, all the lymph ultimately drains into the:
A. Submental lymph nodes
B. Submandibular lymph nodes
C. Deep cervical lymph nodes
D. Retropharyngeal lymph nodes

182. What percentage of dentin is organic?
A. 5–10%
B. 20%
C. 30%
D. 60%

183. Which of the following statements concerning enamel are true?
A. The DEJ is the interface between dentin and enamel, it is also the remnant of the formation of the tooth.
B. Enamel forms more evenly before birth than after birth Deciduous teeth, therefore are almost always uniform in appearance, while permanent teeth show variations in color and degree of calcifications.
C. Ameloblasts enter their first formative state after the first layer of dentin is formed. They secrete enamel matrix as they retreat away from the DEJ, which then mineralizes.

D. Enamel is produced in a rhythmical fashion
E. All of the above statements are true

184. Surrounding each tooth is specialized epithelium known as a
A. Connective tissue attachment
B. Periodontal ligament attachment
C. Junctional epithelium
D. Nasmyth's membrane

185. Which papillae of the tongue listed below are characterized by the absence of taste buds and increased keratinization?
A. Circumvallate papillae
B. Fungiform papillae
C. Filiform papillae
D. Foliate papillae

186. The intrinsic muscles of the thorax are involved in which process listed below ?
A. Laughing
B. Swallowing
C. Breathing
D. Digestion

187. Which muscle of the anterior abdominal wall listed below helps form the cremaster muscle?
A. External oblique
B. Internal oblique
C. Transversus
D. Rectus abdominis

188. The nerve to the mylohyoid muscle is a branch of which nerve listed below?
A. Ophthalmic nerve
B. Maxillary nerve
C. Mandibular nerve
D. Facial nerve

189. Which cells listed below secrete mucus and are abundant in the ileum of the small intestine?
A. Paneth cells

B. Absorptive cells
C. Entero-endocrine cells
D. Goblet cells

190. Which structure listed below is located in the wall of the right atrium near the superior vena cava and acts as a "pacemaker" for the heart?
A. Atrioventricular (AV) node
B. Atrial septum
C. Sinoatrial (SA) node
D. Tricuspid valve

191. Which artery listed below supplies the mucosa of the palate posterior to the maxillary canine?
A. Sphenopalatine artery
B. Greater palatine artery
C. Posterior superior artery
D. Nasopalatine artery

192. Which of the following is the most prominent functional component in the tunica media of small arteries
A. Collagen fibers
B. Elastic fibers
C. Smooth muscle cells
D. Skeletal muscle cells

193. When a tooth first erupts into the oral cavity, where the attachment epithelium derived from?
A. Dental papilla
B. Dental sac
C. Reduced enamel epithelium
D. Dental pulp

194. All of the following are components of a junctional complex, except:
A. Tight junctions
B. Gap junctions
C. Intermediate junctions
D. Desmosomes

195. A tubercle is:

A. A large, rounded roughened process

B. A sharp slender projecting process

C. A small rounded process

D. A prominent elevated ridge or border of a bone

196. Which bone listed below forms the prominence of the cheek and part of the lateral wall and floor to the orbital cavity

A. Sphenoid bone

B. Ethmoid bone

C. Zygomatic bone

D. Occipital bone

197. In the adult, hematopoiesis occurs in which two types of tissue listed below?

A. Nervous tissue

B. Lymphoid tissue

C. Muscle tissue

D. Myeloid tissue

198. The inferior mesenteric artery supplies all of the following organs except the:

A. Sigmoid colon

B. Descending colon

C. Transverse colon

D. Rectum

E. Ascending colon

199. Which of the following cells are found in the seminiferous tubules of the testis?

A. Endothelial cells

B. Interstitial cells

C. Sertoli cells

D. Clara cells

200. Which basic component of a typical cell listed below serves as the cell's external boundary separating it from other cells and from the external environment?

A. Protoplasm

B. Cell membrane

C. Nucleus
D. Golgi bodies

201. The first sign of human tooth development is seen during the:
A. first week
B. third week
C. sixth week
D. ninth week

202. Dislocation of the TMJ is almost always
A. Posteriorly bilateral, and occurs while sleeping.
B. Anteriorly bilateral, and occurs while laughing or yawning
C. Anteriorly unilateral and occurs while chewing food
D. Posteriorly unilateral and occurs while laughing or yawning

203. The sphenomandibular ligament of the TMJ attaches to the spine of the sphenoid bone and
A. The neck of the mandibular condyle
B. The lingula of the mandible
C. The ramus of the mandible
D. The angle of the mandible

204. Which ganglion listed below is located within the facial canal and contains sensory neurons that innervate taste buds on the anterior two-thirds of the tongue?
A. Otic ganglion
B. Ciliary ganglion
C. Semilunar ganglion
D. Geniculate ganglion

205. Which structure listed below is the first formed by the tooth germ and remains in evidence in the formed tooth?
A. Cementoenamel junction (CEJ)
B. Dentinoenamel junction (DEJ)
C. Cementodentinal junction (CDJ)
D. Mucogingival junction (MGJ)

206. The ovaries are:
A. Heart-shaped organs located on either side of the adrenal glands

B. Almond shaped organs located on either side of the uterus
C. Pear-shaped organs situated between the bladder and the rectum
D. Muscular tubes located between the urethra and the rectum

207. Where would you expect to see incremental lines of Retzius?
A. In dentin
B. In cementum
C. In enamel
D. In the pulp

208. Which recurrent laryngeal nerve listed below crossed the arch of the aorta, hooks around the ligamentum arteriosum and ascends in the groove between the trachea and esophagus?
A. Right recurrent laryngeal nerve
B. Left recurrent laryngeal nerve
C. None of the above
D. Both of the above

209. Which muscle listed below is a landmark for locating the glossopharyngeal nerve (CN IX) in the neck?
A. Posterior belly of the digastric muscle
B. Inferior pharyngeal constrictor muscle
C. Stylopharyngeal muscle
D. Anterior scalene muscle

210. All preganglionic and postganglionic neurons of the parasympathetic nervous system release:
A. Dopamine
B. Norepinephrine
C. Acetylcholine
D. Epinephrine

211. Which of the following folds of cranial dura separate the lateral lobes of the cerebellum?
A. Tentorium cerebelli
B. Falx cerebri
C. Falx cerebelli
D. Diaphragma sellae

212. The body contains two types of glands exocrine and endocrine. Which type secrets its products into ducts, where the secretions are then carried to the target site?

A. Exocrine glands
B. Endocrine glands
C. Both of the above
D. None of the above

213. All portions of the pituitary gland listed below are derived from oral ectoderm except

A. Pars distalis
B. Pars tuberalis
C. Pars intermedia
D. Pars nervosa
E. Infundibulum

214. Which gland listed below is often called the "master endocrine gland"

A. Pancreas
B. Thymus gland
C. Pituitary gland
D. Parathyroid glands

215. Which hormone listed below is the most plentiful anterior pituitary hormone?

A. Thyroid stimulating hormone (TSH)
B. Adrenocorticotropic hormone (ACTH)
C. Growth hormone (GH)
D. Follicle stimulating hormone (FSH)
E. Luteinizing hormone (LH)

216. Which muscle listed below flexes, adducts, and medially rotates the arm?

A. Pectoralis major
B. Latissimus dorsi
C. Deltoids
D. Teres major

217. The myofibrils of a skeletal muscle fiber are arranged into the compartments called:

A. Z lines

B. Sarcomeres
C. H bands
D. A bands

218. Which type of joint listed below is characterized by a joint cavity?
A. Fibrous joint
B. Cartilaginous joint
C. Synovial joint
D. All of the above

219. Which of the following is a muscular tube that extends from the pharynx through the mediastinum to the stomach?
A. Pancreas
B. Duodenum
C. Esophagus
D. Large intestine

220. Which of the following cells may be found in the periodontal ligament?
A. Fibroblasts
B. Osteoblasts
C. Cementoblasts
D. Macrophages
E. All of the above

221. Approximately one-third of all principal fibers of the periodontal ligament are:
A. Alveolar crest fibers
B. Horizontal fibers
C. Oblique fibers
D. Apical fibers
E. Inter-radicular fibers

222. All of the following statements concerning cardiac muscle fibers are true except.
A. Make up the thick, middle layer of the heart known as the myocardium
B. Have larger t-tubules and less developed sarcoplasmic reticulums as compared to skeletal muscle fibers

C. In contrast to skeletal muscle fibers, cardiac muscle fibers are short branched, and single or binucleated
D. Their characteristic feature is the presence of intercalated discs
E. Cardiac muscle fibers have less mitochondria between myofibrils and are poorer in myoglobin than most skeletal muscle fibers

223. The lateral wall of the axilla (armpit) is formed by:
A. The clavicle
B. The scapula
C. Serratus anterior muscle
D. The humerus

224. Which chamber of the heart listed below receives blood from the superior and inferior venae cavae and also from the anterior cardiac vein?
A. Right atrium
B. Left atrium
C. Right ventricle
D. Left ventricle

225. The pectinate muscles are located within the heart
A. On the interatrial septum
B. In the right ventricle
C. On the inner surfaces of the right atrium
D. On the sinus venosum
E. On the right side of the interventricular septum

226. Which of the following arteries does not accompany the corresponding nerve throughout its course?
A. Infraorbital artery
B. Inferior alveolar artery
C. Lingual artery
D. Posterior superior alveolar artery

227. Which of the following arteries supply the stomach?
A. Right and left gastric arteries
B. Right and left gastroepiploic arteries
C. Short gastric arteries
D. All of the above

228. The tooth germ is composed of all the structures listed below except

A. Enamel organ
B. Dental sac
C. Dental papilla
D. Hertwig's epithelial root sheath

229. Which stage in the life cycle of a tooth listed below includes final shaping of the tooth?

A. Initiation (Bud stage)
B. Proliferation (Cap stage)
C. Differentiation (Bell stage)
D. Apposition

230. Branches of which artery listed below supply the maxillary and mandibular teeth?

A. Vertebral
B. Occipital
C. Maxillary
D. Subclavian.

231. In a young child, which area of the maxilla listed below grows in height and length to accommodate the developing dentition?

A. Frontal process
B. Zygomatic process
C. Alveolar process
D. Orbital plate

232. Which structure listed below covers the surface of bone and consists of dense regular connective tissue?

A. Diaphysis
B. Endosteum
C. Epiphysis
D. Periosteum

233. The pterygoid plexus of veins surrounds which artery listed below?

A. Maxillary artery
B. Subclavian artery

C. Facial artery
D. Internal carotid artery

234. Which of the following statements concerning the hypoglossal nerve (CN XII) are true?
A. It is a motor nerve supplying all of the intrinsic and extrinsic muscles of the tongue except the palatoglossus, which is supplied by the vagus nerve
B. It leaves the skull through the hypoglossal canal which lie medial to the carotid canal and jugular foramen
C. It passes above the hyoid bone on the lateral surfaces of the hyoglossus muscle deep to the mylohyoid muscle
D. It loops around the occipital artery and passes between the external carotid artery and internal jugular vein
E. In the upper part of its course, it is joined by C1 fibers from the cervical plexus
F. All of the above are true concerning the hypoglossal nerve

235. Which cranial nerve listed below supplies the derivatives of the first branchial arch?
A. Facial nerve (CN VII)
B. Glossopharyngeal nerve (CN IX)
C. Trigeminal nerve (CN V)
D. Vagus nerve (CN X)

236. Which type of cartilage listed below is the most abundant in the body?
A. Hyaline cartilage
B. Fibrocartilage
C. Elastic cartilage
D. All of the above

237. Which structure listed below is a noncellular, protein - polysaccharide layer that anchors an epithelium to the underlying connective tissue
A. Plasma membrane
B. Basement membrane
C. Dermis
D. Tight junction

238. The inferior nasal concha is a part of which bone listed below?

A. Nasal bone
B. Sphenoid bone
C. Ethmoid bone
D. None of the above

239. Which vein listed below is formed by the union of the superficial temporal and maxillary veins within the parotid gland?

A. Hemiazygos vein
B. Left superior intercostal vein
C. Retromandibular vein
D. Subclavian vein

240. What is the function of neutrophils?

A. Transport oxygen
B. Involved in the processes of hemostasis and blood coagulation
C. Involved in the specific immune response
D. Ingest bacterial and other foreign substances

241. Which of the following can be defined as a small pit or depression in bone?

A. Fossa
B. Fissure
C. Fovea
D. Meatus

242. Which cell listed below is committed to differentiate into antibody producing plasma cells?

A. Stem cell
B. Macrophage
C. T cell
D. B cell

243. The liquid portion of the blood is called what?

A. Formed elements
B. Saline
C. Plasma
D. Lymph

244. Which structure listed below associated with the TMJ is fibrous, saddle - shaped and separates the condyle and the temporal bone?

A. Articular fossa
B. Articular disc (meniscus)
C. Articular eminence
D. None of the above

245. Which cell listed below is present in mesenchyme and capable of differentiating into one of the special types of connective tissue or supporting tissues, smooth muscle vascular endothelium or blood cells?

A. Alpha cells
B. B cells
C. Mesenchymal cells
D. Leydig cells

246. If a tooth is being tilted mesially during orthodontics, which two of the following four statements are true?

A. The coronal half of the distal wall will show resorption as a result of osteoclastic activity
B. The coronal half of the mesial wall will show resorption as a result of osteoclastic activity
C. The coronal half of the distal wall will show deposition as a result of osteoblastic activity
D. The coronal half of the mesial wall will show deposition as a result of osteoblastic activity

247. Which part of the urinary system listed below transports urine from the renal pelvis to the urinary bladder?

A. Kidney
B. Ureters
C. Urethra
D. Bowmann's capsule

248. Which of the following is a delicate membrane covering the crown of a newly erupted tooth?

A. Perikymata
B. Primary enamel cuticle

C. Hertwig's root sheath
D. Plasmalemma

249. Which structure listed below is lined with stereocilia?
A. Ovaries
B. Urethra
C. Epididymis
D. Uterus

250. Which cranial nerve listed below passes through the cribriform plate of the ethmoid bone to enter the olfactory bulb where synapses are made?
A. Optic nerve (CN II)
B. Olfactory nerve (CN I)
C. Oculomotor nerve (CN III)
D. Trochlear nerve (CN IV)

251. The urethra is longer in
A. Males
B. Females
C. Is of equal length

252. Which areas of the brain listed below are filled with cerebrospinal fluid?
A. Gray matter
B. Ventricles
C. White matter
D. Pons

253. Which of the following statements concerning the cervical plexus and its branches are true?
A. The motor nerve for most of the infrahyoid muscles are branches of the ansa cervicalis (loop formed by C1, C2 and C3)
B. Cervical nerves C1–C4 contribute motor fibers to the cervical plexus
C. It is positioned deep on the side of the neck, lateral to the first four cervical vertebrae.
D. An important branch of each cervical plexus is the phrenic nerve which supplies the diaphragm.

E. The supraclavicular nerve innervates the skin over the shoulder
F. The transverse cervical nerves provide sensory innervation to the anterior and lateral parts of the neck
G. All of the above statement concerning the cervical plexus and its branches are true

254. The posterior lobe of the pituitary gland consists of which type of nerve fibers listed below?
A. Unmyelinated nerve fibers
B. Myelinated nerve fibers
C. Both myelinated and unmyelinated nerve fibers

255. The peripheral nervous system can be divided into which two divisions listed below?
A. Afferent (sensory) division
B. Afferent (motor) division
C. Efferent (motor) division
D. Efferent (sensory) division

256. All hormones listed below are made in anterior pituitary except —
A. Antidiuretic hormone (ADH)
B. Follicle stimulating hormone (FSH)
C. Luteinizing hormone (LH)
D. Growth hormone (GH)
E. Adrenocorticotropic hormone (ACTH)
F Thyroid-stimulating hormonc (TSII)

257. Which structure listed below can be seen in histologic examination of the submandibular and sublingual glands but not in the adult parotid gland?
A. Myoepithelial cells
B. Serous cells
C. Intercalated ducts
D. Serous demilunes
E. Striated ducts

258. All of the following statements concerning the buccinator muscle are true except:

A. It originates from the outer surface of the alveolar margins of the maxilla and mandible opposite the molar teeth and from the pterygomandibular raphe

B. It is innervated by the buccal branch of the hypoglossal, nerve (CN XIII)

C. It compresses the cheeks and lips against the teeth

D. It inserts at the orbicularis oris muscle and skin at the angle of the mouth

E. It is pierced by the parotid duct

259. The facial nerve, the retromandibular vein, and the external carotid artery lie within which salivary gland below?

A. Submandibular

B. Parotid gland

C. Sublingual gland

260. Synarthroses are:

A. Immovable joints

B. Slightly movable joints

C. Freely movable joints

261. Which muscle listed below is not one of the muscles of mastication?

A. Temporalis muscle

B. Masseter muscle

C. Buccinator muscle

D. Medial pterygoid muscle

E. Lateral pterygoid muscle

262. All of the following statements concerning the respiratory system are true, except:

A. It has two major parts - a branching tree- like set of hollow tubes (the conducting airways) and very thin-walled pouches (the alveoli) at the ends of these tubes

B. The lungs lie in the mediastinum

C. Cartilaginous rings are found in the main bronchi

D. The left lung has a smaller volume than the right lung

E. Alveolar sacs form the functional unit of the lung

263. Lymph leaves the lymph node through the
A. Afferent lymphatic vessels
B. Efferent lymphatic vessels
C. Both of the above

264. All of the following statements concerning the intrinsic muscles of the tongue are true except:
A. They are continued to the tongue and are not attached to bone
B. They are innervated by the pharyngeal plexus
C. They alter the shape of the tongue
D. They are named according to the three spatial planes in which they run

265. Which space listed below should be entered when performing an emergency tracheotomy?
A. Epidural space
B. Medullary space
C. Cricothyroid space
D. Pleural space

266. Which of the following abdominal organs (or viscera) is not located retroperitoneally?
A. Kidneys
B. Aorta
C. Adrenal glands (suprarenal glands)
D. Liver
E. Pancreas

267. Of the muscles listed below that move the forearm, which one is not involved in flexing the forearm?
A. Biceps brachii
B. Brachialis
C. Brachioradialis
D. Triceps brachii

268. All of the following statements concerning the liver are true except:
A. It is the body's largest and most active gland
B. It receives blood from the hepatic artery and portal vein

C. It receives autonomic nerve fibers from the celiac plexus
D. Its function is to store and concentrate bile
E. It is divided into a large right lobe and a small left by the attachment of the peritoneum of the falciform ligament
F. The right lobe is further divided into a quadrate lobe and a caudate lobe by the presence of gallbladder, the fissure for the ligamentum teres, the inferior vena cava and the fissure for the ligamentum venosum

269. All of the following statements concerning the heart are true except:
A. It is hollow muscular organ that is somewhat pyramidal in shape and lies within the pericardium in the middle mediastinum.
B. It is connected at its base to the great vessels but otherwise lies free within the pericardium
C. It contains four hollow chambers: the two upper atria and the two lower ventricles. The atria are separated by the interatrial septum and the ventricles are separated by the interventricular septum.
D. It contains five valves: two atrio-ventrivcular (AV) valves and three semilunar valves.
E. The wall of the heart consists of three layers: the epicardium, myocardium, and endocardium

270. All of the following statements concerning the kidneys are true, except
A. They are located retroperitoneally, the right kidney lies slightly lower than the left kidney due to the large size of the right lobe of the liver.
B. Each kidney is surrounded by a fibrous renal capsule and is supported by the adipose capsule.
C. Each kidney is divided into an outer dark-brown renal medulla and an inner light- brown renal cortex.
D. The renal medulla is composed of renal pyramid separated by renal columns.
E. Each kidney has an indentation, the hilus, on its medial border, through which the ureters, renal vessels and nerves enter or leave.

F. Each kidney receives its blood supply from a renal artery, a branch of the aorta.

271. Which type of connective tissue listed below provides strong, flexible support and is found in tendons and ligaments?

A. Loose (areolar) connective tissue
B. Dense connective tissue
C. Adipose connective tissue
D. Bone tissue

272. Which of the following statements concerning the carotid sinus is true?

A. It is innervated by the facial nerve
B. It is located at the terminal end of the external carotid artery
C. It communicates freely with the cavernous sinus
D. It is stimulated by changes in blood pressure
E. It functions as a chemoreceptor

273. Which vein listed below communicates with the superior ophthalmic vein and thus with the cavernous sinus allowing a route of infection from the face to the cranial dural sinus?

A. Suprascapular vein
B. Facial vein
C. Subclavian vein
D. Transverse cervical vein

274. Hyaline cartilage differs from bone in that hyaline cartilage may grow by which process listed below?

A. Appositional growth
B. Interstitial growth
C. Both of the above
D. None of the above

275. Which of the following is a precursor cell found in the red bone marrow that gives rise to all of the formed elements of the blood?

A. Monoblast
B. Myeloblast
C. Hemocytoblast
D. Lymphoblast

276. Which leukocytes (white blood cells) listed below are the least abundant?

A. Neutrophils
B. Monocytes
C. Eosinophils
D. Basophils
E. Lymphocytes

277. Chromosomes are composed of:

A. RNA and DNA
B. DNA and protein
C. Protein and RNA
D. Lipids and phospholipids

278. The nucleolus of a cell functions to:

A. Synthesize t-RNA
B. Synthesize r-RNA
C. Synthesize m-RNA
D. Synthesize DNA

279. The pterygoid processes or plates are a part of which bone?

A. Temporal
B. Sphenoid
C. Palatine
D. Zygoma

280. Which of the following statements concerning the portal vein is true?

A. It carries half as much blood as the hepatic artery
B. It has also no tributaries superior to its beginning
C. It is formed posterior to the neck of the pancreas by the union of the splenic and renal veins.
D. It ascends anterior to the bile duct and the proper hepatic artery.
E. It passes anterior to the epiploic foramen in the free edge of the lesser omentum.

281. Which of the following are the anatomical and functional units of the kidney

A. Axonemes
B. Nephrons

C. Myofibrils
D. Lobules

282. Which layer of the dermis listed below is a thick, fibrous layer?
A. Papillary layer
B. Reticular layer
C. Both of the above
D. None of the above

283. Which cell junction listed below seems to allow for the passage of ions and small molecules?
A. Tight junctions
B. Hemidesmosomes
C. Gap junctions
D. Intermediate junctions

284. Which of the following substitute for capillaries in the liver, spleen, pituitary gland, adrenal gland, carotid body, pancreas and parathyroid glands?
A. Lymph nodes
B. Venules
C. Sinusoids
D. Lacteals

285. Which artery listed below supplies the brain through its terminal branches—the anterior and middle cerebral arteries?
A. Vertebral artery
B. Coronary artery
C. Internal carotid artery
D. Superior mesenteric artery

286. The primary palate develops as a result of the merger of:
A. The two maxillary processes
B. The two lateral nasal processes
C. The two mandibular processes
D. The two medial nasal processes

287. Teniae coli are characteristic of which organ listed below
A. Stomach

B. Pancreas
C. Large intestine
D. Small intestine

288. Which structure listed below is called the adenoid when enlarged?
A. Lingual tonsil
B. Palatine tonsil
C. Pharyngeal tonsil
D. None of the above

289. Which opening of the diaphragm listed below transmits the aorta, thoracic duct, and azygos vein?
A. Aortic opening
B. Esophageal opening
C. Caval opening
D. None of the above

290. All of the following statements concerning the inguinal canal are true, except:
A. It transmits the spermatic cord in males and the round ligament of the uterus in females; as well as the ilioinguinal nerve in both sexes.
B. It begins at the deep inguinal ring and extends to the superficial inguinal ring .
C. It is much larger in females than in males
D. The interior wall is formed by aponeuroses of the external oblique and internal oblique muscles.

291. Which part of the alveolar process listed below immediately surrounds the root of the tooth and serves as an attachment for the fibers of the PDL?
A. Alveolar bone proper
B. Supporting alveolar bone
C. Lamina dura
D. None of the above

292. Which organ of the male reproductive system listed below produces spermatozoa and secretes sex hormones?
A. Prostate gland
B. Ductus deferens

C. Testis
D. Epididymis

293. Each odontoblast of dentin gives rise to a long slender cytoplasmic extension called
A. Triacetate fibers
B. Tomes fibers
C. Tag fibers
D. Korff's fibers

294. When a patient attempts protrusion, the mandible deviates markedly to the left. Which muscle listed below is unable to contract?
A. Buccinator muscle
B. Temporalis muscle
C. Right lateral pterygoid muscle
D. Left lateral pterygoid muscle

295. During an inferior alveolar nerve block injection, the needle passes through the mucous membrane and the buccinator muscle and lies lateral to which muscle listed below?
A. Masseter
B. Temporalis
C. Medial pterygoid
D. Lateral pterygoid

296. The trachea is a tube that begins below the cricoid cartilage (C6 of larynx) and ends at the level of the sternal angle T5 where it divides into:
A. Terminal bronchi
B. Respiratory bronchi
C. Primary bronchi
D. Tertiary bronchi

297. Which cranial nerve listed below passes through the cavernous sinus, enters the orbit through the superior orbital fissure and supplies the motor functions to the lateral rectus muscle?
A. Trigeminal nerve
B. Facial nerve
C. Abducens nerve
D. Vestibulocochlear nerve

298. The pterygopalatine fossa communicates laterally with the infratemporal fossa by way of which of the following?

A. Sphenopalatine foramen
B. Pterygoid canal
C. Foramen rotundum
D. Petrotympanic fissure
E. Pterygomaxillary fissure

299. Which bones listed below form the floor of the nasal cavity?

A. Ethmoid and palatine bones
B. Nasal bone and maxilla
C. Palatine bone and maxilla
D. Nasal and vomer bones

300. Which two of the following decrease with age in the dental pulp?

A. Number of collagen fibers
B. Number of reticulin fibers
C. The size of the pulp
D. Calcifications within the pulp

301. Which subdivision of the pharynx listed below contains the pharyngeal tonsils in its posterior wall?

A. Nasopharynx
B. Oropharynx
C. Laryngopharynx
D. None of the above

302. Which of the following act to integrate sensory stimuli that give rise to the sensations of heat and pain

A. Substantia nigra
B. Substantia gelatinosa
C. Substantia adamantina
D. Substantia grisea

303. Which of the following statements concerning the spinal cord are true?

A. It is cylindrical, occupies approximately the upper two-third of the vertebral canal, and is enveloped by the meninges.
B. In contrast to the cerebral hemispheres (brain) it has centrally located gray matter and peripherally located white matter.

C. It ends at about the level of L1 in the adult and at the level of L3 in the young child.
D. All of the above statements are true concerning the spinal cord

304. Which structure listed below houses the pituitary gland (hypophysis)?
A. Cribriform plate
B. Crista galli
C. Sella turcica
D. Lacrimal fossa
E. Diaphragma sellae

305. The epiploic foramen (Winslow's foramen) permits free communication between which two structures listed below?
A. The large and small intestine
B. The middle and inner ear
C. The lesser and greater omentum
D. The esophagus and stomach

306. Which structure listed below secretes hormones that are not essential to life?
A. Adrenal cortex
B. Anterior pituitary
C. Adrenal medulla
D. Pancreatic islets of Langerhans

307. Which anterior pituitary hormone listed below controls the production and secretion of hormones called glucocorticoids by the cortex of the adrenal gland?
A. Follicle-stimulating hormone (FSH)
B. Luteinizing hormone (LH)
C. Adrenocorticotropic hormone (ACTH)
D. Thyroid -stimulating hormone (TSH)

308. The area of skin supplied by a single spinal nerve is called a;
A. Fasciculus
B. Dermatome
C. Spindle
D. Bundle

309. Which muscle of the pectoral girdle listed below is innervated by the accessory nerve (CN XI)?

A. Serratus anterior
B. Pectoralis minor
C. Subclavius
D. Trapezius
E. Levator scapulae

310. Which component of the lymphatic system listed below has the following functions: important blood reservoir, phagocytosis of undesirable particles of blood, and manufacturer of mononuclear leukocytes?

A. Thymus
B. Spleen
C. Bone marrow
D. Lymph nodes

311. Which joint listed below allows movement of the head about its vertical axis (rotation to the right or left)?

A. Atlanto-occipital joint
B. Intervertebral joint
C. Atlanto-axial joint
D. Costovertebral joint

312. The nasal cavities are lined by:

A. Stratified squamous epithelium
B. Stratified cuboidal epithelium
C. Pseudostratified ciliated columnar epithelium
D. Pseudostratified cuboidal epithelium

313. All of the following statements concerning the lymphatic system are true except:

A. The main function is to collect and transport tissue fluids from the intercellular spaces in all the tissues of the body back to the veins in the blood system
B. Lymph is a transparent, usually slightly yellow, often opalescent liquid found in the lymphatic vessels
C. It consist of the bone marrow, spleen, thymus gland, lymph nodes, tonsils, appendix. Peyer's patches, lymph, and lymphatic vessels

D. Just like the circulatory system, the lymphatic system has a central heart-like organ to pump lymph throughout the lymph vessels
E. The chief characteristic common to all lymphatic organs is the presence of lymphocytes

314. Which of the following statements is true concerning the triangle of auscultation?
A. It is bounded by the upper border of the latissimus dorsi, the lower border of the trapezius, and the medial margin of the scapula
B. It is the site where breathing sounds can be heard most clearly
C. Its floor is formed by the rhomboid major
D. All of the above statements are true

315. Which tooth tissue listed below has the highest mineral content?
A. Enamel
B. Dentin
C. Cementum
D. Pulp

316. The pharyngeal plexus does not innervate which muscle of the soft palate listed below?
A. Tensor veli palatini
B. Levator veli palatini
C. Palatoglossus
D. Palatopharyngeus
E. Muscularis uvulae

317. Which muscle listed below opens and protrudes the mandible?
A. Temporalis muscle
B. Masseter muscle
C. Medial pterygoid muscle
D. Lateral pterygoid muscle

318. All of the following comparisons between the ileum and the jejunum are correct except:
A. They are both suspended by mesentery

B. The ileum has more plicae circulares (valves of Kerckring) and more villi
C. Less digestion and absorption nutrients occur in the ileum
D. The mesentery of the ileum contains more fat

319. The Spleen:
A. Lies in the lower right inguinal region of the abdominal cavity
B. Lies in the upper right hypochondrium of the abdominal cavity between the stomach and the diaphragm
C. Lies in the upper left hypochondrium of the abdominal cavity between the stomach and the diaphragm
D. Lies in the hypogastrium of the abdominal cavity just below the liver

320. The external carotid artery:
A. Extends from the upper border of the thyroid cartilage to the base of the skull
B. Contributes to form the basilar artery
C. Supplies the occipital lobe of the cerebral hemisphere
D. Gives off the inferior thyroid artery
E. Lies within the substance of the parotid gland

321. The mouth or oral cavity initially appears as a slight depression of the surface ectoderm called the:
A. Medial tongue bud
B. Frontal nasal process
C. Stomodeum
D. Pyramidal lobe

322. Which of the following are found between the basal cells of epithelium and the underlying basal lamina?
A. Focal contacts
B. Hemidesmosomes
C. Desmosomes
D. Gap junctions

323. The small deep penetrating arteries of the basal ganglia known as the lenticulostriate arteries are branches of which of the following?
A. Middle cerebral artery

B. Internal carotid artery
C. Anterior choroidal artery
D. All of the above

324. Three pair of veins return most of the venous blood from the head and neck regions to the heart. Which pair listed below does not?
A. Right and left internal jugular veins
B. Right and left external jugular veins
C. Right and left vertebral veins
D. Right and left gastric veins

325. What bones form the floor of the nasal cavity?
A. Nasal and vomer bones
B. Ethmoid and palatine bones
C. Maxilla and nasal bones
D. Palatine and maxilla bones

326. A patient was in a bau car accident and received a severe blow to the head that fractured his her optic canal. Which of the following pairs of structures are most likely to be injured?
A. Ophthalmic artery and ophthalmic vein
B. Optic nerve (CN II) and ophthalmic vein
C. Optic nerve (CN II) and ophthalmic artery
D. Ophthalmic nerve (CN V-1) and ophthalmic artery

327. Parasympathetic effects
A. Prepare the body to resist stress
B. Lead to acceleration of body activity
C. Cause rage and emotional reactions
D. Maintain normality of body functions
E. All of the above

328. Which extrinsic tongue muscle listed below depresses the tongue?
A. Genioglossus muscle
B. Hyoglossus muscle
C. Styloglossus muscle
D. Palatoglossus muscle

329. Which structure listed below is the functional unit in salivary gland?

A. Nephron
B. Microfilament
C. Adenomere
D. Lobule

330. Which of the following arteries does not accompany the corresponding nerve throughout its course?

A. Lingual
B. Infraorbital
C. Inferior alveolar
D. Posterior superior alveolar

331. What muscles are elevators of the mandible?

A. Medial pterygoid, digastric-both anterior and posterior belly and lateral pterygoid
B. Digastric-both anterior and posterior belly-and lateral pterygoid
C. Medial pterygoid, temporalis, and masseter
D. Digastric-both anterior and posterior belly, temporalis, and masseter

332. All of the following structures are found in dentin except:

A. Globular dentin
B. The neonatal line
C. Contour lines of Owen
D. Tome's granular layer
E. Intertubular matrix

333. What of the following may cause "dead tracts" in dentin.

A. Caries
B. Erosion
C. Cavity preparation
D. Odontoblastic crowding
E. All of the above

334. What group of periodontal ligament fibers has a cementum-to - cementum attachment?

A. Oblique
B. Horizontal

C. Trans-septal
D. Apical
E. Alveolar crest

335. Where are circular fibers found?
A. Free gingiva
B. Attached gingiva
C. Mucogingival junction
D. Epithelial attachment

336. Which of the following structures transmits the internal carotid artery and the greater petrosal nerve?
A. Petrotympanic fissure
B. Sphenopalatine foramen
C. Foramen lacerum
D. Mandibular foramen

337. Permanent teeth move in what direction when erupting?
A. Occlusally and buccally
B. Occlusally and lingually
C. Occlusally and mesially
D. Occlusally and distally

338. Apical abscesses of which teeth listed below have a marked tendency to produce cervical spread of infection most rapidly?
A. Mandibular central and lateral incisors
B. Mandibular canine and first premolar
C. Maxillary first and second molars
D. Mandibular second and third molars

339. The oculomotor nerve (III) enters the orbit through what opening?
A. Sphenomaxillary fissure
B. Superior orbital fissure
C. Pterygomaxillary fissure
D. Optic canal

340. Tropocollagen is a protein molecule found in which fibers?
A. Collagen
B. Elastic
C. Reticular
D. A and C, only

341. What connective tissue cell is most concerned with defense against bacterial invasion?

A. Macrophage
B. Basophil
C. Plasma cells
D. Mast cells

342. Which blood element is a fragment of megakaryocytic cytoplasm?

A. Erythrocytes
B. Platelets
C. Leukocytes
D. Plasma

343. Cyclic DNA is associated with what organelle within a cell?

A. Smooth endoplasmic reticulum
B. Nucleus
C. Mitochondrion
D. Vacuole

344. Which of the following cells is most likely to have an abundant amount of rough surfaced endoplasmic reticulum?

A. Osteocyte
B. Macrophages
C. Osteoblast
D. Mesothelial cell
E. Small lymphocyte

345. What muscle divides the maxillary artery into three parts?

A. Buccinator
B. Lateral Pterygoid
C. Masseter
D. Superior constrictor m of pharynx.

346. Which of the following structures is formed from the first branchial arch?

A. Hyoid bone
B. Buccinator muscle
C. Stylopharyngeus muscle
D. Lateral pterygoid muscle
E. Superior parathyroid gland

347. Which branchial arches are concerned with the development of the tongue?

A. First and second
B. First, third and fourth
C. Second and third
D. First, second, and third

348. What is the first part of the face to form in the embryo?

A. Maxilla
B. Mandible
C. Nasal prominence
D. None of the above

349. Which of the following has no lymph sinuses or crypts and is surrounded partly by connective tissue and partly by epithelium?

A. Thymus
B. Peyer's patch
C. Lingual tonsil
D. Palatine tonsil
E. Pharyngeal tonsil

350. Where would you find valves of Kerckring?

A. Duodenum
B. Jejunum
C. Ileum
D. Appendix

351. Metabolically active follicular colloid in the usual thyroid follicle stains how?

A. Basophilic
B. Acidophilic
C. Variable
D. None of the above

352. What is the average capacity of a stomach?

A. 0.5 liters
B. 0.7 liters
C. 1.0 liters
D. 1.4 liters

353. In what band on transmission electron microscopic preparations of skeletal muscle, would thick myofilaments be observed?

A. I - band
B. Z - band
C. A-band
D. None of the above

354. Alveolar bone proper consists of what type of bone?

A. Woven bone
B. Cortical bone
C. Bundle bone
D. Lamellar bone

355. The splanchnic nerve arise from which region?

A. Pelvis region
B. Lumbar region
C. Thoracic region
D. Sacral region

356. Which ofthe following structures can be seen in histologic examination of the submandibular and sublingual glands but not in the adult parotid?

A. Striated ducts
B. Serous demilunes
C. Intercalated ducts
D. Myoepithelial cells
E. Grandular serous cells

357. What muscle inserts on the mastoid process of the temporal bone?

A. Digastric (posterior belly)
B. Sternocleidomastoid
C. Longus capitis
D. Geniohyoid

358. Which fissure divides the mandibular fossa into two parts?

A. Petrotympanic fissure
B. Sphenomaxillary fissure
C. Tympanomastoid fissure
D. Pterygomaxillary fissure

359. What two muscles form a sling around the angle of the mandible?

A. Medial pterygoid and lateral pterygoid
B. Posterior belly of digastric and lateral pterygoid
C. Masseter and medial pterygoid
D. Buccinator and anterior belly of digastric

360. The eustachian canal, salpingopharyngeal fold, pharyngeal recess, and pharyngeal tonsils (adenoids) are located in which of the following?

A. Nasopharynx
B. Palatopharynx
C. Oropharynx
D. None of the above

361. The middle nasal concha is part of which bone?

A. Sphenoid
B. Ethmoid
C. Maxilla
D. Nasal

362. The nasolacrimal duct drains into what?

A. Inferior meatus
B. Middle meatus
C. Superior meatus
D. Lacrimal meatus

363. Which nerve supplies motor innervation to the mylohyoid muscle?

A. Nerve to mylohyoid (branch of V-3)
B. Hypoglossal
C. Glossopharyngeal
D. Phrenic

364. Which nerve provides major sensory innervation to TMJ?

A. Masseteric nerve
B. Auriculotemporal nerve
C. Facial nerve
D. Maxillary nerve

365. What is the only direction in which the TMJ can be dislocated?
A. Laterally
B. Medially
C. Anteriorly
D. Posteriorly

Answer Key to MCQs in Anatomy, Histology and Embryology

1	C	2	C	3	C	4	B
5	E	6	D	7	B	8	B
9	C	10	C	11	G	12	C
13	D	14	D	15	C	16	B
17	B	18	D	19	B	20	C
21	A	22	D	23	B	24	B
25	D	26	B	27	B, D	28	C
29	D	30	C	31	A	32	E
33	B, D	34	D	35	B	36	D
37	B	38	C	39	C	40	B
41	B	42	C	43	A	44	C
45	C	46	B	47	C	48	B
49	A	50	B	51	C	52	C
53	B	54	B	55	A	56	C
57	B	58	C	59	B	60	C
61	A	62	B	63	B	64	D
65	C	66	C	67	B	68	B
69	C	70	A	71	C	72	C
73	B	74	B	75	C	76	B
77	C	78	C	79	D	80	E
81	A	82	D	83	E	84	B
85	A	86	A	87	C	88	C
89	B	90	E	91	F	92	B
93	B	94	C	95	C	96	B
97	B	98	C	99	B	100	D
101	C	102	C	103	B	104	D
105	C	106	D	107	D	108	E
109	B	110	C	111	F	112	A, C

113 B	114 C	115 F	116 B
117 C	118 D	119 C	120 C
121 C	122 C	123 B	124 B, D
125 A	126 D	127 D	128 D
129 C	130 A	131 C	132 C
133 D	134 B	135 D	136 A
137 C	138 A, D	139 C, E	140 C
141 B	142 B	143 D	144 B, C
145 A	146 B	147 A	148 C
149 B	150 C	151 C	152 B
153 D	154 B	155 A	156 B
157 C	158 D	159 B	160 B
161 B	162 C	163 C	164 A
165 B	166 C	167 C	168 C
169 B	170 B	171 B	172 B
173 B	174 D	175 A, C	176 C
177 B	178 C	179 A	180 A
181 C	182 B	183 E	184 C
185 C	186 C	187 B	188 C
189 D	190 C	191 B	192 C
193 C	194 B	195 C	196 C
197 B, D	198 E	199 C	200 B
201 C	202 B	203 B	204 D
205 B	206 B	207 C	208 B
209 C	210 C	211 C	212 A
213 D, E	214 C	215 C	216 A
217 B	218 C	219 C	220 E
221 C	222 E	223 D	224 A
225 C	226 C	227 D	228 D
229 C	230 C	231 C	232 D
233 A	234 F	235 C	236 A
237 B	238 D	239 C	240 D
241 C	242 D	243 C	244 B
245 C	246 B, C	247 B	248 B
249 C	250 B	251 A	252 B
253 G	254 A	255 A, C	256 A
257 D	258 B	259 B	260 A
261 C	262 B	263 B	264 B

265 C	266 D	267 D	268 D
269 D	270 C	271 B	272 D
273 B	274 B	275 C	276 D
277 B	278 B	279 B	280 E
281 B	282 B	283 C	284 C
285 C	286 D	287 C	288 C
289 A	290 C	291 A	292 C
293 B	294 D	295 C	296 C
297 C	298 E	299 C	300 B, C
301 A	302 B	303 D	304 C
305 C	306 C	307 C	308 B
309 D	310 B	311 C	312 C
313 D	314 D	315 A	316 A
317 D	318 B	319 C	320 E
321 C	322 B	323 A	324 D
325 D	326 C	327 D	328 B
329 C	330 A	331 C	332 D
333 E	334 C	335 A	336 C
337 A	338 D	339 B	340 D
341 A	342 B	343 C	344 C
345 B	346 D	347 D	348 B
349 E	350 B	351 A	352 C
353 C	354 C, D	355 C	356 B
357 B	358 A	359 C	360 A
361 B	362 A	363 A	364 B
365 C			

5

Physiology

HORMONES

1. **ADH/vasopressin** = increases permeability of the collecting ducts to water, so passive Movement of water is facilitated. Acts on DCT/CD
2. **Adrenal cortex hormones** = aldosterone = reabsorption of NaCl is controlled in the kidney tubules.
3. Adrenal cortical insufficiency = K^+ loss and Na^+ retention.
4. Hormones of adrenal Medulla are not essential to life.
5. Main effect of **aldosterone** is that = it acts on DCT.; increases permeability of DCT and CD, i.e. facilitates reabsorption of Na^+.
6. **Aldosterone** = is under the control of angiotensin II.
7. Primary effect of **calcitonin** = to inhibit bone resorption, i.e. decreases the serum Ca^{2+} level.
8. **Cholecystokinin** = contraction of gallbladder
9. **Secretin** = helps in digestion of proteins by increasing flow of pancreatic juice.
10. Principal action of **insulin** = to enhance cell permeability to glucose.
11. Nature's antacid = **secretin**
12. **Pancreozymin** and **secretin** = elaborated by intestinal Mucosal cells
13. **Progesterone** = prevents uterine contraction during pregnancy
14. During menopause = decreased estrogen and increased FSH levels

15. **Parathyroid H** = from chief cells, increase the Ca levels in blood
16. Diurnal secretory rhythm = shown by **cortisol**
17. Pancreatic alpha cells = **glucagon**
18. Pancreatic beta cells = **insulin**
19. **Steapsin** / pancreatic lipase = most imp. enz for digestion of fats
20. Bile salts = aid in digestion of fats
21. **HCl** = secreted by parietal cells of stomach
22. Chief cells secrete = histamine and **serotonin**
23. Salivary **amylase cannot** = hydrolyse sucrose; it can act on starch, dextran, glycogen
24. **Carbonic anhydrase** = contains ZINC; all the Zn in RBCs is associated with this enzyme. It splits carbonic acid in CO_2 and H_2O.
25. **Enterokinase** = secreted in intestinal juices; activates trypsinogen; *not found* in pancreatic juice
26. **Trypsinogen** and **chymotrypsinogen** in = pancreatic juice
27. **Lipase** acts in alkaline media in the intestine
28. Fe^{++} is absorbed from intestine by = facilitated diffusion
29. Myasthenia gravis is associated with = hyperthyroidism
30. Vit D is a steroid derivative

VARIOUS IONS

1. Cl^- is necessary for activation of ptyalin / amylase of saliva.
2. K^+ in blood is found predominantly in RBCs
3. K^+ is the principal *intracellular* cation
4. Na, Cl = principal *extracellular* cations
5. Na = affects the size of action potential directly.
6. Mg^{++} = cofactor in myosin ATPase activation
7. HCO_3 in blood is found predominantly in plasma; helps in *chloride shift* and as buffer.
8. Ca^{++} = in muscles interacts with TROPONIN to trigger contraction

9. Ca^{++} = low conc. = increases excitability of membrane
10. Ca^{++} = high conc. = stabilises the membrane
11. Zn = helps in function of carbonic anhydrase

ACTIVE TRANSPORT = mimp. factor to maintain animal cell volume.

Rate of diffusion = (area × temp × conc grad) / (distance × m. wt.)

Abnormal cardiac rhythm precipitates = HYPOPOTASSEMIA

Majority of Abs have half life of = 1 month

1 gm of Hb can combine with 1.34 ml of O_2 gas.

Factors common to both the clotting pathways = 1, 2, 4, 5, 10

Carotid sinus = has baroreceptors. The increased pressure increases activity of cardiac vagal fibres.

Pulse pressure = SBP – DBP = i.e. 3 : 2 : 1 = SBP: DBP: PP

Parasympathetic stimulation = decreases HR (vagus)

Sympathetic innervation to SA node = increases HR

Decrease in O_2 – conc. causes = arteriolar constriction

Increase in CO_2 – conc. causes = bronchiolar dilation

At normal PP of O_2 in alveoli = Hb is 98 % saturated.

Cardiac and smooth ms = are *electrical* syncytium

Skeletal ms = are true *anatomical* syncytium

In skeletal ms , the contractile Ca^{++} is stored in = sarcoplasmic reticulum (SR)

Skeletal ms fibres are innervated by = anterior / ventral horn cells (motor)

In concussion = BP decreases; pulse increases

In hematoma = BP increases; pulse decreases

Vasovagal shock = activation of symp. N. S (SNS)

Neurogenic shock = blockage of SNS

Primary ms involved in breathing = diaphragm and sterno-cleidomastoid

UNITARY SMOOTH Ms = found only in vasculature; are under the control of SNS.

Immediate source of fuel in skeletal ms = CREATININE PHOSPHATE

Immediate source of energy for nerve conduction = IONIC GRADIENT (Na^+)

Acetylcholine stimulates the secretion of watery saliva (p-symp.)

Nor-epinephrine stimulates the secretion of viscous saliva (symp.)

Total daily vol. of GI secretions = 7 litres; in it daily vol. of gastric secretion is 2 litres; saliva is 15–20%.

Heparin prevents conversion of prothrombin to thrombin, i.e. antithrombin.

Utricles in CNS = tell about the position of head wrt gravity

Glycine is found in collagen/dentin and keratin in enamel

Actinomyosin (myosin : actin = 3:1) is main contractile protein of muscles

Major site of formation of plasma proteins = liver

Normal values

Entity	**Volume**	**PH**
Blood	Is 8% of total body weight	7.4
Saliva	1200–1500 ml/day	6.02–7.05, isotonic
Gastric juices	2000 cc/day	0.9–1.5
Pancreatic juices	1500 cc/day	8–8.3
Total body water	60% of body wt.	
Intracellular volume	40% of body wt.	
Extracellular volume	20% of body wt.	
Blood volume	8% of body wt.	

1. **Bleeding time**
   1–5 min (Duke's method)
   < 5 min (Ivy method)
   < 6.5 min (Jacobson method)
2. **Clotting time**
   1–7 min (capillary tube method)
   2.5–5 min (Krause-Moses method)
   10 min (Lee-White method)
3. Rumpel-Leede test = For capillary fragility
4. 1 gm of Hb combines with 1.34 ml of oxygen.
5. **Pulse pressure** = SBP – DBP; i.e. 120–80 = 40
6. Circulation time = 12 sec

ECG: times of this in sec.

1. PR interval 0.18 sec; is the gap b/w onset of atrial contraction and onset of ventricular contraction.
2. QRS 0.08–0.1 sec
3. ST 0.32 sec
4. QT 0.4 sec

P – wave	Atrial depolarisation
QRS – complex	Ventricular depolarisation, aka ventricular complex
T – wave	Ventricular repolarisation
PR – interval	Atrial depolarisation and AV conduction; propagation of cardiac impulse through AV – node
QRS – interval	Interval total ventricular depolarisation time.
Q – wave	is due to activity of septum.
ST	Continued ventricular depolarisation
QT	Ventricular depolarisation + v. repolarisation.

- **Sterling's law of heart** = i.e. an increase in end – diastolic volume will produce an increased force of contraction over the normal physiologic range. It is a consequence of the length – tension relation. So the strength of myocardial contraction is a **function of initial length** of the ms fibres.
- **Cardiac output** = stroke volume x heart rate, i.e. 5 litres = 70 ml × 72 / min.
- Total duration of cardiac cycle = 0.8 sec; systole = 0.27 sec; diastole = 0.53 sec.
- Atrial systole = 0.1 sec; ventricular systole = 0.3 sec; (i.e. 3 times)
- When HR increases, the duration of diastole decreases; the duration of systole is fixed.
- Heart ms rest during diastole; pulse is the pressure wave felt in arterial wall.
- **Pulse pressure** is the difference b/w systolic and diastolic pressure.
- **Vagal stimulation** causes fall in BP. Vagus is negative chronotropic (decrease HR); dromotropic (conductivity of bundle); inotropic (force of conduction) and bathmotropic (excitability), i.e. is inhibitory to heart.
- **Baroreceptor** stimulation causes hypotension and bradycardia.
- Chemoreceptors stimulation in carotid and aortic bodies cause vasoconstriction and decrease in HR.
- Beta – 1 receptor stimulation causes tachycardia.
- Heart is most sensitive to = adranaline / epinephrine.
- After hemorrhage, the first reactive change to occur is = vasoconstriction.
- **Maximum conduction velocity** is seen in = Purkinje's fibres system, i.e. 4 m / sec.
- Conduction velocity in bundle of His (right bundle branch is longer than left bundle) and ventricular ms = 1 m / sec.
- Conduction velocity is LEAST in AV node.
- **AV node is supplied by left vagus N, and SA node is supplied by right vagus N.**
- Refractory period is longest in = SA node

- **Maximum surface area** is of = capillaries
- **Main peripheral resistance** vessels are = arterioles
- **Bain Bridge reflex** = aka venous reflex; is the reflex increase in HR on venous engorgement of the right atrium and right great veins.
- **Cardiac index** = is the cardiac output per sq meter body surface area. Average CI is 3.2 litres.
- BP = CO × PR. (i.e. cardiac output × peripheral resistance)
- Systolic BP increases with increase in CO; while diastolic BP increases with increase in PR.

Systemic distribution of CO

1. Blood supply to brain = $1/5^{th}$ of CO, i.e. 1000 ml/min.
2. Blood supply to heart = 5% of CO, i.e. 225 ml/min.
3. Blood supply to kidney = $1/4^{th}$ of CO ; 1300 ml/min
4. Blood supply to liver = $1/3^{rd}$; 1500 ml / min
5. Blood supply to ms = 100 – 200 ml / min.

HEART SOUNDS

- I = due to **sudden closure of AV valves,** i.e. mitral and tricuspid; indicates the onset of ventricular systole; duration is 0.15 sec;
- II = due to **closure of semilunar valves**, i.e. aortic and pulmonary; (after protodiastolic period); duration is 0.12 sec.
- III = **rapid rush of blood from atria** to ventricles, i.e. ventricular filling, (after isometric relaxation period)
- IV = **last rapid filling of blood in ventricle** due to start of atrial systole.
- AV valves = are mitral and tricuspids; produce M1, T1 sounds components
- SL valves = are aortic and pulmonary; produce A2, P2 sounds components
- **Protodiastolic period** is the time b/w the onset of diastole and closure of semilunar valves. It is 0.04 sec.

RESPIRATORY QUOTIENTS

RQ = CO_2 produced / O_2 used = 0.85 is the normal

RQ = 1.0 for carbohydrates

= 0.8 for proteins

= 0.7 for lipids

IMPORTANT POINTS

Greatest **cross section** area	Capillaries
Greatest **resistance** to blood flow	Arterioles and pre – capillary sphincters
Least **velocity** of blood	Capillaries
Least **hydrostatic** pressure	Vena cava
Lowest **B.P.** in	Venules
Widest **range of BP** is in	Left ventricle
Largest part of blood is in	Veins
Slowest rate of conduction is in	AV – node
Fastest rate of conduction	Purkinje fibres
Vagus nerve is	Inhibitor to heart
Sympathetic nerve is	Activator/stimulator to heart
Saliva is	Hypotonic to blood
Parasympathetic fibres stimulation causes secretions of	Watery saliva
Sympathetic stimulation causes	Viscous saliva
Normal intrapleural pressure	– 2.5 mm Hg, which decreases to – 6 mm Hg at the end of inspiration
Normal intrapulmonary pressure	Zero, which decreases to – 2 mm Hg at the end of inspiration

DEFINITIONS

1. **Resistance vessels** = i.e. arterioles and small veins which offer major resistance to blood flow.
2. **Capacitance vessels** = are veins which influence the cardiac output.
3. **Refractory period**, RP = after stimulation, there is a brief period during which muscle is not excitable to a second stimulus.
4. **Absolute refractory period** = during the first part of RP, the muscle remains inexcitable to any strength of stimulus.
5. **Relative RP** = in the later part of the RP, the muscle may be excitable to only a stronger stimulus.
6. **Protodiastolic period** = it is a short interval between onset of ventricular diastole and closure of SLV. It is the last $1/4^{th}$ of ventricular systole.
7. **Diastasis** = longest phase of ventricular diastole but amount of filling during this period is minimum. It is middle 3rd part of ventricular diastole.
8. **Frank – Sterling law** = i.e. an increase in end-diastolic volume will produce an increased force of contraction over the normal physiologic range, i.e. heart will pump out the volume of blood that returns to it.
9. **Rigor mortis** = after death, skeletal muscles go into a state of contracture, due to non-availability of ATPs.
10. **Chronotropic** = deals with heart rate
11. **Dromotropic** = deals with conductivity of bundles
12. **Inotropic** = deals with force of contraction
13. **Bathmotropic** = deals with excitability of heart

IMPORTANT CELLS AND SECRETIONS

Stomach	Secretions
1. Chief cells/peptic cells	♦ Pepsin / pepsinogen
2. Oxyntic/parietal cells	♦ HCl (stimulated by GASTRIN)
3. Argentaffin cells	♦ Serotonin
4. G – cells	♦ Gastrin

IMPORTANT CELLS AND SECRETIONS (Contd.)

Duodenum	**Secretions**
1. Brunner's glands	♦ Secretin
Jejunum = chief function is secretion. It has neither Brunner's glands nor Peyer's patches	
Ilium = has mostly Peyer's patches. Its chief function is ABSORPTION.	
♦ PANETH CELLS ♦ GOBLET CELLS ♦ KUPFFER CELLS	♦ In small intestine only ♦ In large intestine only ♦ In liver; are phagocytic
Kidneys ♦ JG cells	♦ Renin
Testes ♦ Leydeg cells ♦ Sertoli cells	♦ Testosterone ♦ For nutrition
Thyroid = parafollicular/ C – cells	♦ Calcitonin
Pituitary gland ♦ Alpha – cells/acidophils ♦ Beta – cells / basophils ♦ Weakly basophils	♦ GH, ACTH, Prolactin ♦ LH, FSH, TSH ♦ MSH
Parathyroid gland = chief cells	PTH
Pancreas ♦ Alpha cells ♦ Beta cells ♦ Delta cells	♦ Glucagon ♦ Insulin ♦ Gastrin

IMPORTANT CELLS AND SECRETIONS (Contd.)

Pineal glands	Melatonin
Adrenal cortex	
♦ Zona glomerulosa	♦ Mineralocorticoids, aldosterone; deal with SALT
♦ Zona fasciculata	♦ Glucocorticoids; deal with SUGARS
♦ Zona reticularis	
ADRENAL MEDULLA	
♦ Chromaffin cells	♦ Some sex hormones; deal with SEX
	♦ Adr, N-Adr; deal with SURVIVAL

Vitamins

Fat soluble = A,D,E,K

Water soluble = B,C

Vitamins	**Synonym**	**Deficiency**
Vit A	Retinol	Xerophthalmia
B_1	Thiamine	Beri – beri
B_2	Riboflavin	
B_3	Pantothenic acid	
B_6	Pyridoxine	
B_{12}	Cyanocobalamine	Pernicious anemia
Niacin		Pellagra
Folic acid		Megaloblastic anemia
H	Biotin	
C	Ascorbic acid	Scurvy
D	Calciferol	Rickets, osteomalacia
E	Tocopherol/ an antioxidant	
K	Naphthoquinone	Hypoprothrombinemia

Vit B_{12} is not found in foods of plant origin; but in animal foods like meat, fish, etc.

IONS

K	Main **intracellular** cation
Na , Cl	Main **extracellular** cations
Ca^{++}	Interacts with TROPONIN to **trigger muscle contraction**; (ATP is for muscle relaxation)
Mg^{++}	Cofactor in myosin ATPase activation
Ca^{++}, low conc.	Increases the excitability of membrane
Ca^{++}, high conc.	Stabilises the membrane
Na^{+}	Affects the size of **action potential**
Zn^{++},	Helps the functions of **carbonic anhydrase** enz.
K^{+}	Mainly in **RBCs**
HCO^{3-}	Mainly in **plasma**

STRUCTURE OF NEPHRONE

- In BOWMAN'S capsule — urine is **isotonic** to blood
- In proximal convoluted tubule — **isotonic**
- In loop of Henle — **hypertonic**
- In distal convoluted tubule — **hypotonic**

STRUCTURE OF MUSCLES

- Z – band — only actin fibers
- H – band — only myosin fibers
- Z – band — junction of 2 I – bands
- A – band — both actin and myosin fibers
- H – band — disappears in contracted muscle

PRECURSOR CELLS

- Megaloblasts — of RBCs
- Myeloblasts — of WBCs; granulocytes

♦ Monoblasts	of monocytes; RE tissue
♦ Megakaryocytes	of platelets

Life span of cells

• RBCs	120 days
• Transfused RBCs	60 days
• Granulocytes	2 – 3 days in tissues; 6 – 8 hrs in circulation
• Lymphocytes	100 – 300 days
• Platelets	10 days
• Mean circulation time	60 sec

Macrophages in different tissues are

• Liver	Kupfer cells
• Lymph nodes; spleeen; marrow	Reticulum cells
• Alveoli in lungs	Alveolar macrophages
• S/c tissues	Tissue histiocytes; clasmocytes
• Brain	Microglial cells
• Blood	Macrophages; Neutrophils

IgA deficiency = is the **most common immune deficiency**; leads to increased susceptibility to infection esp URTI.

Swallowing is triggered by 9th and 10th cranial Ns.

Gastrin = produced by G – cells of duodenum and antrum; stimulates HCl secretion by parietal cells.

CCK = stimulates pancreatic enz secretion; stimulates gallbladder contraction; decreases gastric emptying.

Secretin = stimulates HCO^{3-} secretion from liver and pancreas; released from S – cells in mucosa of upper intestine;

GIP = produced by K – cells in duodenum and jejunum; stimulates pancreatic insulin secretion.

5 TYPES OF COLLAGEN

Type	Location
I	**Most abundant**; found in dermis, bone, tendon, dentin, fascia, fibrous cartilage, organ capsule
II	Mainly in hyaline and elastic C
III	Mainly in reticular fibres; in smooth ms; As; liver; spleen; kidneys; lungs
IV	Basal lamina of **basement membrane**
V	In fetal membrane

Neutrophils are divided in 5 groups according to the no. of nuclei in them as – I, II, III, IV, V as having 1, 2, 3, 4, 5 nuclei respectively.

Group III cells are maximum in no., fully mature and functionally most efficient.

Shift to Left = i.e. increased immature cells, i.e. I, II and so less efficient defense mechanism.

Shift to Right = decreased leucopoiesis and increase no. of hypermature and senile cells.

Stages of RBC development

- Proerythroblast
- Early normoblast
- Intermediate normoblast
- Late normoblast
- Reticulocytes
- Erythrocytes

HEMOGLOBIN

- Normal Hb content is 16 gm % in males and 14 gm % in females.
- Per hour synthesis and destruction of Hb = 0.3 gm.
- Heme part of Hb is synthesised from **glycine and succinyl CoA**.
- **Serum** = plasma minus fibrinogen and other clotting factors.
- Hb → choleglobin → hemosiderin and ferritin + biliverdin.

- Plasma = Blood minus formed elements.
- Biliverdin → bilirubin → in liver → bilirubin glucuronide → in intestine → stercobilinogen → stercobilin.
- Bilirubin glucuronide → urobilinogen → kidneys → urobilin.
- In Hb, iron content is 0.34%.
- 3 gm of Fe is present as Hb in total amount of blood in an adult.
- **Fetal Hb** = HbF = greater affinity for oxygen; takes CO_2 more readily.
- HbF = 2 alpha and 2 beta. It is 70% saturated at 20 mm of O_2 pressure whereas adult HbA is only 20% saturated at 20 mm of O_2 pressure.
- It is a conjugated protein.
- Fe is oxidised and converted to Fe^{3+}; this condition is ka **methemoglobinemia** and O_2 cannot release itself. Met – Hb reductase keeps the iron in the ferrous state.
- **4 heme** join to 1 globin molecule to form one molecule of Hb.
- Hb appears **first in intermediate normoblast** late erythroblast stage.
- Fe is transported through **transferrin**; stored in liver;
- In **bronze diabetes** / hemochromatosis = increased hemosiderin occurs.
- In normal adults, only about 2 % of Hb is HbA_2 type.
- HbS = **glutamic acid in 6th position is replaced by valine** in beta-chain. (Sickle cell anemia)
- CO has almost 250 times stronger affinity for Hb than that of oxygen for Hb.

PLASMA PROTEINS

1. Albumin 4 gm %
2. Globulin 2.5 gm %
3. Fibrinogen 0.3 gm %
4. Prothrombin 0.03 gm %
5. Albumin and proteins concerned with clotting are synthesized in liver.

BLOOD

Specific gravity = 1.055 – 1.060; clinical average in males is 1.057 and in females is 1.053.

Blood = 55 % plasma + 45 % cells.

Plasma = water 91 – 92 % + proteins 7.5 %.

Proteins = albumin 4.7 – 5.7 % + globulin 1.3 – 2.5 % + fibrinogen 0.2 – 0.4 % + prothrombin.

The albumin / globulin ratio is = 1.5 : 1.0.

Chemical analysis reveals = the arginine / lysine ratio is 10 : 18; this ratio remains more constant than the albumin / globulin ratio.

Fibrinogen is different from other plasma proteins by its property of clotting.

Serum contains only albumin and globulin.

Origin = albumin fraction is the first formed; in the adults all the 4 fractions are formed by the liver. **Fibrinogen, prothrombin and albumin are formed in liver only**. Gamma globulin is formed by RE system.

Grains proteins favor globulin formation but animal proteins favor albumin formation.

Vit K helps in the formation of prothrombin in the liver.

Fibrinogen and prothrombin are required in blood clotting;

- ♦ Prothrombin changes to thrombin in p.o. thromboplastin and Ca^{++}.
- ♦ Fibrinogen changes to fibrin in p.o. thrombin.

Hematocrit value = is the ratio of RBCs to plasma.

Antibodies are gamma – globulin in nature.

Iron / transferrin and copper / ceruloplasmin are **bound to globulin fractions**.

Viscosity of plasma is less than that of whole blood.

RBCs carry negative charge; so any condition which increases the positive charge in plasma accelerates the ESR.

Normal ESR values by Wintrobe's method is 0 – 6.5 mm / hr in males; 0 – 15 mm / hr in females.

ESR is increased in all acute infections.

PH of blood = 7.4; RBCs are less alkaline than plasma.

Coagulation is the property of plasma alone; RBCs and WBCs do not take part in it.

Normal coagulation time = according to Lee and White is 3–4 min in capillary glass tube.

Bleeding time = according to Duke's method = 2 – 5 min.

Prothrombin time = Quick = 11 – 16 sec.; average is 12 sec; it increases in deficiency of factors 5, 7, 10. Prothrombin is manufactured in liver; vit K is essential for formation of prothrombin.

CLOTTING FACTORS: (Mnemonic = *face pe tere chunri lagti nahin sunder, aisi chunri se pareshan hai face*)

1. Fibrinogen
2. Prothrombin
3. Thromboplastin
4. Calcium
5. Labile factor / proaccelerin
6. Not essential / accelerin
7. Stable factor / proconvertin
8. Antihemophilic factor
9. Christmas factor / Plasma thromboplastin component
10. Stuart factor
11. Plasma thromboplastin antecedent (PTA)
12. Hagemen factor
13. Fibrin stabilising factor / Laki–Lorand factor.

- Factor 7 is not used up during clotting; its formation is retarded after administration of dicoumarin and in deficiency of Vit K.
- Factor 8 helps in the formation of intrinsic thromboplastin and prothrombin conversion; it **disappears when the blood clots**. In hemophilia, the **defect is not in the platelets** but it is due to the absence of this factor. CT is abnormally increased.
- Factor 9 deficiency gives rise to **hemophilia – C**.

- Factor 10 synthesis is retarded after administration of dicoumarin.
- Factor 11 ultimately leads to formation of thrombin.
- Factor 12 activates the protein-splitting enzyme *kallikrein* to produce plasma kinins.
- Factor 13 **converts the soft clot in solid clot**; its deficiency leads to **poor wound healing**.
- Extrinsic pathway of clotting = uses 7, 10, 5, 2, 1 factors.
- Intrinsic pathway uses = 12, 11, 9, 8, 10, 5, 2, 1 factors.
- In **obstructive jaundice**, vit K is not absorbed due to absence of bile salts; so prothrombin and factor 7 are not produced in liver; leads to increased PT.
- **Heparin** = secreted by **mast cells**; it is an anticoagulant; chemically it is mucoitin polysulfuric acid. It **inhibits the change of prothrombin to thrombin** with a plasma cofactor albumin X and neutralises the action of thrombin on fibrinogen.
- **Fibrinolysis** = done by a proteolytic enzyme in plasma ka **plasmin or fibrinolysin**.
- Removal of Ca^{++} ions = done by citrates / oxalates of Na or K.
- **Dicoumarin** is antagonist to vit K; **inhibits the synthesis of prothrombin in liver**;
- **Phenindione** = depresses the activity of factor 7 more than the prothrombin.
- **Blood volume** = 90 ml / kg body wt; or 8 % of total body wt;
- **Plasma** = 50 ml / kg body wt; or 5 % of total body wt;
- In males, the blood volume is 7.5 % higher than in females; it is due to greater no. of RBCs; plasma volume is same in both.

RBCs = biconcave shape which allows the infolding of the cells when it passes through the capillaries narrower than its own; **dumb bell** shape; nonnucleated so they are **not the true cells**; mean diameter is 7.2 microns;

RBCs count = 5 million in males; 4.5 millions/cubic mm in females; 6 – 7 millions in infants; 7.8 millions in fetus. Count is lowest during sleep and becomes maximum in evening.

- Abnormal form is ka = **poikilocytosis**.
- The diameter and volume of RBCs **increases in acidic blood**; red cells in venous blood are slightly larger than in the arterial blood. In venous blood, about 7.5 % increase in cell volume occurs which is **due to chloride shift**;

Development of RBCs = the parent cell is extravascular ka **haemocytoblast**; in embryo, they develop from the area vasculosa of yolk sac.

After birth, the **bone marrow is the main site of erythrogenesis**.

Most imp factor **controlling the rate of formation of RBCs is the Oxygen content** of arterial blood, a decrease in oxygen stimulates the erythropoiesis. It is stimulated by **erythropoietin** / hemopoietin which is produced by **the renal tissues**.

Sequence of RBCs formation

Stage	**Features**
Hemocytoblast / endothelial cells	Large nucleus
Proerythroblast / megaloblast	Large nucleus with distinct nucleoli; hemoglobin absent
Early normoblast / early erythroblast	Nucleoli absent or rudimentary
Intermediate normoblast / late erythroblast	Nucleus condensed and eccentric; No nucleoli; Hb **appears** at this stage
Late normoblast / normoblast	Nucleus pyknotic ka **pink – spot** nucleus; Hb amount increases
Reticulocytes	In this form, the RBCs start appearing in **circulation**.

Stimulus for maturation
Hemocytoblast / endothelial cells = Not known
Proerythroblast / megaloblast = **Haematinic principle of Castle** – vit B_{12} and folic acid required for converting megaloblasts into early normoblasts. Intrinsic factor helps in absorption of extrinsic factors.

Early normoblast / early erythroblast

1. Metals = **iron** for Hb formation; Cu/ Mn for converting iron into Hb.; Co as a component of vit B_{12}; Ca for conserving more iron.
2. Bile salts = for absorption of the metals.
3. Hormones = **thyroxine** is very imp; **hypothyroidism** leads to hypochromic, macrocytic anemia; **adrenocortical deficiency** is associated with anemia; polycythemia is associated with Cushing's syndrome.

- **Punctate basophilia** = RBCs appear with discrete blue particles esp seen in cases of **lead-poisoning**.
- **Time taken** = 7 days from the stage of proerythroblast to reticulocyte; and 2 more days from reticulocyte to mature erythrocyte.
- When air with low oxygen tension as on hills is breathed, the RBC count increases due to liberation of erythropoietin.
- **Energy metabolism** of RBCs = RBCs are not capable of synthesising Hb; no nucleus; **Kreb's cycle is absent**; so glucose metabolism occurs through EMP, HMP shunt, etc.
- Normal life = 120 days
- Hexokinase enz = acts in the first step of glucose metabolism.
- G-6-PD enz catalyses the first step of HMP shunt.
- Fate of RBCs = cells are destroyed by RE cells; Hb is released; opening of porphyrin ring occurs ka choleglobin or verdo- Hb; iron present in heme is stored as ferritin and hemosiderin; rest of Hb is converted to bilirubin and biliverdin; which combine with alpha – 1 globulin and go to liver.

HEMOGLOBIN (Also see p. 228)

- It is synthesised in RBCs in the bone marrow.
- **Average value** = 14.5 gm % in an adult; males > females; evening > morning; more at high altitudes; normal variation of Hb is mostly due to alteration in no. of RBCs and not due to change in the quantity of Hb in each cells.

- **Iron content** of Hb is 0.34 %; about 3 gm of iron is in Hb; iron remains as ferrous form; it contains 4 atoms of iron and 8 of sulphur;
- One gm of Hb combines with = **1.34 ml of oxygen,** i.e. 2 atoms of oxygen for each atom of iron. About 1200 ml of oxygen can be carried by the total blood in an adult.
- **Fetal Hb is 70% saturated** at 20 mm of oxygen pressure, but **adult Hb is only 20%** saturated at this pressure so HbF has a greater affinity for O_2.
- In plasma, the Hb remains as Hb – hepatoglobin complex.
- Oxy – Hb i.e. Hb with O_2; iron in ferrous state; O_2 can be removed.
- Met – Hb = Hb with O_2; iron in **ferric** state; O_2 can not be removed.
- Carbo – Hb = Hb with CO_2
- Carboxy – Hb = Hb with CO gas due to **coal gas** poisoning; the affinity of Hb for CO is 210 times more than O_2.
- Sulph – Hb = Hb with H_2S gas;

IRON

- Absorbed from the upper GIT esp duodenum;
- Dietary iron is best **absorbed as ferrous** form;
- **Ferritin is the storage form** of iron;
- Hemostasis of iron in body is maintained not through excretion but by controlling the absorption;
- Saturated apoferritin acts as **mucosal block** to prevent further absorption of iron. **Transferrin is iron binding protein** in plasma and helps in its transfer.
- **Gastric HCl** helps the liberation of iron from the organic compounds in diet. Low gastric acidity retards the absorption.
- Whole blood contains the 45 – 50 mgm of iron / 100 ml;
- Total quantity present in RBCs = 3 gm.
- **Primary function of iron** = formation of Hb; 1 gm of Hb carries 1.34 ml of O_2.

Packed cell volume = ratio of cell : plasma = 45 : 55.

MCV = 87 cubic microns

MCHC = 35 %; its value is never higher than the normal;

Anemias

1. After blood loss = normochromic, normocytic
2. Iron loss = hypochromic, microcytic
3. **Sickle cell anemia** = HbS type of Hb
4. **Mediterranean** / Cooley's / thalassemia = HbF is present
5. Aplastic anemia = normochromic, normocytic anemia.
6. Pernicious anemia/Addison's/megaloblastic anemia = macrocytic, normochromic. In it, there is **demyelination of lateral and dorsal columns of spinal cord** occurs. **Folic acid cures only blood** conditions, the **vit B_{12} cures both blood and nerve** conditions. Vit B_{12} is used for the formation of RNA, i.e. the nucleic acid for the integrity of CNS. The basic cause of pernicious anemia is **atrophy of gastric mucosa.**
7. Nontropical sprue = macrocytic, hypochromic type.

Hemolysis / fragility of RBCs = when placed in hypotonic solution, the cell swells up and bursts; Hb comes out in plasma ka **laking of blood**; in hypertonic solution, the cells become crenated by loosing the water;

Normally, hemolysis starts at 0.48 % and completed at 0.33 % of NaCl solution.

In acidosis, the fragility increase; cells show increased fragility in venous blood than the arterial blood.

FORMATION OF LYMPHOCYTES

From mesenchymal cells present in liver, spleen and wall of yolk sac. → enter bone marrow as stem cells → lymphocytes.

FUNCTIONAL SIGNIFICANCE OF LYMPHOCYTES

Defense of body against invasion of bacteria, etc.

Produce ANTIBODIES (Ig) to destroy them, rather than directly attending them (compared with granulocytes and monocytes).

Abs are produced by B-lymphocytes.

> **Antigen → Stimulates B. Lymphocytes → Change to plasma cells→ antibodies produced.**

T-cells recognise foreign body, e.g. microorganism, infected and tumour cells, etc. and produce LYMPHOKINES to destroy them, which stimulate migration of macrophages, neutrophils and eosinophils (MEN) to areas invaded by foreign cells.

B Cells =Blood borne (Abs), humoral response.

T-Cells = Cell-mediated response

Rejection of graft = by T-cells.

FORMATION OF BLOOD

In embryonic life: Blood cells are first formed - in relation to MESENCHYME surrounding the yolk sac.

After 2 months I.U. = blood formation occurs in LIVER.

Later = blood formation occurs in SPLEEN.

Still later = blood formation occurs in BONE MARROW.

Postnatal = blood formation occurs in BONE MARROW and LYMPHOID TISSUES.

RBCs (Summary)

1. Earliest identifiable precursor of RBC are known as **PROERYTHROBLASTS**.
2. Early erythroblasts - do not contain Hb.
3. **Late erythroblasts** - Hb appears.
4. **Reticulocytes** - Leave the bone marrow to enter the blood stream → change to erythrocytes.
5. **Granulocytes** - from myeloblasts
6. **Monocytes** - from hemopoietic stem cells (monoblast)
7. **Platelets**→ from megakaryocytes.

WBC: are nucleated and so true cells, no Hb, colorless; origin is purely from extravascular tissues.

Normal range = 4000 – 11,000 / cu. Mm.

Average ratio of WBCs : RBCs = 1 : 7,00

Count is lowest in mornings; highest in the evenings.

Injection of Adrenaline increases the count.

In new born, the count is very high; about 20,000 / cu. Mm.

Infections increase the esp neutrophilic count.

Allergies, e.g. asthma, hay fever, etc. increase the **eosinophilic** counts.

Leucopenia occurs esp after **irradiations**;

CLASSIFICATION

Granulocytes – 1 – 2 days only

Neutrophils (60 – 70%) = 2 – 4 days

Eosinophils (1 – 4%), = 8 – 12 days

Basophils (0 – 1%).= 12 – 15 days

Agranulocytes –

Lymphocytes (25–30%) = > a day to 2 – 3 days.

Monocytes (5- 10%); are derived from RE system.

Neutrophils

- 60 – 70 %; 10 – 12 microns in diameter;
- Many lobed, the no. of nuclei increases with degree of maturity of the cells;
- Cells with 3 – 4 lobed nuclei are most numerous.
- Metabolically, more active than RBCs.
- **Drum stick** like appearance of the **sex chromatin** body seen in polymorphs; only in females; absent in males; one less than the no. of X chromosomes.

- **Arneth count** / index =

Group	% age	Nuclei
I	5–10	One lobed
II	25–30	2 lobes
III	45–47 %	3 lobes
IV	16–18%	4 lobed
V	2%	5 or more lobes

- Cells with 3 – 4 lobed nuclei are most numerous; more mature and funtionally most efficient.
- **Shift to the left,** i.e. increase in the immature cells and so less effective defensive system.
- **Shift to the right** = i.e. decreased leucopoiesis with increased senile cells.
- **Schilling's** regenerative shift to the right = i.e. younger forms of the neutrophils come out of bone marrow in the circulation.
- Schilling's degenerative shift to the left = failure of neutrophils to mature.

Eosinophils = 10–12 microns in diameter; 2 lobed nucleus; accumulate in allergies; contain histamine; granules found more in no. than basophils.

Basophils = 8–10 microns diameter; kidney shaped nucleus; granules obscure the nucleus; same as mast cells of CT; contain heparin, histamine and 5 – HT.

Granulocytosis = increased no. of granulocytes.

Granulocytopenia = decreased no. of granulocytes in blood.

Small Lymphocytes = 7.5 microns; large nucleus occupying major part of the cell; basophilic; only thin cytoplasmic ring on periphery.

Large lymphocytes = 12 micron in diameter; are the **younger forms of small lymphocytes**.

Monocytes = 16–18 microns in diameter; nucleus is eccentric and cytoplasm resembles **frosted-glass** (but in large lymphocytes, nucleus is central and cytoplasm is clear).

Development of WBCs

- Stimulus of leucopoiesis = **chemotactic**; nucleic acid derived from dead neutrophils acts as a normal stimulus for formation of fresh neutrophils;
- Granulocytes = from red marrow.
- Lymphocytes and monocytes = from spleen and lymphatic glands.

Stages in the Development of granulocytes

- Reticulum cell / hemocytoblast.
- Primitive WBC = non-granular; large no. of nuclei.
- Myeloblast = round nucleus; many nucleoli; no granules.
- Myelocytes = **granules appear**; **nucleoli disappear**;
- Metamyelocytes = nucleus is bilobed; no multiplication of cells; amoeboid movements appear;
- Leucocytes = maturation is proportional to the no. of the lobes of the nucleus. **Maturation takes place in bone marrow only**; not in peripheral blood.

Development of lymphocytes

- Reticulum cells give rise to lymphoblasts;
- Thymus is the main source; give rise to long, lived-type cells.
- Short lived cells from lymphoid tissues.
- Large lymphocytes are mature cells and do not divide further.
- Small lymphocytes are derived from further maturation of large lymphocytes.

Development of monocytes = as reticulum cells → monoblast → monocytes.

Mainly from the reticulum cells of spleen, lymph nodes; and to some extent from bone marrow.

Functions of WBCs

- Lymphocytes migrate in **chronic inflammation**.
- PMN neutrophils release *trypsin like* enz. which helps to digest the dead tissue and forms pus, i.e. in **acute inflammation**.
- Lympho- and monocytes release *pepsin-like* subs which partially liquefies the solid dead tissue and helps in **phagocytosis**.

- Lymphocytes = form beta and gamma globulins; immunoglobulins are gamma globulins; adrenal cortical steroids dissolve the lymphocytes and increase Ab conc in blood.
- Basophils = are rich in **histamine**; increased in no. in allergies.

Abnormalities

- Leucopenia = i.e. decrease of WBC count; mainly due to neutrophils.
- Leucocytosis = i.e. increase of WBC count; in inflammatory conditions - the neutrophils increase; in allergic conditions – eosinophils increase.
- Leukemia = no. of immature WBCs increase in the circulation.

THROMBOCYTES = PLATELETS

- Average life = 5 – 9 days. Total no. = 250000 – 400000 / cubic mm.
- Nonnucleated; biconvex; 2.5 microns size.
- Microfilaments contain THROMBESTHENIN, causing the change in shape of platelets.
- **Development** = from megakaryocytes.
- Functions = **liberate thromboplastin** which activates prothrombin to thrombin and starts clotting in injury.
- **Clot retraction** = due to contractile protein, i.e. thrombosthenin in p.o. ATP and Mg^{++}.
- Purpura = i.e. decrease in no. of platelets; CT remains normal; BT is increased. Clot does not retract

BLOOD GROUPS

- Agglutinogens = on RBCs; start appearing in the 6th wk i.u.; the adult level is reached at puberty.
- Agglutinin= in plasma / serum.
- Groups O, A, B, AB = A into A1 and A2; group A1 is more frequent;
- Group O = **universal donor**; Group AB = **universal recipient**.

- Rh factor = is the agglutinogen of the Rhesus monkey; 85%; there is no corresponding agglutinin in plasma.
- If fetus in Rh-negative mother is of Rh + type, it may lead to **erythroblastosis fetalis** due to the p.o. anti – Rh factors (which enter in the fetal blood from mother), which destroy the RBCs of fetus.

Group	Agglutinogen on RBC	Agglutinin in plasma
O	O	Alpha and beta
A	A	Beta
B	B	Alpha
AB	A and B	Neither alpha or beta.

CARDIOVASCULAR SYSTEM

- Total blood can carry about 1200 ml of O_2 and this O_2 can meet demands only for 5 min.
- Right atrium receives venous blood from 3 main veins = SVC; IVC and coronary sinus.
- Left atrium receives pure blood from lungs through = pulmonary Vs.
- **Tricuspid valve** = is the **right** atrioventricular opening; T_1 sound.
- **Mitral / bicuspid valve** = is the **left** atrioventricular opening; M_1 sound.
- Opening of aorta (with left ventricle) and pulmonary A (with right ventricle) = by **semilunar valves**; produce second heart sound.
- Apices of the valves are restricted to bulge within the atria during ventricular contraction by = **chordae tendinae**.
- Aortic valve = b/w aorta and left ventricle; A_2 sound.
- Pulmonary valve = b/w pulmonary V and right ventricle; P_2 sound.

- Action of valves = is to make the circulation one-way; the AV valves (M, T) open towards the ventricles and the SLVs open away from the ventricles.
- Precapillary sphincter in the capillaries are controlled by = sympathetic nervous system.
- Elastic recoil of the arteries = helps to maintain the circulation.
- Blood supply to the walls of the arteries = by **vasa-vasorum**.

Difference b/w sinusoids and capillaries

- Capillaries are the connective link b/w the arteries and veins, but the sinusoids are the link b/w the same type of vessels.
- Capillaries have continuous epithelial lining while the sinusoids have no continuous lining.

Junctional tissues of the heart

- **SA node** = situated **in the right atrium** at the junction of SVC and right auricular appendage. Generates normal **cardiac impulse @ 70 – 80 / min**.; acts as a **pacemaker**; the rhythm is ka sinus rhythm. Spread of electric impulse is very slow @ 0.05 m/sec.
- **AV node** = is in **right atrium** at the posterior part of interatrial septum close to the opening of coronary sinus; **cardiac impulse** is **@ 40 – 60 / min**; it receives impulse from SA node and transmits to the ventricles through bundle of His; acts as **reserve pacemaker**.
- **Bundle branch** = conducts the atrial impulse into the ventricles; **cardiac impulse** is **@ 36 / min**.
- **Purkinje fibres** = extend from the interventricular septum directly to the papillary ms and then to the lateral walls of the ventricle ending in the subendocardial network; main **function is to conduct impulse quickly to every part of the ventricular ms fibers; fastest conduction**.
- **Heart beat = starts first from the SA node**; 3 separate components of the heart beat at a descending order of frequency are represented by the sequence: sinus → atrium → ventricle.
- **Rate of rhythmicity** = in SA node is 70 – 80/min; in AV node is 40 – 60/min; in atrium is 60/min; in ventricle is 20 – 40 / min., i.e. maximum in SA node.

- **Conductivity** = conduction in bundle of His and Purkinje fibres is 1 m/sec; in ventricular ms is 0.4 m/s; **least in SA node** 0.05 m/s; in AV node is 0.1 m/s.

CARDIAC CYCLE

- Atrial systole initiates the cycle because the SA node is in atrium.
- Right atrium contracts earlier than the left one; left ventricle contracts earlier than the right one but the **right ventricle** ejects blood earlier and ceases later than the left ventricle (i.e. **contracts for longer duration**).
- **Cardiac cycle** is = 0.8 sec.
- Atrial systole = 0.1 sec; A. diastole = 0.7 sec
- Ventricular systole = 0.3 sec; V. diastole = 0.5 sec.
- **S1 sound** = at the onset of ventricular systole; **Mitral and Tricuspid** components; 0.1–0.17 sec; heard in 5th intercostal space; due to **sudden closure of AV valves** by sharp rise of intraventricular pressure; coincides with **spike of R – wave** in ECG; vibrations are transmitted from the valve to the apices of the ventricles.
- **S2** = i.e. **onset of ventricular diastole due to sudden closure of SLVs; Aortic and Pulmonary**; 0.1–0.14 sec; **just after T – wave** of ECG; vibrations are transmitted from the valve to the arteries; pulmonary component precedes the aortic component; during inspiration but not during expiration the S2 is split into aortic component and later a pulmonary component. Its pitch is directly proportional to BP.
- **S3 = opening of AV valve**; 0.04 sec; at the beginning of ventricular filling.
- **S4** = i.e. contraction of atria; **end of ventricular filling**.
- Both S1 and S2 occur during ventricular phase only. ***Onset of ventricular systole is marked by S1 and its termination by S2.***
- Ventricular systole starts at the end of atrial systole; systole of atrium and ventricle never overlap; diastole of the 2 chambers will always partly overlap by 0.1 sec when it is ka **diastole of the whole heart**.

- **Isometric contraction period** = at the start of ventricular systole, it is the brief period when both the valves are closed and the **ventricles are contracting as closed cavities**; 0.05 sec.
- **Ejection period** = SLV open and blood from ventricles is expelled; maximum ejection period (0.11 sec) + reduced ejection period (0.14 sec); now the ventricular systole ends and ventricular diastole starts.
- **Protodiastolic period** = 0.04 sec; a short interval b/w the onset of diastole and closure of SLV, i.e. S2; so the S2 does not occur at the end of the ventricular systole but after this PDP.
- **Isometric relaxation period** = 0.08 sec during which both the valves are closed and **ventricles are relaxing** as the closed cavities; there is no lengthening of the cardiac ms fibers.
- **First rapid filling phase** = 0.113 sec; largest part of the ventricular filling occurs here and S3 is produced due to rapid rush of the blood.
- **Slow inflow phase = aka** diastasis; 0.167 sec; longest phase of the ventricular diastole; minimum filling occurs during this period.
- **Last rapid filling phase** = is due to atrial contraction; 0.1 sec; S4 is produced due to rapid filling of the blood; so the ***onset of filling period is marked by the S3 and its termination by S4.***
- **Apex beat** = is felt at the left 5th intercostal space about 1.27 cm inside the midclavicular line; occurs at the beginning of the ventricular systole and is parallel to S1.

ECG: times of this in sec.

1.	PR interval	0.18 sec; is the gap b/w onset of atrial contraction and onset of ventricular contraction.
2.	QRS	0.08 – 0.1 sec
3.	ST	0.32 sec
4.	QT	0.4 sec
5.	QRST	0.43 sec
6.	T wave	0.27 sec.

P – wave ; 0.1 sec QRS – complex	Atrial depolarisation Ventricular depolarisation, aka ventricular complex.
T – wave	Ventricular repolarisation
PR – interval	Atrial depolarisation and AV conduction; propagation of cardiac impulse from SA node to ventricle through AV – node.
QRS – interval sec 0.08 – 0.1	Interval of total ventricular depolarisation time.
Q – wave	is due to activity of septum.
ST	Continued ventricular depolarisation
QT	0.36 sec; Ventricular depolarisation + v. repolarisation.
TP interval	Measures the diastolic period of heart.

Bipolar leads / standard limb leads *used in the ECG are*

Leads	**Negative terminal**	**Positive terminal**
I	Right arm	Left arm
II	Right arm	Left leg
III	Left arm	Left leg

- P, R, T waves are positive waves and Q, S are negative waves;
- P = is of atrial origin is ka **atrial complex**; QRST is of ventricular origin is ka **venticular complex**;
- RS is the most constant and conspicuous wave having **tallest amplitude**.
- T – wave = abnormalities in it indicate the serious myocardial damage and is often associated with cardiac hypoxia;

Action of vagus on heart: vagus acts as THE INHIBITOR of heart. In mammalian heart, the vagal fibres do not extend beyond the upper part of the bundle. So the ventricular stoppage is due to the indirect effect of atrial slowing.

- Negative **chronotropic** = HR is decreased.
- Negative **dromotropic** = conductivity of the bundle is reduced.
- Negative **inotropic** = force of contraction is reduced.
- Negative **bathmotropic** = excitability of the heart is reduced.
- Vagus exerts a tonic inhibitory control over all parts of the heart.
- Atropine prevents the action of Ach on cardiac ms and HR is increased.
- **Vagal escape** = i.e. the heart escapes from the inhibitory effect of vagus.
- **Bainbridge's reflex** = due to slowing of HR, the engorgement of great Vs and right atrium occurs which inhibits the vagal tone and also stimulate the sympathetic to some extent and the heart starts beating.

Role of sympathetic nerves: are situated in lateral horn cells of the upper thoracic segment of spinal cord (T 1–5, or 6). Of the vagus and sympathetic – **the former has a much stronger influence on the heart** than the latter. It is stimulatory to heart.

- Positive chronotropic = HR is increased, i.e. accelerator.
- Positive dromotropic = conductivity of the bundle is increased.
- Positive inotropic = force of contraction is increased, i.e. augmentor.
- Positive bathmotropic = excitability of the heart is increased, i.e. ectopic beats.

HEART RATE = it is inversely proportional to age.

- Normal value = 72 / min.
- In fetus = 140–150
- Newborn = 130–140
- > 15 yr = 70–80
- In old age = slightly higher, 75–80

- HR is directly proportional to BMR.
- During inspiration, the HR increases; during expiration it falls. It is ka **sinus arrhythmia**.
- **Marey's law** = HR is inversely proportional to BP.
- **Anoxia** = increases the HR through chemoreceptors.
- **Circulation is more sensitive to O_2 lack and respiration is more sensitive to CO_2 excess.**
- Increased intracranial pressure = decreases the HR by directly **stimulating vagus N**.
- Adr = increases BP; decreases HR; increases force of contraction.
- Thyroxine = increases BMR, stimulates SA node and sympathetics.

CARDIAC OUTPUT, CO = is the amount of blood pumped out by each ventricle per beat in circulation.

Stroke volume; SV = is the output per ventricle per beat; is 70 ml.

Minute volume, MV = is the output per ventricle per minute. MV = SV x HR. and is 5–6 litres.

Cardiac index = CO per min per square meter of the body surface. Is 3.3 litres.

Surface area of an average – sized adult is = 1.7 m^2.

SV index = is the SV per square meter of the body surface; is 47 ml.

Distribution of cardiac output = MV of heart is distributed as follows.

1. Kidneys = 1300 ml / min.
2. Brain = 700–800 ml / min.
3. Coronary = 200 ml / min.
4. Muscles = 600–900 ml / min.
5. Liver = 1500 ml / min.
6. Remaining = in skin, bones and GIT.

STARLING'S LAW = within physiological limits, greater the initial length of cardiac ms, stronger will be the force of contraction.

BLOOD PRESSURE

- Is the lateral pressure exerted by blood on the vessel walls while flowing through it.
- **Systolic BP** = maximum pressure during systole. Average = 110 – 120 mm Hg.
- **Diastolic BP** = minimum pressure during diastole. Average = 70 – 80 mm Hg.
- **Pulse pressure** (PP) = is the difference b/w SBP and DBP.
- In adults, the relation b/w SBP / DBP/ PP = 3/2/1.
- **DBP** = Increase in DBP indicates that the heart is approaching towards failure. It is of **greater prognostic significance**. It is the **measure of peripheral resistance**.
- **Peripheral resistance** = Is the resistance which blood has to overcome while passing through the periphery. The **chief seat of PR is the ARTERIOLES**.
- **VASOMOTOR CENTRE** = is situated on the **floor of the 4th ventricle** in the reticular formation at the level of the calamus scriptorius. It is under the control of cerebral cortex and hypothalamus. Depressor center causes inhibition of vaso-constrictor tone.
- Rise of BP stimulates the **baroreceptors of carotid sinus** and aortic arch; decreases HR.
- Reflex vasoconstriction occurs due to stimulation of **chemoreceptors** during fall of BP.
- **Carotid sinus** = is a dilatation **at the root of ICA** and often involving CCA. These pressor receptors are **sensitive to stretch** being stimulated by increased BP. Sinus nerve passes along **glossopharyngeal / 9th N**; and ends in medulla.
- **Aortic arch** = also has stretch receptors; the aortic nerve is a purely afferent nerve; it mostly passes in the **vagus N** and ends in medulla.
- **Carotid body** = is a small nodule present **on the occipital A**, a branch of ECA very close to the carotid sinus. They are **sensitive to chemical changes** in blood. Afferents lie in **aortic nerves**

and vagus Ns. CO_2 excess, O_2 lack, increased H^+ ion conc stimulate respiration, increase HR and BP.

- **Epinephrine** injected in blood increases BP sharply.
- Histamine = causes dilatation of capillaries.
- Alcohol = dilatation of blood vessels as it depresses VMC (vasomotor center).
- Tobacco = increases both SBP and DBP; and pulse rate.
- Vasopressin = increases BP.
- **Velocity of blood** = is the rate of blood flow through a given vessel. It is inversely proportional to the cross sectional area of the blood vessel.
- **Radial pulse** = is the expansion and elongation of the arterial walls passively produced by the pressure changes during systole and diastole of ventricles. Normal pulse is ka CATACROTIC PULSE.
- **Velocity of pulse wave** = is 6 × the velocity of blood.
- **Pulsus alterans** = i.e. the pulse is alternately large and small;
- **Pulsus paradoxus** = the volume and frequency is more during expiration than during inspiration, i.e. reverse of sinus arrhythmia.

Cerebral circulation

- 4 main vessels = 2 ICA and 2 vertebral A.
- 2 vertebral A = form basilar A; which divides into 2 posterior cerebral As.
- Each ICA = gives 2 br = middle cerebral As and anterior cerebral As.
- These **6 arteries** are joined by communicating As (1 anterior and 2 posterior) to form **circle of Willis**. So in **total, 9 As** form circle of Willis.
- The grey matter is more vascular than white matter.
- **Blood brain barrier** = the capillaries of the cerebral vessels, choroid plexus, etc. are less permeable.
- **Liver circulation** = blood enters the liver through 2 sources viz. Portal V and hepatic A; left lobe of liver gets blood from the spleen and the right lobe from the superior mesenteric vein.

RESPIRATORY SYSTEM

- **Ventilation** = is the passage of air in and out of the lungs.
- Distribution or **gas mixing** = is the distribution of O_2 rich inspired air with the air already present in the lungs.
- **Diffusion** = is the gas transfer across the alveolo-capillary membrane due to tension gradient.
- **Perfusion** = flow of adequate amount of blood through lungs s.t. the diffused gases are taken away.
- Upper respiratory tract = extends from upper nares to vocal cords.
- Lower respiratory tract = extends from vocal cords to the alveoli.
- **Trachea** = 10–11 cm long; has incomplete C-shaped cartilaginous rings in the anterolateral walls; glands are innervated by vagus Ns; ciliar movement is independent of nerves.
- **Cough reflex** = is a protective reflex; the larynx and area of bifurcation of trachea are most sensitive areas; the afferents run in the **vagus N**; the explosive sound comes with a velocity of 100 miles / hr.
- **Sneeze reflex** = is also a protective reflex; afferents are in **TRIGEMINAL Ns**.

RESPIRATORY UNIT = has 4 parts

- Respiratory bronchioles.
- Alveolar ducts
- Respiratory atrium
- **Pulmonary alveoli** = are the **last division** of respiratory tree; are lined by thin layer of squamous epithelium; **surfactant** which is a lipoprotein with **dipalmityl lecithin** prevents their collapse.
- **Most important function of respiration** = to keep arterial PCO_2 at 40 mm Hg, i.e. essential for many vital functions of the body.
- As air passes from trachea to lungs, the **first structure** in which gaseous exchange through the wall of an alveolus may occur is = RESPIRATORY BRONCHIOLE **(the functional unit of lung).**

Pressure changes during respiration

- **Intrapleural pressure** = is negative and is – 2.5 mm Hg at the end of the expiration.
- Inspiration = at the end of inspiration, the Intrapleural pressure becomes more negative, i.e. at – 6 mm Hg.
- Then the **intrapulmonary** pressure also goes down from 0 at rest to – 2 mm Hg at the end of inspiration.
- Negative intrapleural pressure is so responsible **primarily for inflow of the air in the lungs**.
- Expiration is a passive process due to relaxation of inspiratory ms.
- **DIAPHRAGM** = supplied by phrenic nerve (C3, C4, C5); the normal breathing is predominantly diaphragmatic.
- Intercostal ms are innervated by intercostal nerves (T1 – T11 Ns).
- Bucket handle motion and pump handle motions of the ribs occurs during respiration.

Definitions in respiration

Tidal volume; TV	Air inspired / expired in / out in quiet respiration.	500 ml
Respiratory minute volume; RMV	TV × respiratory rate **(12/min)**	6000 ml/ min.
IRV; inspiratory reserve volume	Maximum extra volume of air that can be inhaled after a quiet inspiration.	2.0 – 3.2 liters
ERV; expiratory reserve volume	Maximum air that can be breathed out by maximum expiratory effort after a quiet expiration.	1100 ml
Residual volume ; RV	Air remaining in the lungs despite forceful expiration	1200 ml

Definitions in respiration

Inspiratory capacity	TV + IRV; maximum air that can be inspired from the end – expiratory stage.	3500 ml
Functional residual capacity / relaxation volume	ERV + RV; volume of air in lungs after a quiet expiration.	2300 ml
Vital capacity	TV+IRV+ERV; volume of air which can be max. expiratory effort after a max. inspiration.	4600 ml
Total lung capacity	TV+IRV+ERV+RV; vol. Of air the lung can hold after a maximum possible inspiration.	5800 ml
Maximum breathing capacity	Volume of expired air In Douglas bag multiplied by 5	140 liters/ min.
Dead space	The air which remains confined in the upper respiratory tract with each inspiration and is not available for gas exchange.	150 ml

Normal **ratio** of dead space to tidal volume = 0.2–0.35 during breathing at rest.

Partial pressures in mm Hg

PP	**Alveolar air**	**Arterial blood**	**Venous blood**
PaO_2	100	95	40
$PaCO_2$	40	40	46

Average values of tension of O_2 and CO_2

	PO_2	PCO_2
Alveoli	100 mm Hg	40
Venous blood	40	46

Oxygen transport

	O_2 Content	Oxy-Hb	O_2 in sol	PO_2
Arterial blood	19.3	19	0.3	100 mm Hg
Mixed Venous blood	14.2	14	0.2	40 mm Hg

- 1 gm of Hb combines with 1.34 ml of O_2 on full saturation.
- **O_2 capacity of blood** = since Hb is 15 gm / 100 ml of blood, so the O_2 content of saturated blood is 15 × 1.34 = 20 ml/100 ml.
- **DPG (2,3-diphosphoglycerate)** is formed in the RBCs by glycolysis. The reduced Hb can hold one molecule of DPG b/w its beta – chains and so reduces the affinity of Hb for O_2 and **favours its release** in tissues.
- Synthesis of DPG is favoured in anemia, and at high altitudes, so it has a role in O_2 transport in the body.
- In lungs, the time taken for 50% saturation of Hb is only 0.07 sec., and RBCs take 0.5 sec to pass a lung capillary.

O_2 exchange in lungs

- O_2 tension in alveolar air = 100 mm Hg
- In mixed venous blood = 40 mm Hg; so O_2 comes in venous blood from alveoli.

O_2 transport in tissues

- O_2 tension in tissue fluid = 40 mm Hg
- In arterial blood = 100 mm Hg; Hb is 98 % saturated; so O_2 enters the tissues from blood due to tension gradient.

- Blood leaves the tissues at O_2 tension 40 mm Hg, i.e. same as tissue fluid; and Hb is 75 % saturated.

O_2 and CO_2 in blood

Gases	Tension in arterial blood	Tension in venous blood	Total vol % in venous in blood	In arterial blood
O_2	90–100 mm Hg	40 mm Hg	14.0	19.0
CO_2	40 mm Hg	46 mm Hg	52.1	48.3

- CO_2 is carried in blood **mainly, i.e. > 80 %, as bicarbonates** and the major part of bicarbonate is present in plasma. However most of the **bicarbonate is first formed in RBCs,** mainly due to p.o.of enz **carbonic anhydrase** and then shifted to plasma; only 5% is carried as physical solution;
- **Chloride shift** = HCO_3^- from RBCs comes in plasma and Cl^- from plasma goes in RBCs in exchange of bicarbonates.

CO_2 transport in tissues

- Tension of CO_2 in tissues = 46 mm Hg
- In arterial end of capillary = 40 mm Hg, so CO_2 diffuses along tension gradient.

In the lungs

- Tension of CO_2 in plasma = 46 mm Hg
- In alveolar air = 40 mm Hg, so H_2CO_3 breaks down to form more CO_2; **reverse chloride shift** occurs.

Buffering property of Hb is due to **imidaxole group of histadine** linked with heme which has an ionisable H^+ ion.

- PP (partial pressure) of **N_2 gas is maximum** in the inspired air = 596 mm Hg
- PP of O_2 gas in the inspired air = 159 mm Hg
- PP of CO_2 gas in the inspired air = 0.30 mm Hg

- PP of water vapors in the inspired air = 5.00 mm Hg
- **Alveolar air** is poorer in O_2; and is richer in CO_2.
- After normal inspiration, breath can be held for 30 – 50 sec, ka **breath–holding time**.
- Alveolar ventilation is 4 litres / min; and about 5 liters/ min of blood is perfused through alveoli; so the **ventilation / perfusion ratio** is 4 / 5 = 0.8.
- Total amount of blood in lungs at any moment is = 150 ml.
- **Perfusion** = i.e. blood flow through the lungs; is 5 liters / min.
- Normal rate of respiration = 14–18 / min.
- CO_2 has stimulant action on **central chemoreceptors**, which are located **in medulla**, near entry of 9th and 10th Ns; rise in PCO_2 or fall in pH (increased H^+) stimulate them.
- **Peripheral chemoreceptors** = are in **carotid and aortic bodies**; REFLEXLY stimulate respiration by increased conc of CO_2 in blood.
- **Direct action** of O_2 lack on respiratory center is depression of respiration; but the respiration – stimulating action of O_2 lack is **a reflex** one through sino-aortic chemoreceptors.

Pulmonary ventilation is controlled by 3 factors — i.e.

1. Rise in arterial PCO_2.
2. Fall in arterial PO_2.
3. Increase in arterial conc. of H^+, (acidity).

Anoxia/hypoxia = i.e. inadequate or decreased supply of O_2 to the lungs.

Arterial hypoxia / anoxic anoxia = is characterised by LOW O_2 TENSION in arterial blood.

Anemic anoxia = is by low O_2 content of blood due to decreased quantity of Hb.

Stagnant anoxia / hypokinetic hypoxia = is by decreased rate of blood flow through the tissues; O_2 content of venous blood is very low due to stagnation.

Histotoxic anoxia = is the inability of the tissues to use O_2 and occurs in **cyanide poisoning**.

Anoxemia = i.e. diminished O_2 in blood.

Altitude anoxia = i.e. at high altitude due to low barometric pressure.

Dyspnoea = is difficulty in breathing associated with a sense of distress.

Hyperpnoea = is hyperventilation

Orthopnoea = in severe CHF disease, dyspnoea occurs even at rest; the patient feels more comfortable in sitting position than in lying down; it is ka orthopnoea.

Cyanosis = i.e. in which skin and mm assume a bluish color. It depends on the absolute amount of reduced Hb in blood. **At least, 5 gm of reduced Hb must be present** in blood before cyanosis can be produced.

DIGESTIVE SYSTEM

- Proximal end of stomach is guarded by cardiac sphincter and distal end is by pyloric sphincter.
- Bile duct and pancreatic ducts jointly open through **ampulla of vater**.
- **Lesser omentum** of stomach attaches to liver; **greater omentum** hangs over the intestine to the colon as an apron.
- Tongue = filiform and conic papillae have tactile sensitivity for touch; all the other papillae are gustatory.
- Sensation of taste is in chorda tympani N through 7th N (anterior two-thirds of tongue); in 9th N (posterior one-third of tongue); the general sensation of touch, pain, temperature, pressure, etc., by 5th n; ms by 12th n.
- Duct of parotid gland = duct of Stensen; opens opposite upper 2nd molar.
- Duct of submandibular gland = duct of Wharton.
- Duct of lingual gland = duct of Rivinus.
- **Myoepithelial cells** present in the glands are contractile which help in expulsion of secretions in the ducts.
- Parotid gland = entirely serous; sublingual gland is predominantly mucous; submandibular gland is *mixed* but mainly serous.

- Demilunes or crescents of **Giannuzzi** = i.e. the serous cells get compressed at one end.
- Secretions of serous glands is thin, watery, rich in enzymes, esp. ptyalin / amylase; .
- Mucous glands secretions are thick, viscid.
- Pharyngeal reflex = may be absent in 9th n lesions.
- **Oesophagus** = in upper 3rd, the ms are voluntary; in middle 3rd, the ms are both voluntary and involuntary; in lower 3rd, only plain ms are found.
- **GIT**: In muscularis mucosa: smooth muscles arranged as: Inner layer-Circular, Outer layer-Longitudinal
- **Oesophagus** : 3 portions based on muscular layers (muscularis externa)

In upper 3rd - striated m. only

In mid 3rd - striated + smooth ms.

In lower 3rd - smooth ms. only

- **Muscularis externa** : 3 layers of oblique - circular - longitudinal ms. from inside out (opposite of stomach).
- **Valve of Kerckring**-circular fold in mucosa.
- Terminal part of ileum has NO FOLDS.
- **VILLI are largest and maximum in Duodenum. Increase surface area of small intestine by 8 times.**
- No glands are present in submucosa of jejunum and ileum - but present in duodenum (known as **Brunner's glands** - open in crypts of Lieberkuhn, maximum in proximal part of duodenum).

Gallbladder

- Right and left common hepatic ducts and cystic duct form **Bile duct** which unite with pancreatic duct to form hepatopancreatic duct (or Ampulla), which opens into the duodenum at the summit of the major duodenal papilla,
- **Sphincter of Oddi**: well developed smooth muscles in the region of lower end of bile duct.

- Stomach = 3 layers of ms = outer longitudinal; middle is circular; inner is oblique (opposite of oesophagus).
- Simple tubular glands of stomach = secrete the mucous.
- Cardiac glands = secrete mucus
- Mucous neck cells in fundus = secrete mucus.
- Chief/zymogenic/peptic cells in body = secrete pepsin and gastric rennin.
- Oxyntic / parietal cells = secrete HCl.
- Argentaffin cells = secrete serotonin.
- **Gastrin** = stimulates gastric secretions; **enterogastrone** inhibits gastric secretions and gastric motility.
- Small intestine = outer longitudinal and inner circular layer of ms; in muscularis mucose.
- Crypts of Lieberkühn = secrete intestinal juice.
- Folds of Kerckring = increase the surface area of the intestine esp found in jejunum.
- Chief function of jejunum is secretion; but of ilium is absorption.
- **Peyer's patches** = are lymphoid tissues collection; In ilium only.
- Peneth cells = are **in small intestine only**; secrete proteins.
- In duodenum = Brunner's glands = in the submucous coat.
- In jejunum = absent Brunner's glands and Peyer's patches.
- Large intestine = folds are ka **taenia coli**; there is **no villi** in the mm; in anal area the mucous membrane is in folds ka **recta columns of Morgagni**.

SALIVA

- 1200--1500 ML / 24 HRS; sp. Gr = 1.002–1.012; smoker's saliva is rich in thiocyanates.
- Enz kallikrein in saliva produces a substance ka *bradykinin* which produces the vasodilation of salivary gland during secretion.
- Chief function of saliva = are mechanical functions; mainly due to mucin.

- Ptyalin = splits starch up to maltose; maltase converts it in glucose;
- **Buffer** = due to bicarbonate.

GASTRIC JUICE

- 1200–1500 ml / day; **strongly acidic**; contains pepsin, rennin, lipase enzs; sp gr = 1.002–1.004.
- HCl digests the proteins **up to peptone stage**.
- Rennin coagulates caseinogen of milk.

Pancreatic juice

- 1500 ml / day; alkaline; sp gr = 1.010–1.030.
- It has a **high bicarbonate** content.
- Main enz are = trypsinogen; chymotrypsinogen; lipase, etc.

Intestinal juice

- 1–2 liters / 24 hrs; sp gr = 1.010; reaction = **mildly acidic to mildly alkaline**.
- Bicarbonate content is higher than blood or interstitial fluid.
- Enterokinase / enteropeptidase = activate trypsinogen to trypsin.
- **Arginase** = acts on arginine producing urea and ornithin.
- Sucrase / invertase = digests cane sugar.

Bile

- Formation of bile by liver is an **active process**.
- Common bile duct opens in duodenum through ampulla of Vater.
- 500 – 1000 ml / day; sp gr = 1.010 – 1.011; it is definitely **alkaline**.
- Bile salts = sodium taurocholate and glycocholates are formed in liver; are strongest **cholegogues**; glycocholic acid and taurocholic acids are formed by the combination of glycine and taurine with cholic acids.
- Bile is essential for life; and for complete digestion of fats.
- Bile salts are mostly **reabsorbed in intestine** and are re-excreted.

- Bile pigments = bilirubin and biliverdin; bilirubin combines with albumin in plasma; enz biliverdin reductase catalyses the reduction of biliverdin to bilirubin.
- Bilirubin forms mono- and bi-glucuronides catalysed by enz glucuronyl transferase.
- Liver / Kupffer cells, spleen and bone marrow are chief sites of RE cells; take active part in formation of bilirubin.

Stimuli required for secretion of juices

Secretion	Stimulus	Nature
Saliva	Nervous	—
Gastric juice	Nervous, chemical	Acidic
Pancreatic juice	Nervous, chemical	Alkaline
Succus entericus	Nervous, chemical, mechanical	Mild acidic to mild alkaline
Bile	Chemical	Alkaline

Mechanism of salivary secretion

Salivary gland	Parasympathetic route	Sympathetic
Submand and sublingual	From superior salivatory nucleus (dorsal nucleus of 7th n) → nervous intermedius → 7th n → chorda tympani → lingual n → to submand ganglion → glands.	From T 1 – 3 and/ or T4 → superior cervical gang → walls of arteries → glands. They end in serous part of gland.
Parotid	From inferior salivatory nucleus (dorsal nucleus of 9th n) → tympanic br → tympanic plexus → lesser petrosal n → otic gang → through auriculotemporal br of 5th n → glands.	Supply vasoconstrictor fibres to vessels and to myoepithelial cells.

Mechanism of salivary secretion

	Secrete *watery* saliva; act through Ach so ka cholinergic fibres; produce kallikrein which forms bradykinin to produce vasodilation.	Produce *viscous* saliva; act through Adr ka adrenergic fibres; are vasoconstrictor.
	Atropine blocks action of Ach and inhibits salivation.	

- **Conditioned reflex** = is even the sight or smell of food can stimulate salivation although no food is actually given.
- **Unconditioned reflex** = i.e. food is actually given to the animal.

Secretion of HCl

- By oxyntic / parietal cells;
- **Carbonic anhydrase** enz plays an imp role for HCl formation;
- After meals, there is an increase in pH of blood and urine due to liberated HCO_3 – ions and is ka **alkaline tide**.
- It activates pepsinogen to pepsin.
- Zn is required for action of enz. carbonic anhydrase.

Pancreas

- Mixed i.e. endocrine and exocrine gland.
- Main excretory duct of gland is **duct of Wirsung**; opens with common bile duct at ampulla of Vater in 2nd part of duodenum.
- **Islets of Langerhans** = are the endocrine part; it has alpha and beta cells; beta cells secrete *insulin*; alpha cells secrete *glucagon*.
- **Adenyl cyclase activity** and lipolysis are stimulated by secretin and glucagon; here secretin is more potent than glucagon.
- Hepatocrinin = stimulates liver to secrete bile
- Cholecystokinin = causes contraction of gallbladder
- Enterocrinin = stimulates release of intestinal juices.

Vomiting reflex = afferents arise in sensory nerves 5th and 9th; chemicals act on CTZ.

Segmentation movements of small intestine = does not cause forward passage of food but only mixing; while peristalsis causes forward movement.

MUSCLES

- Contraction of ms = membrane depolarisation → Ca released from sarcoplasmic reticulum → myosin ATP-ase activated → cross bridge formed → myosin slides along actin → tension developed.
- Relaxation = Ca pumped back in SR → myosin ATP-ase depressed → cross bridge broken → myosin pulled back to its resting state → tension disappears.
- **Refractory period** = after stimulation, there is brief period during which the ms is not excitable to a second stimulus.
- **Absolute refractory period** = during the first part of RP, the muscle remains unexcitable to any strength of stimulus is ka ARP.
- **Relative refractory period** = in later part of RP, the ms is excitable only with a strong stimulus.
- The ARP in skeletal ms is shorter than in cardiac ms, and so the skeletal ms can be tetanised or fatigued.
- **Isotonic contraction** = is physical shortening of the ms is allowed;
- **Isometric contraction** = physical shortening of the ms is reduced to minimum by making it contract against a strong spring.
- **Rigor mortis** = starts in second hour and is completed in 3 hrs after death. Ms of body involve in this sequence — lower jaw, face neck, thorax, abdomen, upper limb and lastly the lower limb. It disappears in 24 – 36 hrs after death due to autolysis.
- It is a state of permanent irreversible contraction and is associated with deficiency of ATP causing permanent link b/w actin and myosin.

DEFINITIONS

Facilitated diffusion = This process is used to accumulate glucose inside cells.

Primary active transport = This process is used to maintain high extracellular Na^+ concentration.

Co-transport = This process is used to accumulate natural amino acids inside cells.

Counter-transport =This process is used to keep intracellular Ca^{2+} concentration low.

Counter-transport = This process is used to regulate secretion of H^+ into the lumen of the renal proximal convoluted tubule.

Simple diffusion = This process allows Na^+ to enter the apical surface of intestinal epithelial cells.

Primary active transport = This process allows Na^+ to exit the basal and lateral surface of intestinal epithelial cells,

- **Anaphylactic shock = Due** to massive degranulation of mast cells.
- **Cardiac shock** = Due to inadequate cardiac function following a heart attack.
- **Hypovolemic shock** = Caused by a low blood volume and is related to hemorrhage or blood loss.
- **Primary shock** = Also known as syncope or fainting; Usually caused by a reflex that produces arteriolar dilation and/or cardiac slowing.
- **Septic shock** = Is due to infections in the bloodstream.

ONE WORD ANSWER

1. It stimulates parietal cells in the stomach to secrete hydrochloric acid and increases the constriction of the lower esophageal sphincter = **gastrin.**
2. This product of endocrine cells of duodenum causes smooth muscle in the wall of the gallbladder to contract = **cholecystokinin.**
3. A derivative of tryptophan, functions as local activator of smooth muscle in the mucosa of various parts of the gastrointestinal tube = **serotonin.**
4. In addition to stimulating the release of enzymes from the pancreas, this hormone has mild inhibitory effects on motility of several regions of the gastrointestinal tube = **secretin.**

5. It is produced in small intestine and causes the cells lining pancreatic ducts to release large quantity of water and bicarbonate = cholecystokinin.
6. The vagus nerve regulates its secretion because vagal stimulus causes both increased release of bombazine and decreased release of somatostatin = gastrin.
7. This polypeptide is produced in the duodenum and stimulates strong gastric smooth muscle contraction = motilin.
8. Produced by duodenal enterocytes, this cleaves trypsinogen to form trypsin = enterokinase.
9. Its activity is strongly dependent on emulsification of fats by components of bile = lipase.
10. This enzyme functions to allow the concentration of bile by the gallbladder and of saliva by ducts in the salivary glands = Na^+ - K^+ ATPase.
11. An amylase found in saliva, it begins the degradation of starches while food is in the oral cavity = ptyalin.
12. Its activation is primarily due to the action of trypsin = chymotrypsinogen.
13. Which is the precursor of an enzyme whose activity is maximal in an acid milieu = pepsinogen.
14. Which enzyme removes amino acids from the –COOH terminal of peptides and proteins = carboxypeptidase.
15. Which cells are sensitive to growth hormone inhibitory hormone (somatostatin) = acidophils.
16. Which cells are sensitive to gonadotropin–releasing hormone = basophils.
17. Neurophysins are transported to which site prior to the release of oxytocin = distended axon terminals in pars-nervosa.
18. Which cells secrete thyroid-stimulating hormone and luteinizing hormone = basophils.
19. Which hormone binds to its intracellular receptor, activates hormone-receptor complexes which then activate transcription of certain genes to form mRNA. About 30 minutes after hormone binding, proteins promoting Na^+ reabsorption in renal tubules appear in these cells = aldosterone.

20. When this hormone binds to its receptor located in the cell membrane an increase in cAMP levels occur. This **second messenger** in turn causes mobilization of Ca^{2+} from calcified extracellular matrix by osteoclasts = PTH.

A congenital inability to synthesize this hormone leads to Levi-lorian dwarfism. In normal individual this hormone is thought to mediate the effects of growth hormone = somatomedin-C.

When this hormone binds to its nuclear receptor, activated-receptor complexes then activate transcription of certain genes to form mRNA Many enzymes are now synthesized leading to an increase in carbohydrate metabolism, fat metabolism and an overall increase in basal metabolic rate = thyroxine.

Which hormone binds to its receptor, located in the cell membrane, and causes an increase in cAMP and secrete spermatogenic factors = FSH.

When secreted from the pars nervosa, this polypeptide hormone stimulates contraction of smooth muscle in the uterus and myoepithelial cells in the mammary gland ducts = oxytocin.

Which hormone is secreted by cell in the adenohypophysis. Its titer rises during pregnancy and it is required for milk secretion = prolactin.

Which hormone is secreted by the placenta. It is required for growth and development of the ducts of the mammary glands. It is also secreted by the ovary where it stimulates endometrial glandular growth prior to ovulation = beta estradiol.

The release of which hormone from the pituitary gland is inhibited by dopamine. It shows marked increase in secretion during and after periods of nursing = oxytocin.

This is a glycoprotein hormone secreted by the placenta. Its chief function is to stimulate continued growth of the corpus luteum during pregnancy = chorionic gonadotropin.

Small quantities of which hormone are secreted by the luteal cells of the corpus luteum, it inhibits secretion of FSH from the anterior pituitary = inhibin.

A surge in secretion of this hormone is required for a mature ovary follicle to progress to repute = LH.

Which hormone is secreted by the hypothalamus in a pulsatile fashion. It is a decapeptide = gonadotropin releasing hormone.

This is a location where aqueous channels between cells assure free passage of small molecules = gap junction.

This structure is thought to be involved in intercellular adhesions. Here one finds dense plaques on the cytoplasmic face apposed membranes which serve as insertion sites for tonofilaments = macula adherens.

This is a site fusion of outer leaflets of the plasma membrane. It is tight junction preventing terminal materials from leaving the lumen = zonula occludens.

Chylomicra are synthesized from triglycerides, glycolipids and proteins = Golgi apparatus of intestinal absorptive epithelial cells.

Free fatty acids and monoglycerides are converted into triglycerides = SER of intestinal absorptive epithelial cells.

Chylomicra are transported via these lymphatic vessels to the systemic circulation = lacteals.

Tracheal mucosa = pseudostratified columnar epithelium.

Visceral pleura = simple squamous epithelium.

Proximal convoluted tubule = simple cuboidal epithelium.

Epidermis = stratified squamous epithelium.

Duodenal mucosa = simple columnar epithelium.

Which cell differentiates into an immunoglobulin-secreting cell = lymphocytes?

Which cell is the most abundant granulocyte in blood = neutrophils?

Which cell can differentiate into a microglial cell in the central nervous system = monocytes?

Which cell contains granules rich in heparin = basophils?

Which cell is abundant in patients with schistosomiasis = eosinophils?

Which deep periosteal cell can differentiate into a type I collagen-secreting cell = osteoblasts?

Which perichondrial cell can differentiate into a type 2 collagen cell = chondroblasts?

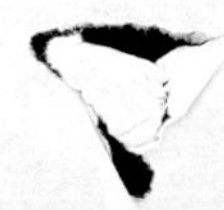

Which cell responds to parathormone by osteolysis = osteocytes?

Which cell type aggregates to form centers of chondrification in embryonic limb buds = mesenchymal fibroblasts?

Which cell is capable of mitotic division when surrounded by type II collagen and cartilage-specific proteoglycan = chondrocytes?

In conjunction with antigen-presenting and antibody producing cell, which cell is required for antibody systhesis = helper T–cells?

Which cell is a bone marrow derivative involved in presentation of antigen to immunoglobulin producing cell = macrophage?

Which cell has an abundant rough endoplasmic reticulum and a prominent nucleolus. It is dedicated to immunoglobulin synthesis and secretion into the blood = plasma cells?

Which cell has a granular cytoplasm with azurophilic granules. It is a different cell which represents the line of defense against foreign cells = natural killer cells?

Which organ is derived from pharyngeal pouches III and IV. It contains reticular epithelial cells and lymphocytes = thymus?

Which organ has a subcapsular sinus. Germinal centers appear in response to antigenic stimulation = lymph nodes?

Which organ is responsible for immune surveillance of the blood and removal of defective erythrocytes from the systemic circulation = spleen?

Which organ is the first major hematopoietic organ in the embryo = liver?

What is the location of the major structures involved in reflexive orientation of the eyes and the head to visual stimuli = midbrain.

What is the location of the decussation of the corticospinal tract = lower medulla?

What is the location of the second order neurons that receive direct synapses from axons of the posterior column of the spinal cord = lower medulla?

What is the location of the motor nucleus for the muscles of facial expression = pons?

What is the location of the portion of the ventricular system called the cerebral aqueduct = midbrain?

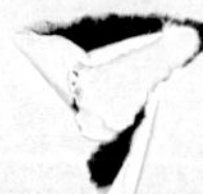

Function of nephron—Selective reabsorption occurs esp. in P.C. tubule - of H_2O, glucose, amino acids, proteins of smaller molecular size and various ions like Na, Cl, PO_4, HCO_3, Ca.

- Axons arise from **anterior grey columns** of spinal cord, are myelinated (are ∝-efferent).
- **Grey matter**-Contains cell bodies of neurons + dendrites / axon starting / ending on cell body. Most of these fibres are UNMYELINATED.
- **White matter** has myelinated fibres?
- **In spinal cord and brain stem = white matter is OUTSIDE**
- In cerebrum, cerebellum = Grey matter is OUTSIDE. Also white matter known as Cortex (inside) has some isolated masses of grey matter which are known as NUCLEI.
- Myelin sheath can be seen if fixed with OSMIC ACID.
- Diameter = 1–22 μm, neuro motor, but some sensory

  Sensory type A = Group I, II, III in decreasing order of velocity and diameter.

  Motor type A = 1. α- fibres - Large diameter, supply skeletal muscles,

  2. Gamma- fibres - Small diameter, supply intrafusal fibres.

- **Medullary cord has both B- and T- cells.**
- Tonsils and Peyer's patches are <u>subepithelial</u> and non-encapsulated.
- T-cells attack foreign cells.

SALIVARY GLANDS

— Contain a digestive enzyme - PTYALIN.

— Are compound tubuloalveolar glands (Racemose glands).

— **SEROUS CELLS** are arranged as round acini, pyramidal shape, e.g. parotid, mixed in submandibular.

— **MUCOUS CELLS** are arranged as TUBULES, e.g. sublingual gland.

— **Smallest duct** = also known as intercalated duct (lined by cuboidal/ flat cells).

— I.C.D. open in = STRIATED DUCT (columnar cells).

— Striated duct open into excretory duct (simple columnar epithelium).

Endocrines

No.	Hormone	Increased	Decreased
1.	Thyroid	Goitre Myxoedema (adults)	Cretinism (Infants)
2.	Pituitary	Gigantism (infants) Acromegaly (adults)	Dwarfism Simmond's dis.
3.	Parathyroid	von-Recklinghansen's dis. of bone; osteitis fibrosa cystica	Tetany
4.	Adrenal cortex	Cushing's synd. (hypertension seen) (hypochromic - anemia)	Acute = Waterhouse - Friderichsen synd. microcystic anemia; atrophy of tongue; etc.) Chronic = Addison dis. (hypotension)

Important points:

- Steroids are used to treat shock and hypotension
- Posterior pituitary and adrenal medulla are controlled directly by NERVOUS STIMULATION
- Hormones of adrenal gland control 4 S's re

(a) Salt = Mineralocorticoids — from zona glomerulosa

(b) Sugar = glucocorticoids—from zona fasciculata

(d) Sex = Androgenic hormones — from zona reticularis

(c) Survival = Adr, n-Adr. — from adr. medulla

Mechanism of action of glucocorticoids is by = Activation of specific genes.

MULTIPLE CHOICE QUESTIONS
Sample Question Paper

1. The Na^+-K^+ pump has which of the most crucial function for all the cells ?

A. It maintains a low extracellular Na^+ concentration
B. It maintains a high extracellular K^+ concentration
C. ATP hydrolysis
D. Maintenance of cell volume.

2. All of the following hormones activate adenylate cyclase when they bind to receptor except

A. Cortisol
B. ACTH
C. TSH
D. Vasopressin

3. Which is the second messenger required for vascular smooth muscle relaxation triggered by atrial natriuretic factor

A. cAMP
B. cGMP
C. Calmodulin
D. Arachidonic acid

4. The second messenger for glucagon is

A. cAMP
B. Calmodulin
C. Inositol triphosphate
D. Arachidonic acid

5. Features in common to Second messengers are

A. Similar chemical structure
B. Activate enzyme cascades
C. Present in sequestered pools in cells
D. Turnover is very slow

6. Calmodulin is most closely related structurally and functionally, to which muscle protein?

A. F-actin

B. Troponin C
C. Tropomysin
D. Alpha - actinin

7. Intracellular Ca^{2+} is normally related to extracellular Ca^{2+} as
A. Equal
B. 1000 fold higher
C. 1000 fold lower
D. 5000 fold lower

8. All of the following statements concerning calmodulin are true except
A. Binds 2 mols ca^{2+}/mol calmodulin at saturation
B. Undergoes a conformational change when saturated by Ca^{2+}
C. Regulates adenylate cyclase
D. Regulates guanylate cyclase

9. The second messenger for insulin is
A. Calmodulin
B. cAMP
C. Ca^{2+}
D. Unknown

10. Neurotransmitters into the synaptic cleft are released by which of the following mechanism?
A. Exocytosis
B. Active transport
C. Diffusion
D. All of the above.

11. Neurotransmitters from the synaptic cleft are removed by which of the following mechanism?
A. Endocytosis
B. Degradation
C. Diffusion
D. All of the above.

12. Enzymatic degradation mechanism inactivates which of the following neurotransmitters?
A. Serotonin

B. Nor-epinephrine
C. Dopamine
D. Acetylcholine

13. For the releases of a neurotransmitter from the presynaptic ending, the influx of which of the following ions is required?
A. Ca^{2+}
B. Na^{+}
C. Cl^{-}
D K^{+}

14. Which of the following is/ are characteristic of the vestibule apparatus?
A. An afferent neural connection with CNS is through 8th nerve
B. The ability to detect linear acceleration via the maculae.
C. The ability to detect angular acceleration via the cristae ampullares of the semicircular canals
D. The ability to detect changes in inertia of rest via the maculae
E. All of the above

15. When a person rotates his head slowly towards the left, then
A. The endolymph moves in the same direction as head movement
B. The hair cells in the crista ampullaris of the horizontal semicircular canal become depolarized
C. Both A and B above
D. Neither A nor B above.

16. The eyes move in which direction with rotation of the head to the left,
A. Move to the left, then rapidly return to the center of the orbit
B. Move to the right, then rapidly return to the center of the orbit
C. Do not move at all
D. Move in the direction of head movement
E. None of the above

17. Efferent connections of the cerebellum originate from the
A. Basket cells
B. Climbing fibers
C. Granular cells
D. Purkinje cells

18. Which of the following are considered to form inhibitory synaptic connection?

A. Climbing fibers
B. Mossy fibers
C. Purkinje cells
D. None of the above.

19. The cerebellum is important in controlling all of the following except

A. Smooth muscle movement
B. Maintaining posture
C. Maintaining balance
D. Initiating voluntary muscle movement
E. Accuracy of muscle movement

20. A patient with intention tremors, scanning speech, " past-pointing" and a drunken gait is expected to have a lesion involving the

A. Vestibulocochlear nerve
B. Red muscles
C. Precentral gyrus
D. Cerebellum

21. One of the reactions in the retinal rods directly caused by absorption of light energy is

A. Transformation of vitamin A to 11-cis retianl
B. Transformation of 11-cis retinal to all-trans retinal
C. Dissociation of scotopsin and vitamin A
D. Combination of 11 - cis retinal with opsin

22. The correct auditory function of the middle ear ossicles is to

A. Amplify the sound
B. Enable the direction of a sound to be detected
C. Filter high frequency sound
D. Protect the inner ear from damage

23. Skeletal muscle CPK is elevated because of

A. Degeneration of neuromuscular junctions
B. Mitochondrial degeneration

C. Muscle fiber degeneration
D. Myosin autoantibody accumulation

24. Muscle spindles have all the following features except:
A. Stretching muscle excites the receptor
B. They are sensitive to degree of stretch
C. They are sensitive to rate of stretch
D. The rate of stretch alters both the primary and secondary response

25. Golgi tendon organs have all the following features EXCEPT:
A. They respond primarily to changes in muscle length
B. They are located near muscle insertion into tendons
C. They are innervated by fast fibers
D. Their outputs are conveyed in the spinal cord.

26. Muscle mass increases with strenuous physical activity due to
A. An increase in blood supply
B. An increase in number of neuromuscular junction
C. Hypertrophy of individual fibers
D. An increase testosterone rcccptors

27. The chief cause of rigor mortis is
A. Decline in ATP production
B. Decrease in muscle Ca^{2+}
C. Release of lysosomal enzymes
D. Death of neuromuscular junctions

28. Calmodulin is most similar structurally and functionally, to which of the following skeletal muscles protein?
A. Actin
B. Myosin
C. Tropomyosin
D. Troposin C

29. Hematopoiesis is most active in the normal adult in:
A. Liver
B. Spleen
C. Thymus
D. Bone narrow

30. Erythropoietin has all of the following features except:
A. Production increases in hypovolemic states
B. Production increases in polycythemia
C. Produced in kidneys
D. Production increases in hypoxic states
E. Production increases in high altitudes

31. Pernicious anemia has all of the following features except:
A. Due to lack of gastric intrinsic factor
B. Ameliorated by vitamin C
C. Associated with folic acid deficiency
D. Associated with vitamin B_{12} deficiency
E. Seen in patients with sprue

32. All of the following are true concerning erythroblastosis fetails except:
A. Leads to hepatomegaly and splenomegaly
B. Common in Rh positive fetuses carried by Rh positive mothers
C. Due to fetal destruction of RBCs
D. Leads to fetal jaundice

33. Which protein is abnormal in patients with hereditary spherocytosis ?
A. Tubulin
B. Fibronectin
C. Collagen
D. Spectrin

34. If pressure is increased in the carotid sinus, all of the following can occur except:
A. A decrease in aortic pressure
B. Atrial tachycardia
C. Reflex bradycardia
D. Vasodilation of arterioles

35. Parasympathetic nervous system stimulation has which effect on the heart?
A. Slowing of the heart
B. Increased activity of the SA node

C. Increased activity of the AV node
D. All of the above.

36. Normal stroke volume of an average adult is close to:
A. 0 ml
B. 50 mL
C. 80 mL
D. 100 mL

37. A major factor that controls the force of heart contraction is
A. The initial length (preload) of cardiac muscle fibers
B. The degree of depolarization of the SA node
C. The number of gap junction between cardiac muscle fibers
D. The length of the bundle of His

38. The sympathetic receptors found in myocardium are of the type of :
A. α_1-adrenergic
B. β_1-adrenergic
C. β_2-adrenergic
D. Gamma amino butyric acid (GABA)

39. What happens on administration of a cholinergic blocking agent:
A. Decreased heart rate
B. No change in heart rate
C. Increased heart rate
D. None of the above.

40. Administration of a β-adrenergic blocking drug causes:
A. Reduce heart rate
B. Reduce cardiac contractility
C. Reduce cardiac output
D. All of the above.

41. An alpha -adrenergic agonist causes:
A. Increase peripheral resistance
B. Decrease peripheral resistance
C. Decrease arterial blood pressure
D. Cause a reflex increase in heart rate

42. Which of the following can excite both the alpha- and β – adrenergic receptors equally?

A. Epinephrine
B. Acetylcholine
C. Gamma aminobutyric acid
D. Norepinephrine
E. Atropine

43. Muscle most important for inspiration is

A. External intercostals
B. Diaphragm
C. Internal intercostals
D. Sternocleidomastoid

44. Most likely cause of death of a person in a fire but not as a result of thermal injury is :

A. Chronic hypoxia
B. Acute hypoxia
C. Fulminate hypoxia
D. Ischemic hypoxia

45. In myocardial infarction, damage to the heart muscle occurs due to:

A. Hyperventilation
B. Chronic hypoxia
C. Ischemic hypoxia
D. Hypoventilation

46. Diffusion of O_2 from alveoli to plasma occurs primarily due to

A. Differences in hemoglobin CO_2 affinity
B. Difference in hemoglobin O_2 affinity
C. Difference in PO_2
D. Difference in PCO_2

47. The enzymes which cause the breakdown of foodstuffs in the lumen of the small intestine

A. Require a strongly acidic environment to function
B. Are all secreted by mucosal glands of the stomach
C. Degrade large molecules by hydrolysing them
D. Are synthesized in response to vagal stimuli

48. Carbonic anhydrase
A. Is secreted by cells in the lining of the esophagus
B. Forms carbonic acid, thus acidifying the contents of the intestine
C. Is responsible for activating salivary amylase
D. Generates H^+ in pancreatic duct cells and gastric parietal cells

49. Most common site of Peptic ulcers is:
A. Esophagus
B. Ileum
C. Duodenum
D. Jejunum

50. All of the following are true concerning renin except:
A. It cleaves angiotensinogen to angiotensin I
B. When blood pressure falls, its secretion is stimulated
C. It is secreted by the macula densa
D. It has indirect effects on aldosterone secretion

51. The GFR for normal 70 kg male is
A. 75 ml/min
B. 125 ml/min
C. 200 ml/min
D. 250 ml/min

52. Plasma is what percentage of the total extracellular fluid mass of the normal human body?
A. 5%
B. 15%
C. 20%
D. 25%

53. The most abundant cation of plasma is
A. Na^+
B. K^+
C. Ca^{2+}
D. Mg^{2+}

54. Respiratory acidosis in chronic respiratory disease is primarily due to:
A. Decrease in HCO_3 concentration in plasma
B. Failure of the lungs to transport O_2

C. Failure of the lungs to excrete CO_2
D. Failure of the lungs to retain H_2O

55. Most important buffer system for maintaining plasma pH is:
A. Phosphate buffer
B. Protein buffer
C. Ammonium buffer
D. Bicarbonate buffer

56. One of the most common causes of proteinuria in diabetes mellitus is
A. Thickening of the glomerular basement membrane
B. Increased ADH secretion
C. Increased insulin secretion
D. Hypoglycemia

57. Ketoacidosis in diabetes mellitus is a consequence of
A. Accelerated fat breakdown
B. Hyperglycemia
C. Renal failure
D. Decreased insulin and increased glucagons

58. A woman having profuse sweating, increased HR, tremors, irritability, elevated BMR, and exophthalmos is having:
A. Hashimoto's thyroiditis
B. Graves' disease
C. Iodine deficiency
D. Cretinism

59. The pathophysiology of Grave's disease is :
A. Activation of adenylate cyclase
B. Hyposecretion of T_3
C. Hyposecretion of T_4
D. Precipitation of TSH

60. The decreased serum Ca^{2+} is most likely due to a decline secretion of?
A. TSH
B. Calcitonin
C. Parathyroid
D. ACTH

61. Which disease is most likely related to malfunction of the insulin receptor?
A. Insulinoma
B. Type II diabetes (NIDDM)
C. Zollinger-Ellison syndrome
D. Atherosclerosis

62. All of the following are physiologic effects of decreased glucocorticoid secretion except:
A. Muscle weakness
B. Increased gluconeogenesis
C. Hypoglycemia
D. Decreased fat mobilization

63. The most accurate statement regarding oxytocin is
A. Inhibits cervical dilation
B. Stimulates uterine smooth muscle contraction
C. Secreted by the adenohypophysis
D. Decreases uterine irritability

64. Following changes occur in the fetal circulatory pattern immediately associated with birth except
A. Closure of the ductus arteriosus
B. Decrease in blood flow through the ductus venosus
C. Increase in blood pressure in the right atrium
D. Increase in blood pressure in the left atrium

65. The most abundant nonaqueous constituent of human breast milk is
A. Lipid
B. Lactose
C. Sucrose
D. Lactalbumin

66. The cells most affected in scurvy are
A. Eosinophils
B. Fibroblasts
C. Liver parenchymal cells
D. Plasma cells

67. The most appropriate cause of fetal hepatosplenomegaly in erythroblastosis fetalis is

A. Due to destruction and production of fetal red blood cells
B. Maternal IgGs cause stimulation of Kupffer cells
C. Show hypertrophy to substitute for compromised placental function
D. To facilitate removal of hemoglobin degradation protects

68. The second heart sound is produced by the near-simultaneous closure of which two valves?

A. Aortic and pulmonary valves
B. Tricuspid and mitral valves
C. Aortic and mitral valves
D. Pulmonary and mitral valves

69. Vagus nerves supplies preganglionic parasympathetic innervation to the large intestine as far distally as the region

A. Near the border between the cecum and ascending colon
B. Near the border between the descending colon and sigmoid colon
C. Near the splenic flexure
D. Near the border between the sigmoid colon and rectum

70. The jaw jerk tests motor fibers of the

A. Mandibular division of the trigeminal nerve
B. Facial nerve
C. Glossopharyngeal nerve
D. Hypoglossal nerve

71. Parkinson's disease is related to dysfunction in the production or release of the neurotransmitter

A. Acetylcholine
B. Adrenaline
C. Dopamine
D. Serotonin

72. Contraction of a muscle occurs because of the action of:

A. Calcium on tropomyosin
B. Magnesium on actin
C. Sodium on actin
D. Sodium on tropomyosin

73. The negative membrane potential is due to:
A. Anions
B. Both a+b
C. Cations
D. Sodium only

74. The time for which human body can store oxygen is:
A. 4–10 minutes
B. 15–20 minutes
C. 25 minutes
D. 30 minutes

75. The enzyme Pepsinogen- I is secreted from:
A. Parietal cells
B. Chief cells
C. G-cells
D. Mucous cells

76. Epinephrine helps in causing :
A. Glycogenolysis
B. Gluconeogenesis
C. Renal tubular acidosis
D. Respiratory alkalosis

77. Autoregulation of blood flow is not a property of:
A. Brain
B. Skin
C. Kidney
D. Muscles

78. Which is the most potent stimulator of haemopoiesis among the following:
A. Tissue hypoxia
B. Infection
C. Malignancy
D. Trauma

79. Which of the haemoglobin appears first in fetus:
A. HbA
B. HbA_2

C. HbF
D. Hb-Gowers

80. An index of GFR can be assessed by:
A. Creatinine clearance
B. Blood urea
C. Sodium clearance
D. PAH clearance

81. Minimum conc. of Meth - Hb required in the blood to produce cyanosis is:
A. 1.5 gm%
B. 1.8 gm%
C. 2.0 gm%
D. 3.5 gm%

82. The minimum amount of reduced hemoglobin in blood for cyanosis to be manifested clinically should be:
A. 3 gm%
B. 5 gm%
C. 8 gm%
D. 10 gm%

83. Widest cross-section area is of which vessel:
A. Arteriole
B. Artery
C. Capillary
D. Vein

84. After absorption, the form of iron in blood is:
A. Apoferritin
B. Ceruloplasmin
C. Ferritin
D. Transferrin

85. The hormone level found decreased in hypoglycemia is of:
A. Epinephrine
B. Growth hormone
C. Steroid
D. Thyroxine

86. Permeability of which of the following ions increases during action potential:

A. HCO_3^-
B. K^+
C. Na^+
D. Cl^-

87. Satiety center is found to be located is:

A. Dorso-median nucleus of hypothalamus
B. Lateral hypothalamus
C. Perifornical region
D. Ventromedian nucleus hypothalamus

88. Pulmonary wedge pressure shows the:

A. Right atrial pressure
B. Right ventricular pressure
C. Left atrial pressure
D. Left ventricular pressure

89. The function of Angiotensin II is to:

A. ↑ Na^+ excretion
B. Aldosterone antagonist
C. Facilitates noradrenaline release
D. Relaxes myogenic control of arterioles

90. CO_2 transport in blood is facilitated mainly by:

A. High solubility of CO_2 in water
B. Presence of carbonic anhydrase in RBC
C. Combinations with hemoglobin
D. Binding with plasma proteins

91. Auditory impulses get relayed to this part of the brain:

A. Inf. geniculate
B. Medial geniculate body
C. Medial leminiscus
D. Sup. colliculus

92. The largest fraction of CO_2 (Carbon Dioxide) gas in blood is present as:

A. Bicarbonate
B. Dissolved

C. In the RBC
D. With CO_2 as carbaminio Hb

93. Blood-brain barrier is not present in this area of the brain:
A. Area posterma
B. Cerebral cortex
C. Corpus callosum
D. Corpus striatum

94. Fetal RBCs differ from adult RBCs by all of the following except:
A. Fetal RBCs are bigger in size
B. Fetal RBCs have shorter life span
C. Less of carbonic anhydrase
D. More 2,3-DPG is present in fetal RBCs

95. Variation in Pulse pressure is seen as the blood flows to the extremities due to:
A. Change in velocity
B. Change in vessel wall
C. Change in viscosity
D. Cross sectional area

Answer Key to MCQs in Physiology

1	D	2	A	3	B	4	A
5	B	6	B	7	D	8	A
9	D	10	A	11	D	12	D
13	A	14	E	15	B	16	B
17	D	18	C	19	D	20	D
21	B	22	A	23	C	24	D
25	A	26	C	27	A	28	D
29	D	30	B	31	B	32	B
33	D	34	B	35	A	36	C
37	A	38	B	39	C	40	D
41	A	42	A	43	B	44	C
45	C	46	C	47	C	48	D
49	C	50	C	51	B	52	D
53	A	54	C	55	D	56	A
57	B	58	B	59	A	60	C
61	B	62	B	63	B	64	C
65	B	66	B	67	A	68	A
69	C	70	A	71	C	72	A
73	C	74	D	75	B	76	A
77	D	78	A	79	D	80	A
81	A	82	B	83	C	84	D
85	D	86	C	87	B	88	C
89	C	90	B	91	B	92	A
93	A	94	D	95	B		

6

Biochemistry

1. HENDERSEN–HASSELBACH EQUATION = pH = pka + log $(A^-) / (HA)$
2. MICHALIS–MENTEN THEORY = $v = v_{max}\ (S) / k_m + (S)$
3. **Ketone bodies** are = acetone, aceto acetic acid, beta-hydroxy butyric acid.
4. **Essential fatty acids** = linoleic acid, linolenic acid, and arachidonic acid (ALL)
5. Holoenzyme = apoenzyme + coenzyme
6. Apoenzyme = protein part
7. Coenzyme = non-protein part
8. Prosthetic group = coenzyme which is covalently bound.
9. **Nucleotide** = base + sugar + phosphate group, i.e. nucleoside + phosphate group (BSP)
10. **Nucleoside** = base + sugar
11. Inductive enzyme = which can be detected in presence of specific substrate only.
12. **Plasma** = **B**lood minus the **F**ormed elements (PBF)
13. **Serum** = **P**lasma minus **F**ibrinogen (SPF)
14. **Serum** = blood minus the formed elements minus fibrinogen
15. G – 6 Pase = is absent in muscles but present in liver
16. Glucagon = increases glycogenolysis in liver; anti-insulin effect.
17. Epinephrine = increases glycogenolysis in muscles

18. CAMP = ka **second messenger**
19. 6 substances formed *from tyrosine* are = DOPA, dopamine, nor – epinephrine, epinephrine, melanin, thyroxin, (DDT MEN).
20. Leucine = is **only ketogenic**
21. Glycine = is **simplest amino acid**, has no optical activity, no asymmetric C – atom.
22. **Lipotropic substances** = methionine, choline, lecithin (MLC)
23. Diet rich in **tryptophan** offsets the deficiency of = NIACIN
24. **Avidin** causes deficiency of = BIOTIN
25. Blood glucose can be decreased **in diabetes mellitus** by removal of the = anterior pituitary
26. **Vitamin K** is required for = production of 2, 7, 9, 10 clotting factors.
27. Daily caloric intake is = 3000 cals.
28. Proportion of protein : fat : carbohydrate in daily requirement = 1 : 1 : 4
29. **Non –sense codons** / stop codons are = UAA, UAG, UGA
30. **Calories generated** form carbohydrate, fats and proteins is 4 k.cal/ gm; 9 k cal/ gm ; and 4 k cal / gm respectively.
31. DNA contains A, T, G, C. A is double bonded with T (with U in RNA), and G is triple bonded with C (A = T, G / C).
32. **Purines** are =adenine, guanine
33. **Pyrimidines** are = cytosine, thymine, uracil
34. Fish = is the highest source of proteins. To maintain good health, fish should be eaten 2 – 3 times / week.
35. Body has 187 joints.
36. At rest, heart pumps out 5 litres / min blood.
37. Glucose = 60–90 mg% fasting; 100–140 mg% after carbohydrate intake.
38. CPK /LDH / SGOT = increased in MI (Myocardial infarction).
39. SGPT/ SGOT = increased in *liver damage;* but SGPT increases more.

40. Specific gravity of blood = 1.060
41. pH of blood and CSF = 7.4
42. CSF has no bilirubin.

SITES OF OCCURRENCES

Citric acid cycle (TCA)	Mitochondria
De novo fatty acid synthesis	Cytoplasm
Electron transport system (ETS)	Mitochondria
Fatty acid oxidation	Mitochondria
Glycolysis (EMP)	In cytoplasm
Glycoprotein synthesis	Golgi body
HMP	Cytoplasm
Hydrolytic enzymes	Lysosomes
mRNA synthesis	From DNA
Oxidative phosphorylation	Mitochondria
rRNA synthesis	Nucleolus
tRNA	In cytoplasm

In cytoplasm = FA synthesis, glycolysis, HMP In mitochondria = TCA, ETS, FA oxidation, oxidative phosphorylation

TRANSFER AGENTS

ALBUMIN carries	Bilirubin, calcium, steroids, free fatty acids
Ceruloplasmin	Copper ions, Cu^{++}
Transferrin	Ferrous ions, Fe^{++}
Alpha – globulins	Thyroxin
Hemopexin	Heme
Hepatoglobulin	Hemoglobin, to prevent its urinary loss
Hemoglobulin	Oxygen, O_2

FUNCTIONS

Thiamine	In decarboxylation reactions
Riboflavin	For transfer of electrons and H^+ ions, i.e. in **redox reactions**
Niacin	In **dehydrogenase** and redox reactions
Pyridoxin	In **amine transfer** reactions/transamination
Biotin	In carbonate / CO_2 carrier reactions
Folic aid	In one – carbon transfer reactions

BONDS in

- Proteins = peptide bonds
- Carbohydrates = glycosidic bonds
- Nucleoproteins = phosphodiester bonds
- DNA – helices = hydrogen bonds

Buffer = a buffer solution is one which resists a change in pH when an acid or base is added to it . It is made up of a mixture of a weak acid and its conjugate base, i.e. salt of that weak acid.

Boyle's law = at a constant temperature, the volume of a given weight of a gas varies inversely as the pressure, i.e. PV = constant

Charles law = at constant pressure, the volume of a given weight of a gas is directly proportional to its absolute kelvin temperature. V/T = constant

Dalton's law of partial pressure = in a mixture of 2 or more gases, the total pressure exerted by mixture is the sum of individual partial pressures P = P1 + P2 + P3 + ————

Osmosis = when 2 solutions of different particle concentration are separated by a semipermeable membrane, a flow of solvent particle occurs from one side of lower particle concentration to the higher conc. till the conc. of solute is equalised.

Vulcanisation = heating the rubber in p.o of sulfur.

Emulsion = dispersion of oil droplets in water or vice versa.

Gibb's principle = i.e. substances which decrease the surface tension tend to concentrate in cell membrane, e.g. phospholipids, soaps cholesterols, etc. are found in higher conc. in cell membrane than the cytoplasm. There exist a potential difference b/w external and internal surfaces of cell membrane which persists as long as the cellular oxidation is occurring; it disappears under anaerobic conditions.

Donnan membrane equilibrium = concentration of diffusible +ve ions is greater on the side of SPM where there is a non-diffusible negative ion; conversely the conc. of the diffusible negative ions will be greater on the side of the membrane which does not contain the non-diffusible negative ions.

D-glucose/ dextrose = biologically it is the most imp sugar; is the **carbohydrate currency** of the body; all the carbohydrates are digested to form glucose before they can be absorbed in blood.

D-fructose = is levorotatory; found in fruit juice/ honey; inulin; cane sugar

D-galactose = in lactose/ milk sugar

D-mannose = in some plant products

Chair form is more stable than the boat form.

Disaccharides = formed of 2 monosaccharide units; by glycosidic linkage, i.e. linkage b/w the first C of one monosac with 2nd or 4th C of another monosac.

Maltose = glucose + glucose; formed during the digestion of starch.

Lactose = glucose + galactose; in milk; hydrolysed by enz lactase.

Sucrose = glucose + fructose; non-reducing sugar; does not form osazones; hydrolysed by enz sucrase; aka **invert sugar.**

Inversion = i.e. phenomenon by which D-sucrose is converted to L-mixture of glucose and fructose; enz sucrase is aka invertase.

Polysaccharides = forms colloidal solutions when heated with water.

Homopolysaccharides = i.e. formed of several units of one monosaccharide only, e.g. starch; glycogen; cellulose; dextrans.

Heteropolysaccharides = i.e. when it contains more than one monosac, e.g. pectin; mucopolysaccharides.

Starch	Made of glucose units;, e.g. amylose; amylopectin; it is hydrolysed by enz amylase
Glycogen	Aka **animal starch;** as it is the main polysac occurring in animal tissues esp liver and ms; Made of glucose units
Cellulose	**Most abundant carbohydrate** in nature; only Made of **glucose units;** hydrolysed by enz cellulase but it is found in **bacteria only**, so cellulose is not used by man and adds to the bulk of feces.
Dextrans	Produced by yeast and bacteria; polymers of glucose; not metabolised by tissues and are thus useful when *given I/V* in retaining water in circulation for long periods, i.e. as **plasma substitutes;** present in plaque also
Inulin	Made of D-fructose; used to **assess GFR** for kidney functions
Agar	Made of sulfated galactose units; used as **culture medium** for bacteria and as treatment of constipation; not used by man and adds to the bulk of feces.

Proteoglycans, i.e. mucoproteins; and GAG, i.e. mucopolysaccharides = proteoglycans are polysaccharides combined with small amounts of proteins, i.e. 95% carbohydrates and 5% proteins. It forms the ground substance of connective tissues. Carbohydrate moieties are aka GAG (glycos amino glycans).

E.g. hyaluronic acid = found in skin; CT; cartilage

Chondroitin sulfate = in cartilage; bone; skin

Heparin = in mast cells of lungs; liver; skin; blood group substances.

LIPIDS

- Fatty acids = have even no. of **C** atoms.
- **Saturated** fatty acids = simplest is the acetic acid; formula is $CH_3\ (CH_2)_n$ COOH; e.g. palmitic acid has 16 C and stearic acid has 18 C atoms.

- **Unsaturated fatty** acid = contains one or more double bonds; e.g. linoleic acid (has C18 – 2, i.e. 18–C atoms and 2 double bonds); linolenic acid (C18–3); arachidonic acid (C 20–4).
- Linoleic and linolenic acids are present in plant sources. Arachidonic acid is *in mammalian tissue only* and is synthesised from linoleic acid. Prostaglandins are synthesised from arachidonic acid. So LA → AA → PG.

Prostaglandins

1. Are derived from PUFA (Poly unsaturated fatty acids).
2. Facilitate the fertilisation of ovum.
3. Exert the stimulant action on smooth ms; smooth ms contraction.
4. Vasopressors; decrease the BP.
5. Functions as regulators of metabolism.
6. Derived from the AA by enz PG synthetase.
7. Ring structure joined at C_8- C_{12} = ka *prostanoic acid.*
8. Required for hormonal stimulation of **enz adenylate cyclase.** But also inhibit the adenylate cyclase of intestinal cells and diminish gastric HCl secretion, e.g. PGE_2 analogues are used for treatment of peptic ulcers.
9. PGE_2 and PGE_2 alpha = for inducing the abortion.
10. Enz phospholipase act on phospholipids → PUFA → PGs in p.o. enz PG synthetase.
11. PGI_2 aka **prostacycline** and TXA_2 / thromboxane are formed by enz prostacycline synthetase and Tx synthetase, with PGH_2 as the common precursor.
12. Leucotrienes are formed in WBCs and are constrictors of bronchial ms.

Rancidity = partial hydrolysis of fat and some oxidation of UFA at double bond; in p.o. moisture and temperature in p.o **enz lipase**.

Saponification No. = no. of mgs of KOH required to saponify the free and combined fatty acids in 1 gm of a given fat. High No. means fat is made of low m.wt fatty acids.

Iodine no. = no. of gm of I_2 required to saturate 100 gm of a given fat. High I_2 no. means high degree of unsaturation in fats.

Acid no. = no. of mgs of KOH required to neutralise the free fatty acids in a gm of fat. It indicates the degree of rancidity of the given fat.

Reichert–Meissel no. = no. of ml. Of 0.1 N alkali required to neutralise volatile fatty acids in 5 gm of fat.

Lecithin

1. Hydrolysed by enz lecithinase; contains **choline.**
2. Rich in liver.
3. Choline prevents accumulation of abnormal amount of fat in liver, i.e. **lipotropic action.**
4. Also a constituent of **acetylcholine**, i.e. transmission of nerve impulses.
5. Aids in emulsification of lipid–water mixtures which is a prerequisite in digestion and absorption of lipids from GIT.

Sphingomyelins = are present in large amounts **in brain and nervous tissues.** In Neimann-Pick's disease, large amounts of sphingomyelins are accumulated in spleen and liver besides brain.

Glycolipids; glycosphingosides and cerebrosides are = present in large amounts **in white matter of brain** and in **myelin sheaths.**

In **Gaucher's dis** = they accumulate in large amounts **in liver and spleen.**

Gangliosides

1. In gray matter of brain;
2. Has N–acetyl neuraminic acid NANA for blood group specificity; for tissue organ specificity; for tissue immunity.
3. Abundant in nerve endings.
4. Accumulate in brain in Tay-Sach's disease; due to lack of enz for its degradation.

Cholesterol = insulating mechanism for nerve impulses; 150 – 250 mg % in blood.

Ergosterol = calciferol is precursor for Vit D_2; and 7- dehydro-cholesterol is precursor to vit D_3.

PROTEINS

- Mimp cell constituents.
- Mammalian ms have 20% proteins; blood plasma has 7%.
- N_2 content of proteins is fairly constant and forms approx 16% of the m.wt of proteins.
- Amino acids = all naturally occurring AA are L – configuration **except GLYCINE.** They form the proteins in different sequences; are 20 in no.
- **Sulfur containing** A As are = cysteine, methionine
- **Glycine** = has no asymmetric C-atom, so it is not optically active.
- Proteins have no free amino groups.
- Histidine = has an imidazole ring also.
- Lysine and hydroxylysine = occur in **collagen**
- **Zwitter ions** = A A s are **amphoteric electrolytes** and give anions and cations ka zwitter ions.
- **Isoelectric pH** of A A s = i.e. pH at which equal no. of cations and anions are formed and does not show any migration when subjected to an electric field. Above the isoelectric pH, more no. of negative ions, which migrate towards the anode are produced and vice versa.
- A A s, e.g. tryptophan, tyrosine; and phenylalanine absorb the UV rays at 260 – 290 mu.
- **Alpha – helix** = N- H group of one AA comes into close proximity of C= O group of 4th AA in the chain and a H – bond is formed b/w C = O and N –H; each turn of helix contains 3.6 AA residues and is 5.4 Å long and 6 Å in diameter.
- **Simple proteins** = on hydrolysis they yield only A A s.
- **Conjugated proteins** = proteins are combined with a non – protein group ka the **prosthetic group.**
- **Derived proteins** = are products of denaturation or of partial digestion of proteins.

NUCLEIC ACIDS AND NUCLEOPROTEINS

- NP are conjugated proteins having NA as their prosthetic group.
- DNA = mainly present in nuclei.
- RNA = mainly present in cytoplasm and nucleolus.
- Ribosomes are richest in RNA; next comes the mitochondria.
- **Nucleotide** = base + sugar + phosphoric acid (BSP)
- **Nucleoside** = base + sugar only.
- Base = purines, i.e. adenine, guanine and pyrimidines, i.e. cytosine, thymine and uracil.
- Sugar = in RNA is D – ribose; in DNA is D_2 – deoxyribose.
- Thymine is replaced by uracil in RNA.
- Base combines with sugar by C – N linkage.
- Polynucleotides formed by union of several nucleotides thro a diester with phosphate at 3' – 5' position (Phospho-diester bond); it can be cleared by enz phosphodiesterse,

DNA

1. A with T by a double H – bond ; and G with C by a triple H – bond.
2. 2 right handed **antiparallel** helices.
3. planes of adjacent pairs are 3.4 Å apart.
4. **Pitch of helix** = each turn of helix has a length of 34 Å and has 10 base pairs.
5. Chromatin is made of HISTONES.

RNA = is of 3 types, i.e. M RNA; r RNA and t RNA/s RNA (soluble RNA). The phosphodiester bond is at 3'–5' location. A with U and G with C pairing occurs.

Melting = DNA gets denatured on heating and so the separation of the 2 strands occurs.

Annealing = if heat denatured DNA is *slowly cooled* the denaturation is reversible, the helical structure is reformed and the 2 strands get together.

Quenching = *rapid cooling* of denatured DNA fixes it in a permanently denatured state.

Blood = 6 – 8% of total body mass in adults

Volume = 80 ml / kg body wt in males; 65 ml/ kg body wt in females

Blood cells = 40–45% by volume

Plasma = 50–60% by volume

Specific gravity = 1.060

PH = 7.4

RBCs (Refer Physiology also)

- are biconcave discs, 6–9 microns in diameter; thickness is 1 microns in the centre and 2 microns at the periphery (Dumb-bell shape).
- Contain Hb 31–33 %
- It has 3 proteins = i.e. spectrin; actin; ankrin
- Glycophosin in the cell wall = responsible for ABO blood grouping.
- RBC cell membrane **contains mainly K^+ ions;** only traces of Na ions.
- In plasma = contains mainly Na^+ ions; only traces of K^+ ions.
- Also Mg^{2+} is in cells, while plasma contains Ca^+ ions.

Granular WBCs

1. Polymorphs = contain *alk. Pase;* it is absent in CML (ch. myeloid leukemia).
2. Eosinophils = contain histamine, plasminogens; increase in allergies.
3. Basophils = contain pepsin, histamine, tryptamine. It is aka *mast cells.*
4. Lymphocytes = produced by thymus glands; produce the Igs.
5. B – cells = produce Igs/circulating Abs.
6. T – cells = for cellular immunity; are antigraft; antitumor, etc.
7. Monocytes = originate in bone marrow and spleeen; function as *macrophages;* take up Ags.
8. Platelets = SMALLEST formed element in blood; no nuclei; rich in serotonin which increases the vascular permeability on release; life is 7 – 14 days.

- **0.9 % NaCl** solution is isotonic to RBCs.

Haemoglobin (Refer to physiology also)

- heme containing proteins are characteristic of aerobic organisms; and absent in anaerobes.
- is an iron – porphyrin compound; a tetra pyrrole structure.
- ferrous iron; iron in heme has 6 valancies.
- is heme + globin.
- has 0.34% iron.
- 4 units each containing one heme forms one molecule of Hb with M.wt. 65,000.
- In human Hb, there are 2 alpha and 2 beta chains.
- Alpha chain = **valine** at N – terminal and **arginine** at C – terminal end.
- Beta chain = **valine** at N – terminal end and **histidine** at C– terminal.
- Heme pocket is hydrophobic.
- In normal adult = 90 – 95% Hb is HbA = is 2 alpha and 2 beta chains.
- 2 – 3% HbA_2 = 2 alpha and 2 delta chains.
- **Fetal Hb** = HbF = 2 alpha and 2 gamma chains ; resistant to denaturation by alkali.
- At birth = HbA is 85% and HbF is 15 %.
- **Sickle cell Hb** = 6th amino acid of beta chain is **valine** instead of **glutamic acid.**
- In sickle cell anemia = only HbS.
- In sickle cell trait = HbS + HbA; RBCs are more resistant to malaria than normal.
- HbM, **methemoglobinemia** = i.e. Fe^{++} gets converted to Fe^{+3}. It is due to replacement of histidine or valine by tyrosine or glutamic acid; it **cannot transport the O_2.**
- **Thalassemia** = rate of synthesis of one chain is low and other chain is in excess.
- Thalassemia – alpha = i.e. alpha chain is not synthesised adequately.
- Thalassemia – beta = i.e. beta chain is not synthesised adequately.

- **Hydrops fetalis** = alpha chain is not synthesised at all.
- Hb A 1C = is glycosylated form of HbA1; is an **index of the level of blood glucose;** it gets **increased in diabetics** to 6–15% (normal is 3–5 %).
- Oxy – Hb = oxygenation of Hb occurs. Hb + $O_2 \leftrightarrow HbO_2$. At PO_2 = 100 mm . Hg, the Hb is 95 – 96 % saturated with oxygen in the lungs.
- If arterial blood – PO_2 = 90 mm.Hg; Hb is 90% saturated and carries 19.6 ml of O_2 / 100 ml of blood.
- In tissues = PO_2 is 10%; the PO_2 in venous blood is 40%; so Hb is 75% saturated; carries 12.6 ml O_2 and so 7 ml O_2 is given to the tissues.
- CO has 200 times affinity for Hb as O_2 and forms carboxy – Hb.
- CO_2 combines with Hb to form carbamino – Hb.
- H_2S combines with Hb to form sulf – Hb; is **not a reversible reaction** and so no longer useful for O_2 transport.

Plasma

1. Proteins = 6.3 – 7.8 gm %
2. Albumin = 3.2 – 5 gm %
3. Globulins = 4 types – alpha 1,2; beta, gamma
4. Fibrinogen = 0.2 – 0.4 gm %

Albumin = low isoelectric pH; low m. wt., **migrates fastest in electrophoresis;** transport of FFA, bilirubin; Ca^{++}, steroids; drugs, e.g. sulfonamides, penicillin, aspirin bind to it.

Alpha – globulin = some act as inhibitor of coagulation and of enz like trypsin, chymotrypsin. **Ceruloplasmin** is Cu^{++} containing alpha–2 globulin; and helps conversion of Fe^{2+} to Fe^{3+}; transports Cu^{++};

Haptoglobulins = make complex with Hb and **prevent its urinary loss** when RBCs breakdown.

Beta – globulins = e.g. lipoproteins; e.g. transferrin is Fe – binding proteins; CRP get increased during acute infections; **hemopexin** binds with heme and prevents is excretion.

Gamma - globulins = i.e. Igs; **cellular immunity** is mediated by T – cells; humoral immunity is mediated by B – cells and Abs are formed. 5 classes of Igs, i.e. GAMDE based on H –chains; are the glycoproteins.

IgM = **first Ab formed** in response to an Ag; impermeable to placenta; mainly found in plasma;

IgG = next Ab formed; present **in largest amount in** plasma; rate of synthesis is highest; can **cross placental barrier** and provides immunity to the fetus.

IgA = gets concentrated *at the site of entry of Ag* in the body; main component of **colostrum milk;** provides protection to GIT of new born.

Active immunity = by exposure to Ag/ foreign cells, e.g. polio; typhoid; measles; small pox

Passive immunity = by injecting Abs; e.g. diphtheria; tetanus; is transient / short lived.

Complement system = they complement the functions of Abs in eliminating Ags; are C1 to C9; divided in 3 groups, i.e.

1. C1 complex = is the recognition unit;
2. C2, C3, C4 = activation unit;
3. C5 – C9 = membrane attack unit.

Haptens = small molecule which are poor Ags, when coupled with a carrier protein become potent Ags aka haptens.

Liver is the sole source of fibrinogen and albumin; most of the alpha and beta globulins.

Gamma globulins = Produced from the plasma cells and RE system.

Normal A/G ratio = 2 : 1 by salting – out method; and 1.3 : 1 by electrophoresis method.

In diseases = A/G ratio becomes reversed and/or albumin decreases and globulin increases esp gamma – globulin. E.g. in kidney dis; chronic infections; dis of liver, etc.

Plasma proteins = help to transport substances like bilirubin, steroids; FAs; metals, etc.

Plasminogen = activated to plasmin **by kallikrein** and causes **fibrinolysis**.

Clotting occurs by extrinsic / intrinsic pathways; the final pathway is activation of factor X to Xa is the end reaction. So formation of **factor Xa is the junction point** for the 2 pathways.

Clotting time = depends on all the clotting factors except factors 7, 13.

Inhibitors of clotting

1. Antithrombin III
2. Heparin = by activating antithrombin III.
3. Coumarin drugs = interfere with vit – K dependent conversion of glutamic acid to gamma – glutamyl carboxylate, so production of factors 2,5,7,9,10 is decreased.
4. Oral contraceptives = forms intravascular thrombotic phenomenon.

Anticoagulants = in vitro = are oxalate / citrate / EDTA, etc. remove the Ca^{++} ions by chelation and prevent the clotting.

Normal values of = in blood.

- Ca^{++} = 9 – 11 mg %
- Cholesterol = 150 – 250 mg
- Urea = 12 – 40 mg
- Glucose fasting = 60 – 90 mg

CSF

1. Proteins = 20 – 40 mg %
2. Volume = 100 –150 ml in adults
3. Per day secretion = 100 –150 ml
4. Main function = protection of brain and spinal cord.
5. **Formed by choroid plexus** = comes into lateral ventricles, then goes to 3rd and 4th ventricles and finally to subarachnoid space.
6. pH = 7.4; same as plasma

7. Proteins = **mainly albumin;** very little globulin and no fibrinogen
8. Glucose = 55 – 80 mg%

Lymph

1. Is drained in thoracic duct and right lymphatic duct to the subclavian Vs.
2. 1–2 litres/day is formed.
3. Protein content is less. It is highest in liver lymphatics and lowest in s/c lymphatics.
4. A/G ratio = much higher than in plasma.

ENZYMES

Conjugated proteins = some enzymes combine with nonprotein prosthetic group

Apoenzyme = protein part of enzyme

Coenzyme = non–protein part of the enzyme

Holoenzyme = conjugated active form of enzyme

Enzymes of glycolysis = in cytoplasm

Enzymes of citric acid cycle and of oxidative phosphorylation = in mitochondria.

Hydrolytic enzymes = in lysosomes

Extracellular enzyme = i.e. which get secreted out of the cell and function outside the cell of origin, e.g. digestive enzymes

Mechanism of action of enzyme = it acts by **lock and key mechanism.**

Michaelis – Menten theory = gave theory of enzyme – substrate complex formation; the ES complex is aka **Michaelis complex.**

Coenzyme = some enzymes are only active in p.o. certain organic substances which are ka coenzymes.

Apoenzymes = i.e. the enzymes which are inactive without the coenzymes are ka apoenzymes.

Table of coenz and enzymes

NAD; NADP; FMN; FAD	With dehydrogenase
Coenz A	With thiokinase
Thiamine pyrophosphate	With transketolase; oxidative decarboxylation of pyruvic acid
Pyridoxal phosphate	Transaminases; amino acid decarboxylases
Biotin	Beta – carboxylase
ATP	Hexokinase; triose kinase

Ionic activators required for some enzyme actions

1. Mg^{++} = for phosphorylation
2. Ca^{++} = for coagulation
3. Zn^{++} = for carbonic anhydrase action
4. Cu^{++} / Fe^{++} = for some oxidative reaction
5. Chelation = for electron transport reactions.

Zymogens / proenzymes = i.e. the enzymes produced by living cells in the *inactive form.* They are **activated by some specific ions** or by proteolytic enzymes. E.g. pepsinogen gets converted to pepsin by H^+ in the gastric juice. The trypsinogen is converted to trypsin by *enterokinase* in the pancreatic juice. Also chymotrypsinogen is converted to chymotrypsin.

Isoenzymes/isozymes = some enz. have **similar catalytic function** but obtained from different sources and exhibit different physical and chemical nature, e.g. LDH, creatinine kinase etc.

Turnover no. = no. of substrate molecules transformed per minute by a single enzyme molecule. **Carbonic anhydrase has highest** T.N.

Enzymes = lower the energy barrier of reacting molecules and start the reaction.

MICHALIS – MENTON THEORY = $v = v_{max}$ (S) / k_m + (S)

Michaelis constant = k_m = is the **concentration of substrate** at which the velocity of enzyme reaction is ½ the maximal possible and at which ½ the active sites of enzyme are occupied by the substrate.

Non–specific inhibition = irreversible.

Competitive inhibition = reversible; the inhibitor has **close structural resemblance** to the substrate and forms enzyme – inhibitor (EI) complex.

Uncompetitive inhibition = i.e. when inhibitor *combines with ES complex* instead of E and causes inhibition and ESI complex is formed. It is not reversible.

Allosteric enzymes = some effectors bind reversibly at specific sites other than the substrate binding sites ka allosteric sites. It may be –ve effector causing allosteric inhibition and + ve effector causing allosteric activation.

DIAGNOSTIC APPLICATION: levels of the enzymes in plasma are studied for it.

Enzyme	**Increases in**	**Decreases in**
Lipase	Acute pancreatitis; Ca. Pancreas	Liver disease; vit A deficiency; diabetes mellitus
Amylase	Acute pancreatitis; Inflammatory conditions of salivary glands	Liver diseases
Trypsin	Pancreatic disease	—
Cholinesterase	Nephrosis; poisoning by certain drugs	Liver dis; malnu-trition; anemia
Alkaline Pase	Rickets/ hyper-parathyroidism; obstructive jaundice	—
Acid Pase/ it originates from prostate gland	In prostatic carcinoma	
SGPT / SGOT	Liver damage (SGPT increases more). Myocardial infarction (SGOT increases more)	

Enzyme	Increases in	Decreases in
LDH	MI; acute leukemias; acute hepatitis; generalised carcinomatosis	
ICD, isocitrate dehydrogenase	Liver dis; increased in CSF in meningitis; cerebral tumors	
CPK; creatinine phosphokinase, it is present in skeletal ms, cardiac ms; brain	In MI	
Ceruloplasmin	Hepatic dis; pregnancy; infections	Wilson's dis, i.e. hepato-lenticular degeneration

Classification = 6 groups, i.e. OTHLIL

1. Oxidoreductase = for oxidation – reduction reaactions
2. Transferase = for transfer of a group except H^+.
3. Hydrolase = hydrolysis, e.g. pepsin / amylase / cholinesterase
4. Lyases = removal of groups and usually leave double bonds
5. Isomerase = conversion of other isomeric forms
6. Ligases / synthetases

Active transport system = i.e. when it occurs **against the concentration gradient.** ATP is required; it is unidirectional.

Passive transport = can occur in any direction.

Mediated / facilitated transport = i.e. when intermediate carriers mediate the transport.

A high **intracellular K^+ is required** for biosynthesis of proteins by ribosomes and for maintenance of membrane potential of excitable tissues; the transport is mediated by enz ka Na^+ - K^+ - ATPase.

For every molecule of ATP hydrolysed = 3 Na^+ ions are extruded and 2 K^+ ions are taken in. It is thus **a Na – Pump;** Mg^{++} ions are required for activity of enzyme.

Transport of glucose into cell is intimately linked with simultaneous transort of Na^+ ions in the cell.

Transport of Ca^{++} from sarcoplasm into sarcoplasmic reticulum is necessary **for relaxation of muscle.** It is done by ATPase system of membrane of SR and is coupled with breakdown of 1 ATP for 2 Ca^{++} transport.

High conc of Na^+ in external medium favours transport of glucose and amino acids; glutathione actively participates in transport.

VITAMINS

Fat soluble = A, D, E, K

Water soluble = B,C

Vitamin A

- Occurs only in animal tissues.
- Required for growth and **epithelial function.**
- Carotenoid pigment present in carrots/spinach/sweet potatoes, etc.
- Destroyed by oxidation and exposure to light.
- Carotenes are converted to vit A **by liver** in man.
- Stored in liver as esterified with fatty acids
- Retinal form required for visual function.
- Conversion of carotene to vit A does not occur efficiently in **diabetes mellitus and hypothyroidism.**
- Rods of retina contain a pigment ka **rhodopsin or visual purple,** concerned with vision in dim light.
- Deficiency causes **night blindness** / nyctalopia.
- Ca^{++} required for normal function of visual cycle
- Zn is required for normal plasma conc of vit A
- Cirrhosis of liver = decreased Zn conc in plasma
- In deficiency = impaired oxidative phosphorylation in liver mitochondria; skin keratinisation occurs; **xerophthalmia; Bitot's**

spots on conjunctiva; keratomalacia; decreased osteoblastic activity.

- It is ka **anti infective vitamin** = as its *ability to prevent infections.*

VITAMIN D: calciferol / vit D_2

- Anti–rachitic activity;
- Highest amount present in fish liver oils
- **Main function** = Ca / P metabolism and mineralisation of skeleton.
- Active form of vit is a dihydroxy derivative; liver adds – OH at C – 25 and kidney at C – 1, i.e. 1, 25-dihydroxy cholecalciferol.
- Addition of –OH by kidney is **regulated by serum Ca^{++} levels** = low levels increase the function / high levels inhibit the reaction, i.e. feedback inhibition.
- Vit D promotes absorption of Ca and P from intestines.
- Facilitates normal function of PTH and increases renal excretion of phosphate.
- Deficiency = *rickets* in infants and osteomalacia in adults.

Rickets

Soft bones; deformed bones, e.g. bow legs and knock knees.

Fontanelles do not close properly = HOT CROSS BUN APPEARANCE OF HEAD.

RICKETY ROSARY = ribs present a beaded appearance at costochondral junction.

Pigeon breast appearance of chest.

Osteomalacia

Rare b'coz skin can synthesise it from 7 – dehydrocholestrol in p.o UV rays.

Normal Ca^{++} levels = 9 – 11 mg %

Ca^{++} levels decrease in serum in this condition.

Urinary excretion of P is increased due to decreased tubular reabsorption

Increased serum alk. Pase occurs.

VITAMIN E = tocopherol

Vit is concerned **with normal childbirth.**

Is an **antioxidant;** found mainly in vegetable oils; also present in vegetable like spinach and lettuce; prevents formation of free radicals.

Its deficiency in rats/chicks causes **brownish discoloration** of adipose tissues and yellowish **discoloration of enamel** of teeth due to oxidation of unsaturated fatty acids.

Protective action in **preventing massive hepatic necrosis** produced on diets deficient in sulfur containing amino acids.

Helps in synthesis of coenz Q, i.e. **ubiquinone,** which is a component of electron transport system.

VITAMIN K = naphthoquinone

Absorbed with fats in p.o. bile salts

Not stored in body, so constant supply is required.

Can **cross placenta** and milk.

Required for formation of clotting factors in **liver, i.e. 7,9,10, prothrombin** (2, 7, 9, 10)

In deficiency = increased PT occurs

Role in clotting, phosphorylation reaction, electron transport system.

Synthesised by bacteria in GIT

Deficiency occurs by = antibiotics (kill the bacteria); obstructive jaundice (absence of bile salts).

Dicoumarol = vit K antagonist = acts by **competitive inhibition.**

WATER SOLUBLE VITAMINS (Refer section of oral-pathology also)

THIAMINE / B1

1. Aka **anti beri – beri** substance / aneurine
2. **TPP is active coenz form** of this vitamin.
3. TPP is required for oxidative decarboxylation reactions and transketolation.
4. Deficiency causes = beri beri; peripheral neuritis

5. **Pyrithiamine** = is its antagonist.

RIBOFLAVIN / B_2

1. FMN and FAD are the 2 coenzymes forms of this vitamin; used in various **H – transfer reactions.**
2. Destroyed on exposure to light.
3. Deficiency causes = **magenta colored tongue;** cheilitis. etc.;
4. *Antagonist* = is dichloro-riboflavin and iso-riboflavin.

NIACIN = aka P-P factor; **pellagra** preventing factor; **nicotinic acid;**

- NAD and NADP are its biologically active forms; act as coenz for **H – transfer** enz, i.e. dehydrogenases.
- It can be synthesised from TRYPTOPHAN.
- NAD is used with lactic acid dehydrogenase, etc.
- NADP is used with G-6-P dehydrogenase. etc.
- Either may be used with glutamic acid dehydrogenase.
- **Deficiency** = pellagra = i.e. 3 D's, i.e. dermatitis; dementia; diarrhoea; and then death occur.
- Niacin causes vasodilation with flushing and sensation of warmth in face / neck/arms; blood flow to skin increases and plasma lipid conc decreases; so it is **used to treat HYPERLIPEMIA.**

PYRIDOXINE: B6 / vit H / adermine

- Its active form is **pyridoxal phosphate.**
- Mainly concerned with metabolism with Amino acids.
- Acts as coenz in **transamination** reactions.
- Required for conversion of **tryptophan** to niacin.
- Required for interconversion of glycine and serine where it functions along with folic acid.
- Deficiency causes = **hypochromic microcytic anemia**; homocysteinuria and cystathioninuria due to impaired metabolism of methionine;
- Isoniazid, an antitubercular, causes its deficiency.
- Antagonist is = **deoxypyridoxine.**

PANTOTHENIC ACID

- Its richest source is honey.

- Acts as a component of coenz – A.
- **Acetyl CoA** is the form in which 2 – C fragment enters the citric acid cycle for oxidation.
- **Deficiency** = adrenal cortical function is depressed b'coz acetyl CoA is required for synthesis of steroid ring and adrenal cortical hormones.

BIOTIN: aka vit H/ **anti egg white** injury factor.

- Antivitamin in egg white = **avidine,** which deprives availability of the vitamin.
- Contains sulfur.
- Large amounts **synthesised by intestinal flora** including man.
- Lost during treatment with antibiotics and sulfonamides.
- It is a coenzyme involved in CO_2 transfer reactions / CO_2 fixation, e.g. acetyl CoA changes to malonyl CoA; pyruvic acid changes to oxaloacetate.
- Deficiency = **spectacled eye** appearance; dermatitis; GIT and CNS symptoms appear.

FOLIC ACID: aka vit M / SLR factor / folacin / B_{10} / B_{11}.

- Widespread presence in green leafy vegetables;
- **Tetrahydrofolic acid is active form** of this vitamin. PABA is an important constituent.
- Some antibiotics and sulfonamides block the incorporation of PABA in folic acid synthesis by competitive inhibition.
- Folic acid changes to THFA in p.o. folic acid reductase and NADPH as coenz and vit C.
- Role in **metabolism of one – C group moieties**.
- Transfer of hydroxymethyl / formyl/ methylene and methylidine groups is mediated by tetrahydrofolate.
- Transfer of carbonyl groups is mediated by BIOTIN.
- **Folate cycle** = involves vit B_{12} and folic acid.
- **Deficiency** = most affected function is **cell multiplication**, e.g. hemopoietic system; *macrocytic anemia;* leucopenia; **figlu** is excreted in urine in large amounts in the deficiency state.

- Folic acid is required during first trimester of frequency to prevent development of neural tube defects.
- **Antagonists** = inhibit cell division and multiplication and so used in treatment of leukemia, malignant growth etc., e.g. aminopterin, amethopterin, etc.
- Trimethoprim inhibits enzymic conversion of DHF to THF by G (–) bacteria and **inhibit the bacterial growth.**
- **Methotrexate** = inhibits the enz in bacteria and mammals.

VITAMIN B_{12} : aka *cobalamine* / anti-pernicious anemia factor/ extrinsic factor of Castle.

- Contains cobalt; concerned with **hemopoiesis;**
- Structure resembles heme = tetra pyrrole ring structure ka **corrin ring** system.
- Only found in liver/eggs/meat/fish/milk/kidneys; **not of vegetable origin**, i.e. its deficiency may occur in strict vegetarians.
- **Primary source of vit** is **microbial synthesis** in intestine.
- Absorbed in intestine only in p.o. **intrinsic factor.**
- Acts as coenz in several reaction, e.g. in conversion of methyl – malonyl CoA to succinyl CoA; homocysteine to methionine; ribonucleotide to deoxyribonucleotide.
- **Deficiency** = urine contains large amounts of methyl – malonic acid; macrocytic anemia = CNS lesions ka subacute combined degeneration;
- **Pernicious anemia** = deficiency of intrinsic factor leads to def of Vit B_{12}; associated with absence of HCl / *achylia* and enzymes in gastric juice.

VITAMIN – C : aka ascorbic acid; found in citrus fruits;

- Rat etc. can synthesise it thro uronic acid pathways;
- Intimately concerned with **metabolism of mesenchymal tissue,** bones, dentin and collagen.
- Maintains the **redox potential** of the cells.
- Formation of hydroxyproline from the proline in collagen synthesis.

- Helps in **absorption of iron** by converting Fe^{3+} to Fe^{2+}.
- *Adrenal cortex* shows high conc of vit C; stimulation of gland by ACTH causes rapid depletion of vitamin indicating that it is **required for normal function** of the **gland.**
- **Deficiency** = *scurvy;* main defect is a failure to deposit intercellular cement substance; delayed wound healing due to deficiency of collagen formation. Dentin and bone are poorly mineralised; on tourniquet test = several petechiae appear.

HCl = secreted by the *parietal cells;* activates pepsinogen to pepsin; facilitates absorption of Fe^{++}.

Fats = inhibits gastric secretion (also by enterogastrone secreted by duodenal mucosa)

Gastrins = secreted by pyloric mucosa; it stimulates HCl secretion.

Secretin and somatostatin inhibit the gastrin secretion.

Histamine = stimulates HCl secretion by *stimulating adenylate cyclase* and cAMP formation.

In pancreatic juice = **trypsinogen** and chymotrypsinogen enz, i.e. zymogens / inactive form which get activated by enz **enterokinase**. Pancreatic lipase / steapsin present are lipolytic.

Important Points

- For each pair of electron transferred or for every atom of O_2 used in respiratory chain = 3 ATPs are generated.
- ATP is formed by ADP in p.o. **adenylate kinase** enz.
- Creatine phosphate is main storage form of energy in muscles.
- Electron transport chain is aka = *respiratory chain* of reactions.
- An intact mitochondrial membrane is needed for effective oxidative phosphorylation.
- ATP – ADP carrier is inhibited by ATRACTYLOSIDE.
- Cyanides act by tightly combining with cytochrome oxidase enz and prevent final step in electron transport chain.
- Dinitrophenol/ionophores, etc. prevent formation of ATP by preventing formation of *proton gradient.*
- NAD^+ is used in reactions leading to substrate oxidation and ATP generation.

- $NADP^+$ is used in reactions where reducing power is to be used for synthetic reactions.
- **Coenz Q** aka **ubiquinone**, has structure similar to Vit K.
- **Cytochromes** = carry electrons only from coenz Q; are Fe – containing hemoproteins; present in all aerobic organisms; their content is **proportional to the respiratory activity** of tissues; heart ms contain the maximum and skin / lung have minimum amounts.

CARBOHYDRATE METABOLISM

1. All carbohydrates get converted in *glucose* = which is ka **carbohydrate currency of the body.**
2. Surplus glucose is converted to glycogen and **stored in liver,** e.g. glycogenesis.
3. About 40 % glucose is converted to fat = lipogenesis
4. G-6-Pase is absent in muscles but present in liver.
5. Glucose = 60 – 90 mg % in peripheral blood normally.
6. **Glycogenolysis** = i.e. glycogen to glucose, in liver in p.o. **enz G-6–pase**
7. In ms = glycogen changes to pyruvic / lactic acid; which goes to blood, to liver, gets converted to glucose to maintain blood glucose level.
8. **Cori's cycle** = i.e. cycle of liver glycogen through blood sugar to ms glycogen and back thro blood lactic acid to liver glycogen.
9. **Gluconeogenesis / glyconeogenesis** = i.e. synthesis of glucose / glycogen by liver from the substances which are **derived from non-carbohydrate sources**, e.g. amino acids, e.g. during prolonged starvation.
10. Glucose changes to CO_2 + H_2O + maximum energy available.
11. In ms, pyruvate / lactate + oxaloacetate → citric acid cycle → CO_2 + H_2O + energy.
12. Hepatocytes , RBCs and brain cells **do not require INSULIN** for entry of glucose into the cells, but ms and adipose tissues require the insulin.
13. Insulin suppresses glycogenolysis and gluconeogenesis in liver, i.e. blood glucose level to kept under control.

14. Some antidiabetic drugs act by increasing insulin production of a functioning pancreas by stimulating beta --cells, e.g. tolbutamide, chlorpropamide, etc.
15. Some drugs, e.g. phenformin, cause uncoupling of oxidative phosphorylation in tissues and enhances glycolysis and glucose uptake by the tissues (ANTI-DIABETICS).
16. **Adrenaline** = secreted in response to hypoglycemia; **antagonize the action of insulin**; stimulates the glycogenolysis in liver and ms by **activating enz phosphorylase (ANTI-INSULIN).**
17. **Glucagon** = stimulates liver glycogenolysis by activating **liver phosphorylase;** increases gluconeogenesis in liver; **no action on ms – phosphorylase (ANTI-INSULIN).**
18. **Glucocorticoids = increase gluconeogenesis in liver** by increasing protein breakdown in tissues; decrease glucose uptake by tissues; so **increase the blood sugar** level (ANTI-INSULIN).
19. **Anterior pituitary H** = e.g. GH /ACTH are **diabetogenic;** GH increases lipolysis.
20. **Thyroid H = enhances absorption of glucose** from GIT and increase glycogenolysis in liver; but also enhances metabolism of glucose.

GLUCONEOGENESIS

- Formation of glucose/glycogen from **non–carbohydrate sources**, e.g. aminoacids, fats, etc.
- not **In adipose tissues** = because enz **fructose 1,6–diphosphatase is absent** there.
- during starvation = **chief amino acid** transported from ms to liver is ALANINE.
- Reversal of glycolysis and citric acid cycle occurs.
- Also **enz G – 6 – Pase** is present in liver and kidney but **absent in ms**, so **ms cannot add glucose to bloodstream directly** (cori cycle)
- It is stimulated by adrenal cortical hormone and so excessive breakdown of proteins occurs. N_2 part is excreted in urine as urea = so **–ve N_2 balance.**

HMP SHUNT / PPP (Pentose-Phosphate pathway)

- Occurs in **cytoplasm**
- F – 6 – P is formed from G – 6 – P thro HMP; that is why it is aka shunt pathway.
- Glucose oxidation occurs here **without intervention of preliminary glycolysis.**
- Coenz used in oxidative reactions of this pathway is $NADP^+$.
- Here C 1 of glucose is oxidised first, whereas in glycolysis it is C3 and C4 which are oxidised first.
- **First step** involves **enz G-6-P dehydrogenase;** this enz is inhibited by sulphonamides and quinacrine.

GLYCOLYSIS / ANAEROBIC PATHWAY / EMBDEN – MEYERHOFF PATH (EMP)

- Here pyruvic acid is changed to lactic acid;
- Change of glucose / glycogen to pyruvic / lactic acids is ka EMP.
- Only **one step is oxidative step** / dehydrogenation when NAD+ changes to NADH.
- **Glucagon** = decreases F-2,6–DP; causes an **increase in gluconeogenesis** while inhibits glycolysis.
- Pyruvic acid changes to lactic acid in anaerobic conditions by the action of **enz lactic dehydrogenase.**
- PA changes to acetate and goes in citric acid cycle in aerobic conditions.
- All enzymes required in glycolysis are in cytoplasm/**extra-mitochondrial**.
- **Energy production** = if glycolysis stops at pyruvic acid then 8 ATPs are gained; if PA changes to lactic acid then only 2 ATPs are gained.
- **Fluoride** inhibits the enz ENOLASE.
- Inhibition of glycolysis in p.o. O_2 = is ka **Pasteur effect**.
- **Mammalian RBCs** metabolise glucose by glycolysis only = b'coz **enz required for oxidation of pyruvate are not present in them**.

KREB'S CYCLE / CITRIC ACID CYCLE

- Is the **aerobic** pathway; occurs **in mitochondria** along with respiratory chains, i.e. it starts by conversion of pyruvate to acetate ka oxidative decarboxylation and enz pyruvate dehydrogenase is required and acetyl CoA/active acetate molecule is formed.
- Cycle starts with condensation of a molecule of acetyl – CoA with oxaloacetate to form citric acid in p.o. enz citrate synthetase.
- 12 ATPs are produced for each acetate molecule.

Total energy output from glucose = 36 ATPs as shown below:

- during glycolysis from each glucose molecule = 8
- conversion of 2 pyruvate to 2 acetate molecules = 6
- oxidation of 2 acetates in citric acid cycle = 24
- - 2 ATPs used in glycerophosphate shuttle = 2 ; so net = 36 ATPs

GLYCOGENESIS

- Glycogenesis is formation of glycogen in ms and liver esp.
- **Liver is the only organ** which can synthesis glycogen from monosaccharides other than glucose.
- **First step** = **phosphorylation** of glucose to G-6-P in p.o. **glucokinase** / hexokinase enz.
- Glucokinase acts only on D-glucose.
- In liver = glucokinase predominates; it is **absent in ms;** and deficient in livers of diabetics.
- **Fetal liver** contains **only hexokinase;** glucokinase appears at birth.
- Glucokinase decreased in fasting and in DM.
- Glycogen synthetase is a specific enz for glycogenesis.
- Glucose units are linked by 1,4 – glycosidic linkages.
- Glucose + ATP → G-6-P + ADP
- G-6-P → G-1-P
- G-1-P + UTP → UDP-glucose + glycogen
- Glycogenolysis is intimately **related to ms contraction** .
- In the resting ms = synthetase I predominates.
- In contracting ms = synthetase D predominates.

- **Adrenaline inhibits** glycogen synthesis thro the production of cAMP.

GLYCOGENOLYSIS

- Is breakdown of glycogen to glucose.
- Phosphorylase is the key enzyme in it.
- cAMP is formed from ATP by **enz adenyl cyclase**.
- **Adr and glucagon** stimulates **adenyl cyclase** and so stimulates the *glycogenolysis in liver.*
- **cAMP** increases glycogen breakdown and decreases glycogen synthesis in liver.
- **Galactosemia** = i.e. inability to convert galactose to glucose due to deficiency of enz galactose – 1 – phosphate uridyl transferase.
- Conversion of fructose to glucose can occur **only in the liver** and intestines. **Fructose can be used by liver and adipose tissues; but brain and ms can use only glucose.**
- Absence of aldolase-B enz → causes hereditary fructose intolerance.

LIPID METABOLISM

- Fat absorbed mainly in lymphatics in the form of **chylomicrons**; transported with albumin in plasma.
- **Apoprotein** = protein component of plasma lipoproteins; 3 groups, i.e. A group = in HDL; B group = is in LDL / VLDL/ chylomicrons; C – group is in HDL /VLDL/chylomicrons
- **Liver is the main source** of endogenous plasma lipoproteins.
- Fatty acids from blood and synthesised in liver are incorporated in VLDL and secreted back in the circulation.
- **Insulin and ethanol favour** increased synthesis of VLDL by liver.
- Liver also converts cholestrol to bile acids and thus plays an important role in homeostasis of blood cholesterol.
- Liver has 5 % of lipid content; body has 15% of the lipids.
- Substances, e.g. choline; methionine; etc. which prevent fatty liver aka LIPOTROPIC SUBSTANCES; e.g. inositol; pyridoxine; vit E etc.

- In choline deficient animal = plasma VLDL are absent.
- Diabetes mellitus = leads to **fatty liver.**
- Injection of **anterior pituitary hormones** = have **ketogenic factors;** it mobilises lipids from tissues to liver and causes fatty liver.
- Lipoprotein lipase enz hydrolyses the lipids of chylomicrons and helps their passage into the tissues = this enz is **activated by HEPARIN**. Its activity is enhanced by insulin and glucose; inhibited by GH, Adr, ACTH, etc.
- Formation of triglycerides from fatty acids /glucose = enhanced by insulin.
- Breakage of triglycerides to FA and released in blood is = enhanced by glucagon, Adr, Nadr, ACTH, GH, thyrotropic hormones, DM, starvation.
- **Insulin** = decreases cAMP levels by **inhibiting enz adenyl cyclase** and stimulating phosphodiesterase. Nicotinic acid and PGE **accentuate insulin effect.**
- FFAs are transported in plasma by forming a loose **complex with plasma albumin.**
- **Adipokinin from anterior pituitary** = also enhances plasma FFA levels by increasing lipolysis of depot fats.
- FFAs are used in liver for their incorporation in VLDL which are then returned to plasma.
- **First step in oxidation** of FA involves THIOKINASE / ACYL CoA synthetase and forms acyl-CoA.
- Acetyl CoA / active acetate can be formed from carbohydrate / lipids / fats/ F A s / ketogenic A Acids / ketone bodies and can be oxidised in citric acid cycle (complete metabolism of fat occurs to give energy) and for synthesis of FA/cholesterol/ketone bodies, etc.
- **Total energy gained** from palmitic acid = 129 ATPs.
- **Ketone bodies** = acetoacetic acid; beta – hydroxy butyric acid; acetone (ABHA).
- In DM/starvation = increased amount of fat is metabolised which increases ketone bodies in the blood and urine; thus leading to ketosis and ketonuria.

- Synthesis of FA can occur both in mitochondria and cytoplasm;
- **Mitochondrial synthesis** = long chain FA esp stearic and palmitic are formed; pyridoxal phosphate / **biotin** is required in the initial step of condensation of acetyl CoA to acyl CoA.
- **Extramitochondrial system** = FA are produced from acetyl CoA; acetyl CoA is formed in mitochondria, in which enz. **pyruvate dehydrogenase** is present. Then to come out of the mitochondria, acetyl CoA has to **combine with oxaloacetate** to form citrate. Then in cytoplasm, the acetyl CoA is released from this in p.o. enz **ATP – citrate lyase**. Mainly palmitic acid is formed.
- **Essential FA** = linoleic, linolenic (C–18 acids, derivatives of stearic acid); arachidonic acid (C–20 , derivative of arachidic acid) (ALL).
- Mammalian tissues can convert linoleic to linolenic and arachidonic acid in p.o. PYRIDOXINE; so **only LINOLEIC ACID is the only FA which is absolutely indispensable**.
- Prostaglandins are formed from arachidonic acid.
- Their deficiency causes fatty liver; and high cholesterol level in blood.

Abnormalities of lipid metabolism

1. Gaucher's disease = **cerebrosides** increased in brain/liver/spleen.
2. Niemann-Pick disease = **sphingomyelins** increased in liver/ spleen/ bone marrow.
3. Tay-Sachs disease = **glycosides** increase in brain.

GENETICS AND NUCLEIC ACIDS

- Nucleotide = nucleoside + phosphate (BSP)
- Nucleoside = base + sugar
- Purine and pyrimidine are catabolised to uric acid.
- Formation of carbamyl aspartate is a **committed step** in pyrimidine biosynthesis.

URIC ACID METABOLISM

- Normal level = 2–6 mg %
- Mainly excreted in urine by glomerular filteration.
- In *gout* = uric acid levels increase in blood and abnormal deposition of uric acid occurs in tendons, joints and bursae. The deposits are ka TOPHI.
- **Primary gout** = due to overproduction of PRPP and altered kinetics of enz PRPP – synthetase.
- Sec. Gout = due to increase in **purine catabolism**, e.g. in leukemia; renal failure, etc.
- **Uricosuric drugs** = e.g. salicylates, concophen, adrenal cortical hormones, etc. cause **increase in urinary excretion** of uric acid by decreasing its reabsorption, so given in **treatment of gout.**
- **Allopurinol** = competitive inhibition of xanthine oxidase and decreased production of uric acid.
- In von–Gierke's dis = increased production of uric acid due to **deficiency of G - 6 - Pase** and leads to overproduction of PRPP and uric acid.

Biosynthesis of nucleic acids

- DNA forms RNA in p.o. **enz DNA dependent RNA polymerase** by the process ka **transcription**. Synthesis of RNA is ka transcription.
- RNA forms proteins by the process of **translation**.
- DNA forms DNA by the process of **replication** in p.o. enz DNA – polymerase.
- DNA can guide its own synthesis but RNA cannot. It is guided by DNA.
- Replication of DNA requires enz DNA – polymerase.
- **Okazaki piece** = DNA containing approx 100 nucleotides and attached to a small RNA molecule of 10 nucleotides is ka okazaki piece.

PROTEIN METABOLISM

- Amino acids in blood = 30–50 mg %
- Amino acids are **actively transported** into tissues, **pyridoxal phosphate** is one of the requirements for normal uptake.
- GH, insulin, testosterone favour the uptake of amino acids by tissues.

Protein synthesis

- Mainly occurs in **ribosomes of** RER; ribosomes have 2 components, i.e. 30 S and 50 S.
- It is specifically guided by genes / DNA carried by mRNA to the site of protein synthesis.
- Part of DNA strand which is concerned with the synthesis of any single polypeptide chain is ka CISTRON.
- Replication of a mRNA from DNA is ka **transcription** and is mediated by enz RNA – polymerase II.
- 4 bases, i.e. AGTC can form 64 different triplets.
- **Non-sense/terminator codons** = UAA, UGA, UAG; they do not code for any amino acids.
- A. acids join thro peptide bond/3' – 5' linkage to form polypeptide chain.
- 3 ATPs are required for synthesis of a peptide bond (1 ATP + 2 GTP); and for initiation process, one more GTP is required.
- **mutation** = transition, i.e. if one purine changes to another purine or one pyrimidine to other pyrimidine.
- **Transversion** = i.e. if purine changes to pyrimidine or vice versa.
- **Operon concept** = genes concerned in the synthesis of proteins with related functions are located as a single unit in one region of chromosome is ka operon.
- **Operator gene** = is at the beginning of operon units; it regulates the activity of other genes in the unit.
- **Structural genes** = are directly concerned in the synthesis of mRNA.

- **Regulator gene** = has a controlling effect on operator gene.
- **Attenuator** = located just proceeding the structural genes.

Inhibitors of protein synthesis

1. Mitomycin = prevents replication of DNA strands.
2. Actinomycin – D = prevents the formation of mRNA.
3. Tetracycline/streptomycin/chloramphenicol = selectively combine with one or more ribosome components and prevent combination at initiator site.
4. Cycloheximide = inhibits formation of peptide bonds by inhibiting the enz peptide synthetase.
5. Rifamycin = specific inhibitor of enz DNA dependent RNA polymerase.
6. Diphtheria toxin = blocks elongation phase of protein synthesis by its effect on elongation factor, EF 2.

Essential amino acids = threonine; valine, leucine, isoleucine, lysine, methionine, phenylalanine, tryptophan, arginine, histidine. In them, arginine and histidine are not absolutely essential.

Methionine and phenylalanine are mainly required for synthesis of cysteine and tyrosine.

If deficiency of amino acids = then negative N_2 balance in body occurs.

Oxidation of amino acids

- Urea is formed by transamination and oxidative deamination,
- A A s may be glycogenic/ketogenic or both.
- Only LEUCINE is **ketogenic.**
- Isoleucine, lysine, phenyl alanine, tyrosine, tryptophan are both, i.e. ketogenic and glycogenic.
- **Transamination** = occurs by enz transaminases or amino-transferases which is present in liver, kidney, and brain. **Pyridoxal phosphate is required as coenzyme.**
- Lysine, threonine, proline and hydroxyproline cannot be aminated from their respective keto acids.

- Urea formation occurs in liver by **kreb – Henseleit cycle**.
- Enz **arginase** which is required in final step of producing urea from arginine is **present only in liver** and absent in all other tissues.
- **First step** = is formation of carbamyl phosphate from CO_2 and NH_3.
- Formation of carbamyl phosphate and citrulline (from ornithine) occurs in mitochondria.
- Now, citrulline leaves mito- and remaining steps up to the formation of urea and ornithine occur in cytosol.
- Now, ornithine re-enters mitochondria to repeat the cycle.

Glucose – alanine cycle

- Glucose from liver enters ms; forms pyruvate, which forms lactate and alanine.
- Lactate and alanine go to liver to form glucose; it is ka Glucose – alanine cycle.

1. Tyrosine can be synthesised from **phenylalanine.**
2. Adr/ N adr/ melanin are formed from DOPA which is formed from tyrosine / phenylalanine.
3. In **phenyl ketonuria** = the enz **phenyl alanine hydroxylase** is absent in liver and so phenyl alanine gets converted to phenyl pyruvic acid which is excreted in urine.
4. In **alkaptonuria** = enz **homogentisic acid oxidase** is absent in liver, so HGA/ alkapton is excreted in urine and urine darkens on standing.
5. In **albinism** = inability to convert DOPA to melanin due to absence of **tyrosinase** in melanocytes.
6. **Tryptophan** = from every 60 mg of tryptophan, about **1 mg of niacin** is formed. Also forms 5 HT/ serotonin in platelets/ intestinal mucosa, which is vasoconstrictor and smooth ms constrictor and stimulates cerebral activity.
7. MAO inhibitors prolong serotonin action on brain and produce psychic stimulation.
8. Reserpine = releases 5 HT and produces depression of cerebral activity.

9. **Hartnup's disease** = defect in renal and intestinal transport of tryptophan; **pellagra – like s/s appear.**
10. **Melatonin** = hormone of **pineal body** and peripheral Ns; it is synthesised **from serotonin.**

Porphyrin metabolism

- Condensation of succinyl CoA and glycine in p.o. ALA – synthetase.
- ALA – synthetase required = it is a **rate – limiting enz** in heme – synthesis.
- ALA – synthetase requires **pyridoxal phosphate** for activation and reaction occurs **in mitochondria.**
- About 8 gm of Hb is synthesised and degraded per day.
- **Erythropoietic porphyria** = enz ferrochelatase / heme synthetase is deficient which adds iron to protoporphyrin IX.
- **Acute intermittent porphyria** = enz uroporphyrinogen I synthetase is deficient in liver.
- **Lead poisoning** = lead inhibits the enz uroporphyrinogen I synthetase and ferrochelatase enz.

WATER AND ELECTROLYTE BALANCE

- Water content of human body = 50 – 70 %; 55 % of body weight in males; 50 % of body wt in females.
- Plasma = 5 % of the body wt.
- Daily output = 2000 – 2500 ml as —

1. Urine = 1000 – 1500 ml.
2. Sweat = 400 ml
3. Feces = 200 ml
4. Respiration = 400 ml

- Sensory nerves responding to dryness of mouth and pharynx = are 9th and 10th Ns.
- **Thirst centre** = located in 3rd ventricle; stimulated by *osmoreceptors* and sensory nerves of mouth/pharynx during dehydration.

- ADH = helps reabsorption of water in distal convoluted tubules.
- During dehydration = along with water, intracellular K^+ pass out and extracellular Na^+ passes in the cells.
- Chief ions of body fluid = Na; K; Cl; HCO_3^-.
- **Chief cations** of intracellular fluid = K, Mg
- Chief cations of extracellular fluid = Na
- Total conc. of ions in extracellular fluid = 310 m.osmols/ litre which is 155 m.eq of cations + 155 m.eq of anions.
- **Sodium – potassium pump** = maintains the high gradient of Na and K on either side of cell membrane; is **energy requiring** pump; requires enz Na – K – ATPase which breaks one ATP, pumps 3 Na out and 2 K ions in the cell against the conc gradient and requires Mg for its action.

RESPIRATION

- Average adult man uses 250 ml O_2 and eliminates 200 ml of CO_2/min.

		Solubility in plasma and RBC fluids
PO_2 in alveolar air	100 mm Hg	
PO_2 in arterial blood	100	
PO_2 in venous blood	40	
PO_2 in interstitial fluid	30	
PCO_2 in alveolar air	40	
PCO_2 in arterial blood	40	2.7 ml/100 ml
PCO_2 in venous blood	46	3.2 ml/100 ml
O_2 in arterial blood	19.6 ml/100 ml	Hb is 97% saturated
O_2 in venous blood	12.6 ml/100 ml	Hb is 70% saturated

- Time required for saturation of blood with O_2 = 0.7 sec.
- Myoglobin = has only one heme per molecule; 95 % saturated at PO_2 100 mm Hg.; 80 % saturated at PO_2 20 mm Hg.
- Hb = 4 subunits, i.e. alpha 1,2; beta 1,2. S –shaped dissociation curve of O_2 for Hb.

Diphosphoglycerate / DPG

- Allosteric regulator of Hb activity
- Present in RBCs.
- Affinity for reduced Hb is 2 × that of oxy-Hb.
- Helps in more efficient release of O_2.
- **Increased levels in people at high altitudes**.

CO_2 = allosteric regulator; 6.6 ml/100 ml of CO_2 is added to venous blood; Hb has higher affinity for CO_2 than oxy-Hb; forms carbonic acid in solution.

Fetal respiration = O_2 dissociation curve of HbF is considerably shifted to left cp. to adult Hb. It is due to **low affinity of HbF to DPG**.

Carbonic anhydrase enz facilitates formation of H_2CO_3 and its dissociation to form bicarbonate. It is present in RBCs. It require Zn^{2+} for its action.

Modes of transport of CO_2 = total 6.6 ml/100 ml.

1. 7–8% = as physical solution
2. 4% = by plasma proteins (as H^+ and HCO_3^- ions)
3. 20% = as carbamino Hb
4. 70% = by isohydric transport; **maximum**; no change in pH.

Haldane effect = binding of O_2 to Hb displaces CO_2 from it is ka Haldane effect.

Chloride – bicarbonate shift

- 90% CO_2 taken up by RBCs.
- HCO_3^- content of venous plasma is increased.

- Corresponding decrease of chloride content of venous plasma and an increase in RBCs chloride content, i.e. HCO_3 shifted out of RBCs and **Cl^- shifted in the RBCs.**
- Reverse occurs in the lungs.

Respiratory centre = present in **medulla oblongata;** stimulated by increase in PCO_2 and H^+ conc.; depressed by decreased PCO_2 and H^+ conc.

Chemoreceptors = stimulated by **decreased PO_2** and increased PCO_2 and H^+ conc of arterial blood; main stimulus is decreased PO_2.

IONS OF THE BODY

Na^+ = chief **extracellular** cation

Cl^- = chief extracellular anion; conc. in CSF is higher than in plasma.

K^+ = chief **intracellular** cation

Na pump = is an **energy requiring** mechanism.

Addison's dis is due to deficiency of ACTH = it leads to increased renal excretion of Na^+; so decreased in blood Na level occurs. (hyponatremia)

Cushing's dis / due to increase of adrenal cortex function; increased aldosterone levels = increased blood Na.

Normal nm irritability depends on = Na, K / Ca, Mg, H ions ratio and balance.

A deficiency of K^+ = depressed cardiac ms

A gross increase in K^+ = paralysis of skeletal ms.

Hyperfunction of adrenal cortex ; Cushing's disease = increased loss of K in urine and so decreased in plasma levels.

Hypofunction of adrenal cortex/**Addison's dis** = increased plasma K–level, i.e. opposite of Na.

Tissue protein synthesis causes an uptake of K = approx 2 mg / gm of protein.

Synthesis of glycogen in liver and ms = K required is 3 – 4 mg/gm of glycogen

Hypokalemia = occurs in alkalosis; dehydration; Cushing's syndrome.

Hyperkalemia = occurs in crush synd; Addison's disease.

Condition	pH	HCO_3^-
Respiratory acidosis	Decreased	Increased
Resp alkalosis	Increased	Decreased
Metabolic acidosis	Decreased	Increased
Metabolic alkalosis	Increased	Decreased

Calcium = plasma levels are 9–11 mg%.

- Most abundant ion in body
- Depressant effect / regulatory on nm irritability.
- **Calmodulin** = acts as a receptor molecule for Ca^{++} and helps to regulate a large no. of function but it is inhibited by phenothiazine drugs.
- Present in **milk** in maximal amounts
- Metabolism is regulated by vit D and PTH.
- High protein diet favors its absorption, while high cereal diet diminishes it
- An acidic pH of intestine and vit D favors its absorption.
- A Ca : P ratio of not more than 2:1 and not less than 1:2 is necessary for its absorption.
- It is chiefly **bound to albumin**
- **RBCs do not contain any Ca**.
- Ca in glomerular filtrate is absorbed completely in PCT; it is associated with Na^+ reabsorption.
- In DCT = Ca^{2+} active reabsorption occurs unrelated to Na^+; PTH stimulates it in DCT.
- **Hyperparathyroidism** = plasma Ca increased; by **bone demineralisation**. And decreased P due to decreased tubular reabsorption of P.

- **Hypoparathyroidism** = plasma Ca decrease; P increased; if < 7 mg% then **tetany** occurs; Carpopedal spasm;
- Plasma Ca × P product is 10 × 4 = 40 in normal adults.
- **Renal rickets** = increased urinary excretion of phosphate, i.e. hyperphosphaturia; and decreased blood Ca / P levels; aka vitamin – D resistant rickets (VDRR).
- It is excreted in feces / P is excreted in urine.

PHOSPHORUS: PTH increases P excretion in urine by decreasing its reabsorption.

Bone

- Osteoblasts are rich in alkaline Pase.
- Vit C ar d A are required for normal activity of osteoblasts.
- Vit K s required for formation of gamma – carboxyglutamate and so has a role in metabolism of bone and teeth.

TEETH

- Enamel is more dense and hardest tissue of the body.
- Enamel **in embryonic tooth** is made of **high proline content**.
- Enamel in **adult tooth** = much of the protein disappears; but only **few keratin** remains.
- Turnover rate of PO_4 in dentin is = $1/6^{th}$ of the bone and T. O rate in enamel is $1/100^{th}$ of the bone.
- Lack of vit A = causes hypoplastic enamel.
- Lack of vit C = affects calcification of dentin.
- Vit D is required for absorption of Ca/P from the gut and its deposition in bone and teeth.
- Saliva rich in mucin has less cleaning action on teeth and so more caries occurs.
- **F inhibits enolase** enz and so decreases the acid formation and so caries.

MAGNESIUM

- With Ca and H^+, it depresses N M activity and balances the action of Na and K.
- Useful in postmenopausal osteoporosis.
- Reduces leg cramps during pregnancy; improves bone Ca^{++} use;
- Increased plasma levels = depress nervous system; can cause anesthesia and **paralysis of skeletal** ms.
- Mg and K are normal cations of intracellular fluid.
- Decreased plasma levels lead to = *tetany*
- In hypoparathyroidism = Ca and Mg decrease
- Aldosterone = increased urinary excretion of Mg.

Sulphur = is present in cysteine and methionine, heparin; insulin.

Zinc = Avoids complication of congenital malformation; offsets the detrimental effect of calcium on zinc absorption. Helps in action of enz. carbonic-anhydrase; required for epithelial integrity.

IRON

- Required for O_2 transport; found very less in milk.
- Its deficiency leads to = hypochromic microcytic anemia.
- Only 10 % of food iron is absorbed esp in stomach and duodenum; depends on *mucosal load* of iron.
- Fe^{+2} form is readily absorbed in stomach and duodenum.
- Deficiency of HCl and high phosphate diet = decreases Fe absorption.
- **Transport form of iron** = is **transferrin**; has 2 atoms of iron/ Fe^{3+}. It moves with beta – globulin.
- **Storage form of iron** / Fe^{3+} = (Fe + *apoferritin*) = is **ferritin**; has approx 4300 atoms of iron.
- **Erythropoietin** promotes rapid transfer of mucosal iron to transferrin.
- If excess iron load, the ferritin gets denatured and forms **hemosiderin**.
- A **deficiency of vit C** favours the formation of hemosiderin.

- For iron to enter / leave the cell, it should be in the Fe^{2+} form.
- **Synthesis of Hb requires = 27 mg Fe/day.**

COPPER

- Is bound to **ceruloplasmin** in serum; is associated with *alpha – globulin.*
- Favors the transport of iron from intestines.

COBALT = is found in vit B_{12}.

ZINC

- NECESSARY FOR Maintaining plasma conc. of vit A
- Component of enz **carbonic anhydrase**; alcohol dehydrogenase, etc.
- Zn content of **WBCs decreases** to 10 % of the normal levels in **leukemias**.
- Zn deficiency causes **delayed wound healing** and impaired taste.

MULTIPLE CHOICE QUESTIONS
Sample Question Paper

1. The test done to check urine urobilinogen is:
A. Tri-iodine test
B. Ehrlich's aldehyde test
C. Rothera's test
D. Benedict's test

2. 2 strands of DNA are held by which bonds:
A. Covalent
B. Coordinate
C. Metallic
D. Hydrogen

3. Normal serum potassium level (mEq/L) is:
A. 1.5–2.5
B. 2.5–3.5
C. 3.5–5.5
D. 5.5–7.5

4. Tertiary structure of a protein can be seen with:
A. Enzyme degradation
B. Electron microscopy
C. X-ray diffraction technique
D. Immunoassay

5. The enzyme HMG-COA is useful in the synthesis of:
A. Porphyrins
B. Hemoglobulin
C. Fatty acids
D. Cholesterol

6. Which is a metabolite of androgenic hormone:
A. 17-OH steroid
B. 17 ketosteroid
C. 17 ketogenic steroid
D. Progantriol

7. The chains present in Adult hemoglobin are:

A. $2\alpha + 2\beta$
B. $2\alpha + 2\gamma$
C. $2\beta + 2\gamma$
D. $2\alpha + 2\delta$

8. Ammonia in the Kidney cells is synthesized from:

A. Glutathione
B. Purine
C. Glutamine
D. Glycine

9. The template used in reverse transcription by messenger RNA is:

A. Single stranded DNA
B. Double stranded DNA
C. Ribosome
D. r-RNA

10. In plasma, the cholesterol is carried by:

A. LDL
B. VLDL
C. HDL
D. Chylomicrons

11. Cystinuria is characterized by:

A. Generalised aminoaciduria
B. Systemic acidosis
C. Cysteine calculi in renal tubular cells
D. Recurrent cysteine calculi

12. Urine test can be helpful in determining of the following disorder:

A. Galactosemia
B. Cretinism
C. Neonatal tetany
D. Mucoviscidosis

13. Body fat in cold water channel swimmers is:

A. Accumulated around the abdominal viscera
B. Concentrated retroperitoneally

C. Deposited preferentially in the liver
D. Differentially deposited in subcutaneous tissue

14. The following statements about enzymes are true except:
A. At substrate conc, the initial rate of an enzyme catalysed reaction increases conc. only with increasing substrate concentration.
B. Enzymes affect the equilibria of the reactions they catalyze.
C. In the presence of an appropriate enzyme, the free energy required to reach the transition rate of a chemical reaction is decreased.
D. The V_{max} value for substrate is not altered by a competitive inhibitor.

15. The following are important features of genetic code except:
A. Each amino acids specified by only one triplet codon.
B. The genetic code is degenerate.
C. The reading frame should be correctly set at the beginning of mRMA
D. Three of the possible 64 nucleotide triplets do not code for any amino acids.

16. The sixth coordination position of Fe^{2+} in deoxy hemoglobin is:
A. Occupied by O_2
B. Occupied by glycine.
C. Empty.
D. Occupied by serine.

17. The precursor of Melatonin is:
A. Tryptophan
B. Tyrosine
C. Phenylalanine
D. Histidine

18. Which of the following contributes the flexibility to protein chain:
A. Glycine
B. Tryptophan
C. Proline
D. Serine

19. Which of the following is used as Co-Enzyme in trans-amination reaction:

A. Pyridoxine phosphate
B. NAD
C. Thymine
D. Acyl COA

20. c-AMP increases glycogenolysis by:

A. Contributing phosphate
B. Causing dephosphorylation.
C. Uncoupling.
D. All of the above

21. Compound required for metabolism of Pyruvate:

A. Thiamine
B. Niacin
C. Pyridoxine
D. Riboflavin

22. Abnormal Hb is found in which of the following condition:

A. Hereditary spherocytosis
B. G-6-P-D deficiency
C. Sickle cell anaemia
D. Pernicious anaemia

23. The protein not synthesized in liver is:

A. Fibrinogen
B. Albumin
C. Prothrombin
D. Gamma globulin

24. All of the following are DNA bases except:

A. Uracil
B. Cytosine
C. Adenine
D. Guanine

25. The variable part of the antibody molecule is:

A. N terminal
B. C-terminal
C. Intermediate region
D. Carbohydrate moiety

26. The substance having an affinity but no intrinsic activity is the:

A. Agonist
B. Partial agonist
C. Antagonist
D. Physiological antagonist

27. Most active form of vitamin-D is:

A. 1α - calciferol
B. 1,25 dehydrocholecalciferol
C. 24,25 dehydrocalciferol
D. 25 - dehydrocholecalciferol

28. Ketotic amino acid is:

A. Arginine
B. Methionine
C. Threonine
D. Glycine

29. Aromatic ring is found in:

A. Arginine
B. Proline
C. Phenylalanine
D. Glycine

30. Ions present in Cytochrome:

A. Copper
B. Iron
C. Both
D. None

31. Substance to which Endoplasmic reticulum is not permeable:

A. Malate
B. Phenyl pyruvate
C. Glycopyrole
D. Triacylglycerol

32. High dose of glucose can cause all except:

A ↑Pancreatic Amylase
B. ↑Acetyl Carboxylase
C. ↑ glucose – 6 - phosphatase
D. ↑G-6-PD Levels

33. A patient presenting with slow growth, fever, blue eyes shows following in urine:

A. VMA
B. Methamanic acid
C. Homogentisic acid
D. Phenylpyruvic acid

34. All of the following are Essential Amino acids except:

A. Phenyl alanine
B. Leucine
C. Isoleucine
D. Tyrosine

35. The prosthetic group of an enzyme which is an inorganic ion, it is called a:

A. Coenzyme
B. Cofactor
C. Apoenzyme
D. Holoenzyme

36. Source of energy to heart is:

A. Fatty acids
B. Glucose
C. Glycogen
D. Ketone bodies

37. Cyclic AMP activates glycogenolysis by:

A. Activating protein kinase
B. Activating gluose-1 phosphatase
C. Activating glucose-6 phosphatase
D. ↑ β-oxidation

38. Enzyme which helps to produce urea is:

A. Urease
B. Succinic-dehydrogenase
C. Aspartase
D. Arginase

39. Commonest enzyme deficiency is:

A. G-6-P-D
B. Glucose-6 phosphates

C. Glucose 1,6 diphosphatase
D. Hexokinase

40. Isotope of an element has the same:
A. Atomic weight
B. Atomic volume
C. Atomic number
D. None of the above

41. The test used to diagnose the Thiamine deficiency is:
A. Blood Enol- Pyruvate levels
B. RBC transketolase activity
C. Serum thiamine estimation
D. Acetyl Co A levels

42. Active transport means:
A. Transport across chemical gradient
B. Transport across electric gradient
C. Transport with energy expenditure
D. Transport with no energy expenditure

43. NADPH is used in the:
A. Fatty acid synthesis
B. Glycogenesis
C. Gluconeogenesis
D. HMP shunt pathway

44. Which of the following is not a product of pentose pathway:
A. Sedoheptulose phosphate
B. Glyceraldehyde-3-phosphate
C. CO_2
D. NADPH

45. The chief site of Protein synthesis is:
A. Golgi complex
B. Inside nucleus
C. Mitochondria
D. Ribosomes

46. True essential fatty acid is
A. Arachidonic acids
B. Linoelic acid

C. Linolenic acid
D. Oleic acid

47. The maximum amount of proteins in the Dietary fibers is:
A. Collagen
B. Pectin
C. Proteoglycan
D. Starch

48. Impaired glucose tolerance predisposes to:
A. IHD
B. Nephropathy
C. Neuropathy
D. Retinopathy

49. Due to incomplete Oxidation of Phenylpyruvic acid, which disease occurs:
A. Phenylketonuria
B. Albinism
C. Tyrosinosis
D. Alkaptonuria

50. The enzyme of the glycolytic cycle inhibited by the Fluoride ions:
A. Aldolase
B. Enolase
C. Hexokinase
D. Phospho-Fructokinase

51. Difference in reversible and irreversible reaction is:
A. Entropy
B. Heat production
C. Work done
D. Temp. change

52. The structure of all the proteins is:
A. L-forms
B. D-forms
C. Mostly D-form
D. D as well as L forms

53. The fact true about Unconjugated bilirubin is:
A. Easily excreted by kidney
B. Not lipid soluble
C. More water soluble
D. Bound to serum albumin

54. Gene transmitted but not translated is:
A. Histone
B. Keratin
C. t-RNA
D. Glycosyl transferase

55. Plasma Membranes is mainly composed of:
A. Protein
B. Phospholipid
C. Cholesterol
D. Carbohydrate

56. End product of old chain fatty acid oxidation is:
A. Acetyl CoA (B chain)
B. Propionyl CoA
C. Malonyl CoA
D. Histidine

57. Find the true statement regarding the action of alpha amylase:
A. Breach glucose end of carbohydrate
B. Cleaves only at alpha 1–4,
C. Cleaves only at alpha 1–6
D. Both B and C

58. Which amino acid does not have chirality
A. Lysine
B. Leucine
C. Arginine
D. Histidine

59. The amino acid which can protonate and deprotonate simultaneously at neutral pH is:
A. Histidine
B. Arginine

C. Glycine
D. Leucine

60. Haemolysis seen in the deficiency of the enz. G-6-P-D is due to decrease in:
A. NADPH
B. NADH
C. H^+
D. TPP

61. Gluco-corticosteroids increase the blood sugar levels by:
A. Decreased Peripheral use.
B. Gluconeogenesis
C. Increased glycolysis
D. None of the above

62. Rough E.R. is site of synthesis for:
A. Protein
B. Carbohydrate
C. Cholesterol
D. All of the above

63. Membrane integrity of RBC is due to:
A. Ankyrin
B. Glycophorin
C. P-protein
D. Spectrin

64. Triple helix is seen in the structure of
A. Collagen
B. Elastic tissue
C. DNA
D. All of above

65. The protein providing the Motility to a cell is:
A. Tubulin
B. Keratin
C. Motilin
D. Phorin

66. All of the following can use ketone bodies as source of energy except:
A. Brain
B. Heart
C. Liver
D. Muscles

67. Glucose can be synthesized from all except:
A. Glycerol
B. Lactic acid
C. Alanine
D. Acetoacetic acid

68. Post-translational defect in scurvy is due to non-hydroxylation of:
A. Proline
B. Glycine
C. Isoleucine
D. Leucine

69. Gaucher's disease is caused due to deficiency of:
A. Glucosyl-ceramide
B. Sphingomyelin
C. Terpenes
D. Ganglioside

70. First committed step in Glycolysis is:
A. Hexokinase
B. Glucokinase
C. Phosphofructokinase
D. Aldolase

71. Proof-reading of m-RNA is done by:
A. Peptidyl transferase
B. Aminoacyl transferase
C. Formulas
D. RNA polymerases type–1

72. The enzyme not present in the Skeletal muscles is:
A. Glucose-6-phosphatase
B. Hexokinase

C. Isomerase
D. Phosphofructokinase

73. DNA melting refers to:
A. Splitting of DNA into single strands
B. Breaking DNA into fragments
C. Breaking DNA down to bases
D. Recurrent mutation

74. TCA cycle substrate level phosphorylation occurs at:
A. Succinate dehydrogenase
B. Malonate reductase
C. Thiokinase.
D. Hexokinase

Answer Key to MCQs in Biochemistry

1	B	2	D	3	C	4	C
5	D	6	B	7	A	8	C
9	A	10	A	11	D	12	A
13	D	14	B	15	A	16	D
17	A	18	C	19	A	20	A
21	A	22	B	23	D	24	A
25	B	26	C	27	B	28	A
29	C	30	C	31	B	32	C
33	C	34	D	35	B	36	A
37	A	38	D	39	A	40	C
41	B	42	C	43	D	44	C
45	D	46	B	47	B	48	B
49	A	50	B	51	A	52	A
53	D	54	A	55	B	56	B
57	B	58	C	59	A	60	A
61	B	62	A	63	D	64	A
65	C	66	C	67	D	68	A
69	A	70	C	71	B	72	A
73	A	74	A				

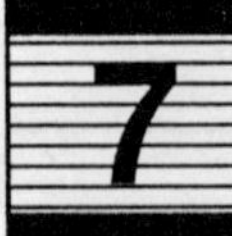

MCQs in Physiology and Biochemistry

1. **The neurotransmitter of the preganglionic sympathetic neurons is:**
   A. Norepinephrine
   B. Acetylcholine
   C. Dopamine
   D. Serotonin

2. **The isoelectric point (p) is the pH at which:**
   A. The number of positive charges outnumbers the negative charges
   B. The number of positive charges equals the number of negative charges
   C. The number of negative charges outnumbers the number of positive charges
   D. None of the above

3. **All of the following are factors that decrease insulin secretion EXCEPT:**
   A. Decrease in blood glucose level
   B. Secretion of somatostatin
   C. Secretion of glucagon
   D. Secretion of either epinephrine or norepinephrine

4. **The primary purine bases in both RNA and DNA are:**
   A. Thymine (T) and Guanine (G)

B. Adenine (A) and Guanine (G)
C. Cytosine (C) and Thymine (T)
D. Guanine (G) and Cytosine (C)

5. Which major type of protein present in the plasma functions to provide colloid osmotic pressure in the plasma?
A. Globulin
B. Albumin
C. Fibrinogen
D. None of the above

6. The largest number of chemoreceptors which are important for detecting changes in oxygen in the blood and help regulate respiratory activity are located in the:
A. Basal bodies
B. Carotid bodies
C. Residual bodies
D. Nissl bodies

7. The processes which take place in the nephrons, ultimately leading to urine formation include:
A. Glomerular filtration
B. Tubular reabsorption
C. Tubular secretion
D. All of the above

8. Proteins that make up the cell membrane serve as:
A. Transporters
B. Enzymes
C. Receptors
D. Mediators
E. All of the above

9. The four structural and functional portions of the cardiac conduction system are listed below. Which portion is called the "pacemaker" of the heart?
A. Sinoatrial node
B. Atrioventricular node
C. Atrioventricular bundle
D. Purkinje fibers

10. Which of the following statements concerning the Frank-Starling law of the heart are true?
A. It is the mechanism that allows the heart to adjust intrinsically to changing demands
B. It is the mechanism that matches cardiac output to venous return
C. The basis for this law is the intrinsic ability of the heart to adapt itself to changing loads of in-flowing blood
D. It is the mechanism that normally allows the heart to pump automatically whatever amount of blood flows into the right atrium from the veins
E. All of the above

11. The major hormone responsible for lactogenesis is:
A. Growth hormone
B. Adrenocorticotropic hormone (ACTH)
C. Prolactin
D. Thyroid-stimulating hormone (TSH)

12. Cortisol (hydrocortisone) has a direct inhibitory effect on which two structures listed below:
A. Adrenal cortex
B. Hypothalamus
C. Anterior pituitary gland
D. Posterior pituitary gland

13. Which of the following is the best known stimuli for increasing the rate of thyroid-stimulating hormone (TSH) secretion by the anterior pituitary gland?
A. Exposure to heat
B. Exposure to cold
C. Exposure to stress
D. All of the above

14. Which of the following is the major regulatory enzyme of cholesterol synthesis?
A. Squalene synthetase
B. Mevalonate kinase
C. HMG CoA reductase
D. HMG CoA synthetase

15. The globin (protein) portion of a hemoglobin molecule consists of:

A. One alpha chain and one beta chain
B. Two alpha chains and two beta chains
C. Three alpha chains and three beta chains
D. Four alpha chains and four beta chains

16. The thick ascending loop of Henle reabsorbs:

A. Potassium ions and water
B. Water only
C. Sodium and chloride ions
D. Potassium and chloride ions

17. Genetic recombination experiments depend heavily upon the action of which two enzymes listed below?

A. Restriction endonucleases
B. Alkaline phosphatase
C. DNA ligases
D. Creatine kinase

18. 84% of the entire blood volume of the body is in the:

A. Pulmonary circulation
B. Systemic circulation
C. Heart
D. Pulmonary vessels

19. Folic acid:

A. Is a coenzyme in carboxylation reaction, in which it serves as a carrier of activated carbon dioxide
B. Is a component of coenzyme A
C. Plays a key role in one-carbon metabolism, and is essential for the biosynthesis of the purines and the pyrimidine, thymine
D. Is a component of the visual pigments of rod and cone cells

20. Inhibitors of enzymes decrease the rate of enzymatic reactions. Which type of inhibitor listed below binds to the enzyme or the enzyme-substrate complex at a site different from the active site?

A. Competitive inhibitors
B. Noncompetitive inhibitors

C. Irreversible inhibitors
D. None of the above

21. Which intraocular structure listed below controls the amount of light that enters the eye by opening and closing like the aperture of a camera lens?
A. Sclera
B. Cornea
C. Iris
D. Pupil
E. Lens

22. All of the following are synthesized from the amino acid tyrosine EXCEPT:
A. Dopamine
B. Serotonin
C. Norepinephrine
D. Epinephrine

23. All of the following statements concerning niacin are true EXCEPT:
A. It is also called nicotinic acid
B. It is a component of NAD and NADP
C. It can be formed from the amino acid arginine
D. High supplemental doses are effective in treating hyperlipidemia
E A deficiency leads to pellagra

24. The Michaelis constant, K_m, is:
A. Independent of pH
B. Numerically equal to – ½ V_{max}
C. Dependent on the enzyme concentration
D. Numerically equal to the substrate concentration that gives half-maximal velocity

25. Which of the following ions has a higher concentration in the intracellular fluid (ICF) than in the extracellular fluid (ECF)?
A. Chloride (Cl)
B. Potassium (K)
C. Sodium (Na)
D. Bicarbonate (HCO)

26. Spatial summation occurs when:
A. Two inhibitory inputs arrive at a postsynaptic neuron within one minute of each other
B. Two excitatory inputs arrive at a postsynaptic neuron simultaneously
C. Two inhibitory inputs arrive at a postsynaptic neuron 10 seconds apart
D. Two excitatory inputs arrive at a postsynaptic neuron in rapid succession

27. All of the following statements are true EXCEPT:
A. Peripheral nerve fibers can sometimes regenerate if the some (cell body) is not damaged and some of the neurilemma remains intact
B. The neurilemma forms a regeneration tube through which the growing axon reestablishes its original connection
C. If the nerve originally led to a skeletal muscle, the muscle atrophies in the absence of innervation but regrows when the connection is reestablished
D. Nerve fibers of the CNS (brain and spinal cord) possess the thickest neurilemma

28. Which of the following affect bone mass, structural integrity, and bone loss?
A. Age
B. Race
C. Gender
D. All of the above

29. Which two amino acids listed below, have sulfur containing side chains (R-groups)?
A. Lysine
B. Cysteine
C. Arginine
D. Glutamate
E. Methionine

30. Which of the following serves as a principal source of carbon for nonessential amino acids?
A. Fats
B. Water

C. Carbohydrates
D. Urea

31. A synapse consists of:
A. An axon terminal
B. A synaptic cleft
C. Postsynaptic membrane
D. All of the above

32. Buffers:
A. Prevent a change in pH when Cl ions are added to or removed from a solution
B. Prevent a change in pH when H ions are added to or removed from a solution
C. Prevent a change in pH when K ions are added to or removed from a solution
D. Prevent a change in pH when Na ions are added to or removed from a solution

33. Which of the following causes the secretion of secretin?
A. High pH in the duodenum
B. Neutral pH in the duodenum
C. Low pH in the duodenum
D. None of the above

34. The most important aspect of the DNA double helix is:
A. The randomness of the pairing of bases
B. The specificity of the pairing of bases
C. The phosphodiester linkages
D. That it forms a double spiral coil

35. Serum contains which of the following?
A. Blood cells
B. Platelets
C. Fibrinogen
D. None of the above

36. Which structure listed below controls or affects body temperature, appetite, water balance, pituitary secretions, emotions, and autonomic functions, (including sleep and wakeful cycles)?

A. Basal ganglia
B. Thalamus
C. Hypothalamus
D. None of the above

37. All of the following will cause a decrease in the glomerular filtration rate (GFR) EXCEPT:
A. Constriction of the afferent arteriole
B. Constriction of the efferent arteriole
C. Increased plasma protein concentration of glomerular capillary blood
D. Ureteral stone

38. Molecules that can easily penetrate a biologic membrane are usually:
A. Large and nonpolar
B. Small and polar
C. Large and polar
D. Small and nonpolar

39. Which of the following represents the standard bipolar limb lead I of the ECG?
A. Right arm (-) and left arm (+)
B. Right arm (-) and left leg (+)
C. Left arm (-) and left leg (+)
D. All of the above

40. The three factors that affect the magnitude of the resistance the blood encounters as it flows through vessels are listed below. Which factor has the most powerful relationship?
A. Blood viscosity
B. Vessel length
C. Vessel radius
D. Thickness of the intimal wall

41. All of the following statements concerning calcitonin are true EXCEPT:
A. It is synthesized and secreted by the parafollicular cells of the thyroid gland
B. Its secretion is stimulated by a decrease in serum calcium
C. It acts primarily to inhibit bone resorption

D. Along with parathyroid hormone and 1.25-DHC, it is a major regulator of calcium metabolism

42. Secretion of growth hormone is increased by all of the following EXCEPT:

A. Sleep
B. Stress
C. Obesity
D. Starvation
E. Exercise
F. Hypoglycemia
G. Hormones related to puberty

43. Which hormone listed below is secreted in response to dilation of the cervix?

A. Parathyroid hormone (PTH)
B. Follicle-stimulating hormone (FSH)
C. Oxytocin
D. Estradiol

44. The cell (plasma) membrane is a fluid mosaic of:

A. Lipids
B. Proteins
C. Lipids and proteins
D. Carbohydrates

45. Erythropoietin:

A. Raises the blood sugar level
B. Controls blood pressure
C. Promotes protein production
D. Stimulates red blood cell production

46. Which mechanism below is essential to the production of an osmotically concentrated urine?

A. Proprioceptive mechanism
B. Association mechanism
C. Countercurrent mechanism
D. Investing mechanism

47. The Nucleic acids (DNA) are complex molecules composed of all of the following EXCEPT:

A. Nitrogenous bases
B. Five-carbon sugars
C. Glycans
D. Phosphate groups

48. Which two forces listed below tend to move fluid out of a capillary membrane?
A. Capillary pressure
B. Interstitial fluid pressure
C. Colloid osmotic pressure of the plasma
D. Colloid osmotic pressure of the interstitial fluid

49. The pH of saliva is:
A. Between 1.0 and 3.0
B. Between 2.5 and 4.5
C. Between 6.0 and 7.0
D. Between 9.0 and 10.0

50. All of the following characterized saliva EXCEPT:
A. High potassium and bicarbonate ion concentrations
B. Low sodium and chloride concentrations
C. It is hypertonic
D. Its production is inhibited by vagotomy

51. Coenzyme A contains:
A. Riboflavin
B. Niacin
C. Pantothenic acid
D. Biotin

52. Enteropeptidase (enterokinase) which is produced by intestinal cells converts:
A. Chymotrypsinogen to chymotrypsin
B. Trypsinogen to trypsin
C. Pepsinogen to pepsin
D. Proelastase to elastase

53. All of the following are water-soluble vitamins EXCEPT:
A. Vitamin B-complex
B. Vitamin C
C. Vitamin E
D. Vitamin H

54. Gastric secretion is regulated by which two mechanism listed below?

A. Counter-current mechanism
B. Neural mechanism
C. Hormonal mechanism
D. Immunological mechanism

55. Action potentials in the skeletal muscle cell membrane initiate depolarization of the T tubules, which opens calcium ion release channels in the sarcoplasmic calcium. The calcium ions that are released from the sarcoplasmic calcium bind to which of the following?

A. ATP
B. Acetylcholine
C. Troponin
D. Tropomyosin

56. The descending (motor) spinal tracts carry impulses from the brain to lower motor neurons that regulate the activity of skeletal muscles. Upper motor neurons originate in the brain and form which two major systems listed below?

A. Pyramidal system (corticospinal tract)
B. Spinothalamic system
C. Extrapyramidal system
D. Reticulospinal system

57. Excitatory neurotransmitters in the CNS include all of the following EXCEPT:

A. Acetylcholine (ACH)
B. Glycine
C. Epinephrine
D. Dopamine
E. Serotonin

58. Which of the following solutions has an osmotic pressure different from the other two solutions?

A. 1 M glucose
B. 1 M sodium chloride
C. 1 M potassium nitrate
D. None of the above

59. Ovulation occurs as a result of:

A. The progesterone-induced LH surge
B. The estrogen-induced FSH surge
C. The progesterone-induced FSH surge
D. The estrogen-induced LH surge

60. All of the following are actions of estrogen EXCEPT:

A. Causes of development of female secondary sex characteristics at puberty
B. Causes of development of the breasts
C. Maintains pregnancy
D. Promotes secretory changes in the uterine endometrium during the latter half of the monthly female sexual cycle, thus preparing the uterus for implantation of the fertilized ovum.

61. All of the following statements are true EXCEPT:

A. Blood is normally slightly acidic, with a pH range of 6.45 to 6.55
B. The blood's acid-base balance is controlled precisely because even a minor deviation from the normal range can severely affect many organs
C. The body uses three mechanisms to control the blood's acid-base balance
D. An abnormality in one or more of these pH control mechanisms can cause one of two major disturbances in acid-base balance acidosis or alkalosis

62. Histones are small proteins that are positively charged at physiological pH due to their high content of which two amino acids listed below?

A. Cysteine
B. Arginine
C. Lysine
D. Glutamine

63. Which of the following would cause the release of norepinephrine and epinephrine from storage vesicles in the adrenal medulla?

A. Response to fright

B. Exercise
C. Cold
D. Low levels of blood glucose
E. All of the above

64. Which enzyme listed below is abundant in the liver?
A. Creatine kinase (CK)
B. Lactate dehydrogenase (LDH)
C. Glutamate-pyruvate transaminase (GPT)
D. Glutamate-oxaloacetate transaminase (GOT)

65. Glycogen, starch, and glycosaminoglycans are classified as:
A. Monosaccharides
B. Disaccharides
C. Oligosaccharides
D. Polysaccharides

66. Jaundice refers to yellow discoloration of the skin, sclera, and tissues caused by:
A. Hyperlipidemia
B. Hyperglycemia
C. Hyperbilirubinemia
D. Hypercalcemia

67. Which fatty acids listed below are essential fatty acids?
A. Lauric and myristic acids
B. Palmitic and stearic acids
C. Linoleic and linolenic acids
D. Butyric and caproic acids

68. During intense exercise, which of the following accumulates in muscle?
A. Glucose
B. Ethanol
C. Lactate
D. Glycogen

69. Which of the following parameters is decreased during exercise?
A. Heart rate (HR)
B. Cardiac output (CO)

C. Total peripheral resistance (TPR)
D. Stroke volume (SV)

70. Which valve below is composed of two cusps that prevent a backflow of blood from the left ventricle to the left atrium during ventricular contraction?
A. Tricuspid valve
B. Mitral valve
C. Pulmonary valve
D. Aortic valve

71. Which GI hormone listed below has the ability to enhance the release of insulin in response to infusions of glucose?
A. Gastrin
B. Gastric inhibitory peptide (GIP)
C. Cholecystokinin (CCK)
D. Secretin

72. End-organ resistance to which hormone listed below results in polyuria and elevated serum osmolarity?
A. Oxytocin
B. Antidiuretic hormone (ADH)
C. Parathyroid hormone (PTH)
D. Aldosterone

73. Aldosterone's primary effect is on the:
A. Liver
B. Heart
C. Kidneys
D. Lungs

74. Which electron-carrier complex of the respiratory chain listed below contains NADH as the electron donor?
A. Complex I
B. Complex II
C. Complex III
D. Complex IV

75. Which of the following glycosaminoglycans is also known as the cement substance of tissues?
A. Chondroitin sulfate
B. Dermatan sulfate

C. Hyaluronic acid
D. Keratan sulfate
E. Heparin sulfate

76. Which of the following are steroids with detergent properties and are used to emulsify lipids in foodstuff passing through the intestine to enable fat digestion and absorption through the intestinal wall?
A. Phospholipids
B. Proteins
C. Bile salts
D. Carbohydrates

77. All of the following statements concerning the backbone of DNA are true EXCEPT:
A. It is constant throughout the molecule
B. It consists of deoxyriboses linked by "phosphodiester bridges" or "phosphodiester linkages"
C. It is hydrophobic
D. It is highly polar

78. The cerebellum functions to:
A. Maintain muscle tone
B. Coordinate muscle movement
C. Control balance
D. All of the above

79. All of the following statements concerning the pentose phosphate pathway are true EXCEPT:
A. It produces carbon dioxide (CO_2)
B. It can produce NADPH
C. It requires ATP for phosphorylation
D. It can produce five-carbon sugars (used for DNA and RNA)
E. It is controlled by inhibition of glucose 6-phosphate dehydrogenase by NADPH

80. Carbonic anhydrase catalyzes the reaction between:
A. Carbon dioxide and oxygen
B. Oxygen and water
C. Carbon dioxide and bicarbonate
D. Carbon dioxide and water

81. All of the following statements concerning vitamin C are true EXCEPT:

A. It is also called biotin
B. It is an antioxidant
C. Diets high in vitamin C reduce the risk of certain types of cancer
D. It is a cofactor required for the hydroxylation of proline and lysine

82. The proteolytic enzyme that dissolves fibrin is:

A. Prothromobin
B. Thrombin
C. Fibrinogen
D. Plasmin

83. All of the following conditions increase the likelihood of edema formation EXCEPT:

A. Inflammation
B. Standing
C. Venous constriction
D. Arteriolar constriction

84. Which of the following are functions of the stretch reflex?

A. To maintain muscle tone for posture
B. To increase efficiency for locomotion
C. To smooth out movements
D. Acts as site of coordination for higher order inputs
E. All of the above

85. A motor neuron and all of the muscle fibers that it innervates is called a:

A. Map unit
B. Svedberg unit
C. Motor unit
D. Kind unit

86. FAD and FMN contain:

A. Folic acid
B. Riboflavin
C. Ascorbic acid
D. Thiamine

87. Alveolar ventilation is expressed as:
A. Respiratory rate × (Tidal volume + Dead space)
B. Respiratory rate + (Tidal volume + Dead space)
C. Respiratory rate × (Tidal volume - Dead space)
D. Respiratory rate + (Tidal volume - Dead space)

88. Which of the following factors influence pulmonary ventilation?
A. Arterial PO_2
B. Arterial PCO_2
C. Arterial pH
D. All of the above

89. In protein, amino acids are joined covalently by:
A. Hydrogen bonds
B. Peptide bonds
C. Ionic bonds
D. Van der Waals interactions

90. Which of the following can be defined as electron or protein-transfer proteins having one or several heme groups?
A. Aminotransferases
B. Cytochromes
C. Isomerases
D. Vitamin B complex

91. The two main types of adrenergic receptors in the autonomic nervous system are:
A. Nicotinic and muscarinic
B. Alpha and gamma
C. Gamma and beta
D. Alpha and beta

92. Rods and cones of the retina are examples of:
A. Mechanoreceptors
B. Photoreceptors
C. Chemoreceptors
D. Thermoreceptors

93. Which enzyme below is an RNA-directed DNA polymerase?
A. RNA ligase

B. DNA polymerase
C. Reverse transcriptase
D. DNA ligase

94. Under normal conditions, oxygen is carried to the tissues almost entirely by:
A. Albumin
B. Hemoglobin
C. Insulin
D. Cytochrome C

95. Which structures listed below are the last small branches of the arterial system and act as control valves through which blood is released into the capillaries?
A. Venules
B. Arteries
C. Arterioles
D. Veins

96. Which of the following are complex lipids similar to fats, but with a phosphorus and nitrogen-containing compound replacing one of the fatty acid molecules?
A. Carbohydrates
B. Phospholipids
C. Steroids
D. Proteins

97. The liver releases glucose back into the circulating blood during exercise. Besides the skeletal muscle, what other organ takes up this extra glucose?
A. Kidneys
B. Heart
C. Brain
D. Lungs

98. The P wave of the normal electrocardiogram (ECG or EKG) represents:
A. Ventricular repolarization
B. Atrial repolarization
C. Ventricular depolarization
D. Atrial depolarization

99. The cardiac cycle is the period from the beginning of one heartbeat to the beginning of the next. How many phases does this cycle have?

A. One
B. Two
C. Three
D. Four

100. After food has become mixed with stomach (gastric) secretions, the resulting mixture that is passed from the stomach to the duodenum is called

A. Bile
B. Chyme
C. Mucin
D. Glycerol

101. Which compound listed below is important in fat metabolism?

A. Heparin
B. Choline
C. Thrombin
D. Serotonin

102. The complex process by which platelets, plasma, and coagulation factors interact to control bleeding is called?

A. Homeostasis
B. Hemostasis
C. Hemotherapy
D. Hemopoiesis

103. All of the following statements concerning chylomicrons are true EXCEPT:

A. They are the smallest of the lipoproteins
B. They are the least dense of the lipoproteins
C. They contain a high proportion of triacylglycerols
D. They are assembled in the intestinal mucosa as a means to transport dietary cholesterol and triacylglycerols to the rest of the body
E. They function to deliver dietary triacylglycerols to adipose tissue and muscle and dietary cholesterol to the liver

104. Black urine is a common finding in people with:
A. Phenylketonuria
B. Alkaptonuria
C. Cystinuria
D. Albinism

105. Which of the following is the most abundant glycosaminoglycan in the body?
A. Keratan sulfate
B. Hyaluronic acid
C. Dermatan sulfate
D. Chondroitin sulfate
E. Heparin sulfate
F. Heparin

106. A severe thiamine deficiency syndrome found in areas where polished rice is the major component of the diet is called
A. Pellagra
B. Beri-beri
C. Scurvy
D. Megaloblastic anemia

107. The enzyme glucose 6-phosphatase is found most abundantly in which organ listed below?
A. Brain
B. Lungs
C. Liver
D. Pancreas

108. Vitamin B is a collective term for:
A. Pyridoxine
B. Pyridoxal
C. Pyridoxamine
D. All of the above

109. The key regulatory enzyme for glycogen synthesis is:
A. Glycogen phosphorylase
B. Phosphoglucomutase
C. Glycogen synthase
D. Phosphofructokinase

110. The pitch of a sound is related mainly to which of the following characteristics of sound wave?
A. Amplitude of waves
B. Frequency of waves
C. Superimposed wave
D. Secondary waves
E. Length of waves

111. Sensory impulses travel via sensory (afferent, or ascending) neural pathways to the sensory cortex in the parietal lobe of the brain where they are interpreted. Which pathway in the somatosensory system listed below processes sensations of temperature, pain and light touch?
A. The fasciculus gracilis and fasciculus coneatus tracts
B. Spinothalamic tract

112. The action potential is an explosion of electrical activity that is created by a:
A. Polarizing current
B. Depolarizing current
C. Repolarizing current
D. All of the above

113. Which intraocular structure listed below contains the nerves that sense light and the blood supply that nourishes them?
A. Iris
B. Pupil
C. Choroid
D. Retina

114. Hyperopia (far sightedness) is corrected with which type of lens?
A. Convex lens
B. Concave lens
C. Cylindric lens
D. Toric lens

115. Which GI hormone listed below is secreted from the G cells (enteroendocrine cells) of the stomach in response to a meal?

A. Gastrin
B. Cholecystokinin (CCK)
C. Secretin
D. Gastric inhibitory peptide (GIP)

116. All of the following are actions of glucocorticoids (cortisol) EXCEPT:
A. Stimulation of gluconeogenesis
B. Anti-inflammatory effects
C. Stimulation of fat deposition and inhibition of lipolysis
D. Suppression of the immune response
E. Maintenance of vascular responsiveness to catecholamines

117. All of the following statements concerning heparin are true EXCEPT:
A. Unlike other glycosaminologycans that are extracellular compounds, heparin is an intracellular component of mast cells that the arteries, especially in the liver, lungs, and skin
B. It serves as a powerful anticoagulant
C. It is used in the treatment of certain types of lung, blood vessel, and heart disorders, and during or after certain types of surgery (open heart or bypass surgeries)
D. Small quantities are produced by basophil cells of the blood
E. It is usually found in large quantities in the blood

118. The most calcified of the dental tissues is:
A. Dentin
B. Enamel
C. Cementum
D. Pulp

119. Elastin is composed of all of the following amino acids EXCEPT:
A. Glycine
B. Hydroxylysine
C. Proline
D. Lysine
E. Hydroxyproline

120. Collagen contains approximately 1000 amino acids, one-third of which are:

A. Arginine
B. Glycine
C. Cysteine
D. Histidine

121. The synapse between axons of motor neurons and skeletal muscle is called a:

A. Gap junction
B. Costochondral junction
C. Neuromuscular junction
D. Mucocutaneous junction

122. Glucagon has all of the following actions EXCEPT:

A. Increases the blood glucose concentration
B. Increases blood fatty acid and ketoacid concentration
C. Decreases blood amino acid concentration
D. Increases urea production

123. The degenerate nature of the genetic code implies what?

A. That many amino acids are designated by more than one codon (triplet)
B. That only one amino acid is designated by one codon (triplet)
C. Neither of the above
D. Both of the above

124. The normal plasma concentration of calcium varies between:

A. 3.0 and 5.0 mg/dl
B. 5.5 and 7.5 mg/dl
C. 8.5 and 10.5 mg/dl
D. 15.0 and 20.0 mg/dl

125. Within the spinal cord, the H-shaped mass of gray matter is divided into horns, which consist mainly of neuron cell bodies. Cell bodies in the posterior (dorsal) horn relay:

A. Voluntary motor impulses
B. Reflex motor impulses
C. Sensory impulses
D. All of the above

126. Ammonia is produced from the metabolism of a variety of compounds. Which compound listed below is quantitatively the most important source of ammonia?

A. Glutamine
B. Amino acids
C. Amines
D. Purines and pyrimidines

127. The ventricles are completely depolarized during which isoelectric portion of the electrocardiogram (ECG)?

A. QRS complex
B. Q-T interval
C. S-T segment
D. T wave

128. Blood flow is directly proportional to the pressure difference between the two ends of the vessel but is inversely proportional to the fractional resistance to the blood flow through a vessel. This relationship can be expressed as:

A. $\text{Flow} = \text{pressure} \times \text{resistance}$

B. $\text{Flow} = \dfrac{\text{resistance}}{\text{pressure}}$

C. $\text{Flow} = \dfrac{\text{pressure}}{\text{resistance}}$

D. None of the above

129. Steroid hormones include all of the following EXCEPT:

A. Cortisol
B. Progesterone
C. Insulin
D. Testosterone
E. Estrogen
F. Aldosterone

130. The granulose cells in the corpus luteum produce which two hormones listed below?

A. Prolactin
B. Progesterone
C. Estrogen
D. Oxytocin

131. Almost all secretions by the pituitary gland are controlled by signals transmitted from which of the following:

A. The Cerebrum
B. The Medulla
C. The Hypothalamus
D. The Pons

132. Caries activity is directly proportional to all of the following EXCEPT:

A. The consistency of fermentable carbohydrates ingested
B. The quantity of fermentable carbohydrates ingested
C. The frequency of ingesting fermentable carbohydrates
D. The oral retention of fermentable carbohydrates ingested

133. Which of the following is considered to be the normal hemoglobin?

A. Hemoglobin A
B. Hemoglobin C
C. Hemoglobin H
D. Hemoglobin S
E. Hemoglobin M

134. The kidneys regulate acid-base balance by the:

A. Secretion of bicarbonate ions (HCO_3) into the renal tubules and the reabsorption of hydrogen ions (H)
B. Secretion of hydrogen ions (H) into the renal tubules and the reabsorption of bicarbonate ions (HCO_3)
C. Secretion of both hydrogen (H) and bicarbonate ions (HCO_3) into the renal tubules
D. Reabsorption of both hydrogen (H) and bicarbonate ions (HCO_3)

135. Hydrolysis of DNA will yield all of the following EXCEPT:

A. Ribose
B. Phosphoric acid
C. Deoxyribose
D. Nitrogenous bases (adenine, guanine, thymine, and cytosine)

136. Changes in blood pressure are due mainly to alterations in resistance by the:

A. Veins

B. Venules
C. Capillaries
D. Arterioles

137. Biotin is :
A. The precursor of FAD
B. Required for the carboxylation of acetyl CoA, an intermediate in fatty acid synthesis
C. A cofactor required for the hydroxylation of proline and lysine
D. A fat-soluble vitamin

138. Osteoblasts that are actively depositing bone matrix secrete large quantities of which enzyme listed below?
A. Creatinine phosphate
B. Hyaluronidase
C. Alkaline phosphatase
D. Acid phosphatase

139. All of the following statements concerning vitamin D are true EXCEPT :
A. It is involved in calcium metabolism
B. 25-hydroxycholecalciferol is the active form
C. Vitamin D and parathyroid hormone both increase serum calcium
D. A deficiency causes a net demineralization of bone resulting in rickets in children and osteomalacia in adults

140. The normal pH of pancreatic juice is :
A. 1.0 to 2.0
B. 4.0 to 6.0
C. 8.0 to 8.3
D. 9 to 10.5

141. Which of the following are sources of high-energy phosphate that keep the ATP pool filled for muscle contraction?
A. Creatine phosphate
B. Glycolysis of glycogen
C. Cellular respiration in the mitochondria of the muscle fibers
D. All of the above

142. All of the following statements are true EXCEPT.
A. Preganglionic neurons have their cell bodies in the CNS and synapse in autonomic ganglia
B. Sympathetic ganglia are located in the paravertebral chain
C. Cholinergic neurons, whether in the sympathetic or parasympathetic nervous system, release norepinephrine as the neurotransmitter
D. The majority of sympathetic postganglionic neurons are adrenergic

143. All of the major anterior pituitary hormones except one exert their effects by stimulating "target glands". Which of the following does not affect a "target gland"?
A. Prolactin
B. Thyroid-stimulating hormone (TSH)
C. Luteinizing hormone (LH)
D. Growth hormone (GH)
E. Follicle-stimulating hormone (FSH)
F. Adrenocorticotropic hormone (ACTH)

144. All of the following are the cardinal symptoms of diabetes EXCEPT:
A. Polydipsia
B. Polyuria
C. High blood pressure
D. Polyphagia
E. Weight loss
F. Loss of strength

145. The basal ganglia consists of :
A. Caudate nucleus
B. Putamen
C. Globus pallidus
D. Substantia nigra
E. Subthalamic nucleus
F. All of the above

146. Which of the following statements concerning the two principal laws of thermodynamics are true?
A. They apply only to closed systems, that is entities with which there can be no exchange of energy

B. The first law says that the total quantity of energy in the universe remains constant (this is the principle of the conservation of energy)
C. The second law states that the quality of this energy is degraded irreversibly (this is the principle of the degradation of energy)
D. The second law, known as Carnot's principle, is controlled by the concept of entropy
E. All of the above statements are true

147. All of the following statements concerning prostaglandins are true EXCEPT:
A. They have a very short half-life
B. They generally act locally on or near the tissue that produced them
C. They are synthesized only in the liver and the adrenal cortex
D. The common precursor of the prostaglandins is arachidonic acid (an unsaturated fatty acid)
E. Their synthesis can be inhibited by a number of unrelated compounds including aspirin and cortisol

148. All of the following statements concerning enamel hypoplasia are true EXCEPT :
A. It is a defect in the mineralization of the formed enamel matrix
B. The enamel of primary and permanent teeth appear pitted
C. Radiographically the enamel is either absent or very thin over tips of cusps and interproximal areas
D. It can be caused by nutritional deficiencies

149. Ovulation occurs :
A. 7 days before menses, regardless of cycle length
B. 14 days before menses, regardless of cycle length
C. 18 days before menses, regardless of cycle length
D. 21 days before menses, regardless of cycle length

150. When the lungs are in the resting position, the pressure within them, which is called the intrapulmonary pressure, is equivalent to which of the following?
A. Blood pressure

B. Critical pressure
C. Atmospheric pressure
D. Transmural pressure

151. All of the following are causes of metabolic alkalosis EXCEPT :
A. Use of diuretics (thiazides, furosemide, ethacrynic acid)
B. Vomiting
C. Chronic renal failure
D. Overactive adrenal gland (Cushing's syndrome or use of corticosteroids)

152. All of the following are signs indicative of a deficiency of proteins EXCEPT :
A. Lack of vigor and stamina
B. Weakness
C. Mental depression
D. Xerostomia
E. Poor resistance to infection
F. Impaired wound healing
G. Slow recovery from disease

153. Epinephrine and norepinephrine are secreted from the
A. Thyroid gland
B. Adrenal medulla
C. Pineal gland
D. Adrenal cortex

154. All of the following statements concerning transamination reactions are true EXCEPT:
A. These reactions involve the transfer of an amino group from one amino acid to an o-keto acid
B. The enzymes that catalyze these reactions are known as transaminases or aminotransferases
C. Glutamate and a-ketoglutarate are often involved in these reactions, serving as one of the amino acid/-keto acid pairs
D. Pyridoxal phosphate (PLP) which is derived from vitamin B, serves as the cofactor for these reactions
E. All amino acids participate in these reactions at some point in their catabolism

155. Glycosaminoglycans are :

A. Disaccharides
B. Homopolysaccharides
C. Heteropolysaccharides
D. Monosaccharides

156. All of the following statements concerning addison's disease (adrenocortical insufficiency) are true EXCEPT:

A. It results when underactive adrenal glands produce insufficient amounts of corticosteroids
B. It usually occurs in young adults and affects males more often than females
C. In 30% of people with Addison's the adrenal glands are destroyed by a cancer, amyloidosis, an infection such as tuberculosis, or another identifiable disease
D. In the other 70% of people with Addison's disease, the cause isn't known for certain, but is suspected that the adrenal glands are destroyed by an autoimmune reaction
E. It is characterized by hypotensed pigmentation of the skin; low levels of serum sodium chloride and dicarbonate with an elevation of serum potassium

157. Fatty acid breakdown (catabolism) occurs where?

A. In the cytosol
B. In the mitochondria
C. In the nucleus
D. None of the above

158. The branch point molecule of glycolysis is :

A. Glucose 6-phosphate
B. Glyceraldehyde 3-phosphate
C. Phosphoenolpyruvate
D. Pyruvate

159. Which of the following contribute adrenergic fibers to the heart and affect the heart's irritability?

A. First four thoracic spinal nerves (accessory nerves)
B. Left vagus nerve
C. Right vagus nerve
D. Trigeminal nerve

160. Which of the following substances is filtered but not reabsorbed by the kidney tubules?

A. Sodium chloride
B. Inulin
C. Para-aminohippurate (PAH)
D. Glucose

161. Somatostatin inhibits are secretion of all of the following hormones EXCEPT:

A. Insulin
B. Glucagons
C. Antidiuretic hormone (ADH)
D. Gastrin

162. Oral contraceptives inhibit:

A. Follicle growth
B. Ovulation
C. Follicle formation
D. Puberty

163. All of the following statements concerning the citric acid cycle (Krebs' cycle) are true EXCEPT:

A. The cycle starts with the 4-carbon compound oxaloacetate, adds 2 carbons from acetyl CoA, loses 2 carbons as CO, and regenerates the 4-carbon compound oxaloacetate
B. The pyruvate that enters this cycle is generated by the glycolysis of glucose or protein catabolism
C. This cycle is controlled by regulation of several enzyme activities. The most important of these regulated enzymes are citrate synthtase, isocitrate dehydrogenase, and "α-ketoglutarate dehydrogenase complex
D. The enzymes involved in the citric acid cycle are found in the cytosol
E. Aspartic acid and oxaloacetic acid are interconvertible (G) For each molecule of glucose metabolized 2 molecules of ATP are formed.

164. Sucrose, lactose, and maltose are common:

A. Monosaccharides
B. Disaccharides

C. Oligosaccharides
D. Polysaccharides

165. The use of fat instead of glucose for energy leads to an excess of ketone bodies. This condition disturbs normal acid-base balance and homeostatic mechanisms, leading to:
A. Glomerulonephritis
B. Megaloblastic anemia
C. Ketosis
D. Scurvy

166. There are three separate types of RNA, each of which plays an independent and entirely different role in protein synthesis. Which type transports activated amino acids to the ribosomes to be used in assembling the protein molecule?
A. Messenger RNA
B. Transfer RNA
C. Ribosomal RNA
D. None of the above

167. Which type of shock listed below is most often associated with severe trauma and reactive peripheral vasodilation?
A. Hypovolemic shock
B. Cardiogenic shock
C. Septic shock
D. Neurogenic shock
E. Anaphylactic shock

168. Which enzyme listed below catalyzes the oxidative deamination of glutamate?
A. Histidase
B. Aspartate aminotransferase (AST)
C. Glutamate dehydrogenase
D. Alanine aminotransferase (ALT)

169. The aerobic breakdown of a single molecule of glucose produces a net profit of how many ATP?
A. 20-24 ATP
B. 30-32 ATP
C. 36-38 ATP
D. 44-48 ATP

170. A major role of proteins is to serve as:
A. Bile salts
B. Enzymes
C. Fatty acids
D. Ketone bodies

171. All of the following are functions of zinc EXCEPT:
A. It stabilizes cell membranes
B. It functions in taste acuity
C. It is needed in collagen formation / healing
D. It is involved in vitamin B_{12} formation
E. It is essential in cell-mediated immunity

172. All of the following statements concerning muscle spindles are true EXCEPT:
A. They are found within the belly of muscles
B. They consists of small, encapsulated intrafusal fibers and run in parallel with the main muscle fibers (extrafusal fibers)
C. The finer the movement required, the lesser the number of muscle spindles in a muscle
D. They detect both static and dynamic changes in muscle length

173. Muscle cells use which of the following to store energy?
A. Creatine phosphate
B. FADH2
C. NADH
D. Phosphoneolpyruvate

174. Which of the following is the active form of vitamin D?
A. Cholecalciferol
B. 25-hydroxycholecalciferol
C. 1,25-dihydroxycholecalciferol
D. 24,25-dihydroxycholecalciferol

175. The factors that determine how rapidly a gas will pass through the respiratory membrane include:
A. The thickness of the membrane
B. The surface area of the membrane
C. The solubility of the gas in the substance of the membrane

D. The pressure difference between the two sides of the membrane
E. All of the above

176. The volume of air remaining in the lungs after a maximal expiration is called the:
A. Vital capacity (VC)
B. Tidal volume (TV)
C. Residual volume (RV)
D. Functional residual capacity (FRC)

177. The plasma protein of the highest concentration in plasma is:
A. Globulins (alpha, beta, and gamma)
B. Fibrinogen
C. Albumin
D. None of the above

178. All amino acids found in proteins are of the:
A. D-configuration
B. L-configuration
C. F-configuration
D. C-configuration

179. Which of the following is the cause of the "positive" afterpotential which occurs for a few milliseconds after the action potential is over?
A. Many sodium channels remain open for several milliseconds after repolarization of the membrane is complete
B. All potassium channels remain closed for several milliseconds after repolarization of the membrane is complete
C. Many potassium channels remain open for several milliseconds after repolarization of the membrane is complete
D. All sodium and potassium channels remain closed for several milliseconds after repolarization of the membrane is complete

180. Which receptors listed below are sensitive to pressure, pain, and chemical changes in the internal environment of the body?
A. Exteroceptors

B. Interoceptors
C. Both of the above
D. None of the above

181. Which blood group listed below has neither antigen A or B?
A. A
B. B
C. O
D. AB

182. The function of arteries is to:
A. Act as control valves through which blood is released into the capillaries
B. Exchange fluid, nutrients, electrolytes, hormones, and other substances
C. Transport blood under high pressure to the tissues
D. Act as conduit for the transport of blood from the tissues back to the heart

183. All of the following statements concerning fatty acid synthesis are true EXCEPT:
A. Fatty acid synthesis involves two carbon additions from acetyl-CoA and an acyl protein (ACP)
B. The important step in fatty acid synthesis is the first one in which acetyl-CoA, carbon dioxide, and bicarbonate form malonyl-CoA
C. Fatty acid synthesis is not a simple reversal of " β-oxidation used for the catabolism of fatty acids
D. Fatty acid synthesis takes place in the mitochondria while fatty acid breakdown (catabolism) occurs in the cytosol (cytoplasm)

184. Gluconeogenesis, which occurs mainly in the liver, is the synthesis of glucose from compounds that are not carbohydrates. Which organ below is a minor contributor of newly synthesized glucose molecules?
A. Appendix
B. gallbladder
C. Kidneys
D. Pancreas

185. Which valve below is composed of three cusps that prevent a backflow of blood from the aorta into the left ventricle during ventricular relaxation?

A. Pulmonary valve
B. Tricuspid valve
C. Mitral valve
D. Aortic valve

186. The stretch receptors of the atria that elicit the Bainbridge reflex transmit their afferent signals through the:

A. Trigeminal nerves to the medulla of the brain
B. Vagus nerves to the medulla of the brain
C. Facial nerves to the medulla of the brain
D. glossopharyngeal nerves to the medulla of the brain

187. Deficiency of which hormone listed below causes hypocalcemia and hyperphosphatemia?

A. Aldosterone
B. Testosterone
C. Follicle-stimulating hormone (FSH)
D. Parathyroid hormone (PTH)

188. Hemoglobin:

A. Carries carbon dioxide to the cells from the lungs and oxygen away from the cells to the lungs
B. Carries carbon monoxide to the cells from the lungs and carbon dioxide away from the cells to the lungs
C. Carries oxygen to the cells from the lungs and carbon dioxide away from the cells to the lungs
D. Carries carbon monoxide to the cells from the lungs and oxygen away from the cells to the lungs

189. Most of the glomerular filtrate is reabsorbed in the:

A. Descending (thin) loop of Henle
B. Distal convoluted tubule
C. Proximal convoluted tubule
D. Ascending (thick) loop of Henle

190. All of the following are clinical features of hyperthyroidism EXCEPT:

A. Restlessness, irritability, and fatigability

B. Heat intolerance (sweating)
C. Tachycardia (a rapid heat rate)
D. Weight gain
E Fine hair
F Diarrhea
G. Tremor (shakiness)

191. The majority of glycosaminoglycans in the body are linked to core proteins, forming:
A. Glycoproteins
B. Glycolipids
C. Proteoglycans
D. None of the above

192. Which cardiac muscle listed below has a longer refractory period?
A. Ventricular muscle
B. Atrial muscle
C. Bundle of his
D. Purkinje fibers

193. All of the following statements concerning thyroid hormone are true EXCEPT:
A. Collectively referred to as thyroid hormone, T3 and T4 are the body's major metabolic hormones
B. It regulates metabolism by speeding cellular respiration
C. T_3 (tri-iodothyronine) has several times the biologic activity of T4 (thyroxine)
D. It stimulates bone maturation as a result of ossification and fusion of the growth plates
E. It decreases glycogenolysis, gluconeogenesis, and lipolysis

194. Which of the following vitamins is required for blood clotting?
A. Vitamin A
B. Vitamin K
C. Vitamin E
D. Vitamin D

195. A Competitive inhibitor of an enzyme;
A. Increases Km without affecting Vmax
B. Decreases Km without affecting Vmax
C. Increases Vmax without affecting Km
D. Decreases both Vmax and Km

196. Vitamin A (retinol) is:
A. Required for blood clotting
B. Required for the hydroxylation of proline and lysine residues in the precursor of collagen
C. Required for formation of the visual pigments of rod and cone cells
D. Required for synthesis of cofactor required for reactions in the oxidation of pyruvate to carbon dioxide and water

197. Gastric secretions include all of them except
A. Mucus
B. Hydrochloric acid (HCL)
C. Pepsinogen
D. Ptyalin
E. Intrinsic factor

198. Isotopes of an element:
A. Have different chemical properties but the same weights
B. Have the same chemical properties but different weights
C. Have different chemical properties and weights
D. Have the same chemical properties and weights

199. The two types of cholinergic receptors in the autonomic nervous system are:
A. Nicotinic and alpha
B. Alpha and beta
C. Nicotinic and muscarinic
D. Muscarinic and beta

200. Saltatory conduction serves to:
A. Increase the velocity of nerve transmission along myelinated fibers
B. Conserve energy since the sodium and potassium pumps have to reestablish concentration differences only at the nodes of Ranvier

C. Allow repolarization to occur with little transfer of ions
D. All of the above

201. Which of the following are heat-generating mechanisms?
A. Increased metabolism
B. Shivering
C. Vasoconstriction of cutaneous blood vessels
D. All of the above

202. Histamine causes all of the following responses EXCEPT:
A. Bronchoconstriction
B. Increased blood pressure
C. Increased vascular permeability (particularly in capillaries and venules)
D. Secretion of HCl
E. Vasodilation (particularly the arterioles)

203. All of the following are formed via the cyclo-oxygenase pathway EXCEPT:
A. Prostaglandins
B. Prostacyclin
C. Leukotrienes
D. Thromboxanes

204. Tyrosine is produced by hydroxylation of the essential amino acid:
A. Histidine
B. Lysine
C. Valine
D. Phenylalanine

205. All of the following statements are true EXCEPT:
A. During early childhood, a boy does not secrete gonadotropins, and thus has little circulating testosterone
B. Secretion of gonadotropins from the adrenal gland, which usually occurs between the ages 16 and 20, marks the onset of puberty
C. These pituitary gonadotropins stimulate testes functioning as well as testosterone secretion

D. During puberty the penis and testes enlarge and the male reaches full adult sexual and reproductive capability
E. Puberty also marks the development of male secondary sexual characteristics

206. Which of the following is a glycoprotein hormone (10% carbohydrate) that is synthesized by the thyroid follicular cell and iodinated once it has been synthesized?
A. Glucagon
B. Cortisol
C. Thyroglobulin
D. Aldosterone

207. The activity level of which enzyme listed below controls the rate of glycolysis?
A. Aldolase
B. Phosphoglucose isomerase
C. Phosphofructokinase
D. Triose phosphate isomerase

208. The quantitative relation between the concentration of a week acid (HA) and its conjugate base (A) is described by the:
A. Arrhenius equation
B. Henderson-Hasselbalch equation
C. Bohr equation
D. Einthoven equation

209. Of the 20 amino acids commonly found in proteins, how many are not essential in the adult diet because they can be synthesized in the body?
A. 5
B. 9
C. 11
D. 18

210. Simple sugars are also called:
A. Monosaccharides
B. Disaccharides
C. Oligosaccharides
D. Polysaccharides

211. Gaucher's disease is a disorder of lipid metabolism caused by a deficiency of:

A. Hexosaminidase A
B. Sphingomyelinase
C. Glucocerebrosidase
D. α-L- iduronidase

212. Which of the following is the major source of Acetyl CoA for fatty acid synthesis?

A. Creatinine
B. Paraaminohippuric acid (PAH)
C. Glucose
D. Cholesterol

213. All of the following enzymes participate in what anaerobic process? Hint: it occurs in the cytosol of all cells of the body:

- Hexokinase
- Phosphoglucose isomerase
- Phosphofructokinase
- Aldolase
- Triose phosphate isomerase
- Glyceraldehyde 3-phosphate dehydrogenase
- Phosphoglycerate kinase
- Phosphoglyceromutase
- Enolase
- Pyruvate kinase

A. Glycolysis
B. Kreb's cycle
C. Respiratory chain
D. TCA cycle

214. Venous return is the blood returning to the heart via the inferior and superior vena cavae. Which of the following assists venous return?

A. The contraction of skeletal muscles
B. The pressure changes in the thorax and abdomen during breathing
C. The presence of valves
D. All of the above

215. The bundle of His arises in the:
A. SA node
B. AV node
C. Right ventricle
D. Left ventricle

216. The peptide hormone principally involved in the digestion of lipids is:
A. Serotonin
B. Enterogastrone
C. Enkephalins
D. Somatostatin

217. The oxidation of one NADH by the electron transport chain leads to the formation of how many ATP?
A. 1
B. 2
C. 3
D. 4

218. All of the following are reducing sugars EXCEPT:
A. Lactose
B. Maltose
C. Sucrose
D. Glucose

219. The kidneys normally excrete:
A. 1 to 2 L of urine per day
B. 10 to 20 L of urine per day
C. 50 to 75 L of urine per day
D. 100 to 150 L of urine per day

220. A complete DNA molecule consists of two polynucleotide chains or strands that:
A. Are parallel
B. Are perpendicular
C. Are antiparallel
D. Are antiperpendicular

221. Which part of the brainstem listed below serves as an autonomic reflex center to maintain homeostasis, regulating respiratory, vasomotor, and cardiac functions?

A. Midbrain
B. Pons
C. Medulla oblongata
D. None of the above

222. Which two situations listed below will excite the respiratory neurons and increase respiration/

A. A decrease in hydrogen ion concentration in the arterial blood
B. A decrease in the PCO_2 of arterial blood
C. An increase in hydrogen ion concentration in the arterial blood
D. An increase in the PCO_2 of arterial blood

223. Which receptors below are stimulated by distension of the lungs?

A. Irritant receptors
B. J receptors
C. Joint and muscle receptors
D. Lung stretch receptors

224. All of the following statements concerning muscle fibers are true EXCEPT:

A. Fast-twitch fibers are about twice as large in diameter
B. Slow-twitch fibers are mainly organized for endurance, especially for the generation of aerobic energy
C. The enzymes of the aerobic metabolic system are considerably more active in slow-twitch fibers than in fast-twitch fibers
D. Fast-twitch fibers contain more mitochondria and myoglobin
E. Fast-twitch fibers can deliver extreme amounts of power for a few seconds to a minute or so, whereas, slow-twitch fibers deliver a prolonged strength of contraction over many minutes or hours

225. Fluoride (fluorine) is found primarily in:

A. Milk

B. Drinking water
C. Seafood
D. Eggs

226. An isotonic solution is:
A. A solution that when placed on the outside of a cell will cause osmosis out of the cell
B. A solution that when placed on the outside of a cell will cause osmosis into the cell
C. A solution that when placed on the outside of a cell will not cause osmosis
D. None of the above

227. A reflex is:
A. A delayed response to a stimulus
B. An automatic response to a stimulus
C. None of the above
D. Both of the above

228. All of the following are major minerals EXCEPT:
A. Calcium
B. Chloride
C. Copper
D. Phosphorous
E. Magnesium

229. Many of the digestive proteases are produced and secreted as inactive:
A. Carbohydrates
B. Lipids
C. Zymogens
D. Ketone bodies

230. ATP is produced via:
A. Substrate-level phosphorylation
B. Electron-transport phosphorylation
C. Photophosphorylation
D. All of the above

231. Which member of the electron transport chain listed below is also called Coenzyme Q?
A. Flavin mononucleotide (FMN)

B. Ubiquinone
C. Cytochromes b and c
D. Cytochromes a + b

232. All of the following statements concerning myoglobin are true EXCEPT:
A. It is a heme-protein present in heart and skeletal muscle
B. It functions both as a reservoir for oxygen and as an oxygen carrier
C. It decreases the rate of transport of oxygen within the muscle cell
D. It consists of a single polypeptide chain that is structurally similar to the individual polypeptide chains of the hemoglobin molecule

233. The difference in electrical charge between the inside and the outside of the cell membrane of an unstimulated (nonconducting) neuron is called the:
A. Relative refractory potential
B. Action potential
C. Resting membrane potential
D. Absolute refractory potential

234. The autonomic nervous system (ANS) is a set of efferent pathways from the central nervous system that innervates and regulates all of the following EXCEPT:
A. Glands (both exocrine and endocrine)
B. Cardiac muscle
C. Skeletal muscle
D. Smooth muscle
E. Visceral organs

235. Glutamate is derived form a-ketoglutarate. All of the following amino acids can be derived from glutamate EXCEPT:
A. Asparagine
B. Glutamine
C. Proline
D. Arginine

236. The sequence of amino acids in a protein is called the:
A. Primary structure

B. Secondary structure
C. Tertiary structure
D. Quaternary structure

237. The cyclic nucleotides cGMP and cAMP are called:
A. Neurotransmitters
B. Second messengers
C. Third messengers
D. Hormones

238. Which cellular structure listed below is composed of rRNA and protein?
A. Mitochondria
B. Golgi apparatus
C. Ribosomes
D. Lysosomes

239. The unpleasant sensation of difficulty in breathing is called:
A. Hypercapnea
B. Dyspnea
C. Apnea
D. Orthopnea

240. Which part of the ear is also called the tympanic cavity?
A. Inner ear
B. Middle ear
C. External ear
D. None of the above

241. Which of the following are the two main types of intrafusal fibers that are encapsulated in sheaths to form muscle spindles?
A. Nuclear bag fibers
B. Nuclear pipe fibers
C. Nuclear chain fibers
D. Nuclear rope fibers

242. The method of measuring heat loss or energy loss is called:
A. Enthalpy
B. Hydropathy index
C. Calorimetry
D. Entropy

243. All of the following will promote the release of oxygen from oxyhemoglobin (the hemoglobin dissociation curve will shift to the right) EXCEPT:

A. Increased carbon dioxide concentration (PCO)
B. Increased body temperature
C. Decrease in the pH
D. Increase in the pH

244. The pulmonary circuit is characterized by:

A. High pressure and low resistance
B. Low pressure and high resistance
C. Low pressure and low resistance
D. High pressure and high resistance

245. All of the following bonds are considered to be weak bonds EXCEPT:

A. Hydrogen bonds
B. Ionic bonds
C. Covalent bonds
D. van der Walls interactions

246. How do local anesthetics effect the nerve membrane?

A. They increase potassium flux
B. They increase the membrane excitability by increasing the membrane's permeability to sodium ions
C. They decrease the membrane's permeability to sodium ions and reduce the membrane excitability
D. They increase the calcium and chloride flux

247. Which vitamin below is synthesized only by microorganisms and is not present in plants?

A. Vitamin A
B. Cobalamin (vitamin B_{12})
C. Vitamin C
D. Vitamin E

248. All of the following statements concerning allosteric enzymes are true EXCEPT:

A. They frequently catalyze a committed step early in a metabolic pathway

B. They often have two or more subunits each with substrate binding sites that exhibit cooperativity
C. Allosteric activators cause the enzyme to bind substrate more readily
D. Allosteric inhibitors cause the enzyme to bind substrate less readily
E. They follow the Michaelis-Mention kinetics

249. The volume of blood pumped per minute by each ventricle is the:
A. Total peripheral resistance (TPR)
B. Cardiac output (CO)
C. Stroke volume (SV)
D. Heart rate (HR)

250. The first heart sound corresponds to the closure of the:
A. Semilunar valves
B. Pulmonary valve
C. Aortic valve
D. Atrioventricular valves

251. Which blood lipoprotein listed below is the most dense?
A. Chylomicrons
B. VLDLs
C. LDLs
D. HDLs

252. All of the following statements concerning the urea cycle are true EXCEPT:
A. The two nitrogen atoms that are incorporated into urea enter the cycle as ammonia and aspartate
B. Urea is produced by the hydrolysis of ornithine
C. The first two reactions leading to the synthesis of urea occur in the mitochondria, whereas the remaining cycle enzymes are located in the cytosol.
D. The urea that is formed in the urea cycle is passed via the blood stream to the kidneys and is excreted into the urine

253. Which mineral listed below is important in the formation of hemoglobin?
A. Sodium

B. Potassium
C. Iron
D. Magnesium

254. Acetyl CoA is used by the liver for the synthesis of:
A. Cholesterol
B. Bile salts
C. Ketone bodies
D. Hormones

255. All of the following statements concerning vitamin E are true EXCEPT:
A. It is also called tocopherol
B. It serves as an antioxidant
C. It prevents free radicals from oxidizing compounds such as polyunsaturated fatty acids
D. It is the most toxic of the fat-soluble vitamins

256. Which amylase listed below converts starch to maltose and dextrins?
A. Alpha-amylase
B. Beta-amylase
C. Glucamylase
D. All of the above

257. Diabetes insipidus:
A. Results from the decreased production of glucagons
B. Results from the decreased production of antidiuretic hormone (vasopressin)
C. Results from the decreased production of growth hormone
D. Results from the decreased production of thyroid hormone

258. Dextrans are:
A. Polysaccharides of fructose obtained from yeast and bacteria
B. Polysaccharides of galactose obtained from yeast and bacteria
C. Polysaccharides of glucose obtained from yeast and bacteria
D. Polysaccharides of ribose obtained from yeast and bacteria

259. Gastric secretion is said to occur in three phases. Which of the following is not one of those phases?

A. Cephalic phase
B. Caudal phase
C. Gastric phase
D. Intestinal phase

260. Important functions of the liver in protein metabolism include:
A. Deamination of amino acids
B. Formation of urea for removal of ammonia from the body fluids
C. Formation of plasma proteins
D. The ability to synthesize certain amino acids and other important chemical compounds from amino acids
E. All of the above

261. Which hormone listed below is often called the "stress hormone?
A. Growth hormone (GH)
B. Thyroid-stimulating hormone (TSH)
C. Adrenocorticotropic hormone (ACTH)
D. Follicle-stimulating hormone (FSH)

262. The volume of blood expelled by the ventricles of the heart is called what?
A. Stroke volume
B. Cardiac output
C. Residual capacity
D. Reserve volume

263. Cardiac output, blood viscosity, blood volume, and peripheral resistance are all factors involved in the maintenance of what?
A. Diastolic arterial blood pressure
B. Aortic blood pressure
C. Systolic arterial blood pressure
D. Pulse pressure

264. Which circulation is most of the blood volume of the body found in?
A. Systemic

B. Pulmonary
C. No difference in blood volume between the two circulations
D. Brain

265. Which structures below act as control valves through which blood is released into the capillaries?
A. Venules
B. Arterioles
C. Veins
D. Arteries
E. Capillaries

266. Where is the resistance the greatest of any part of the systemic circulation?
A. Aorta
B. Arterioles
C. Veins
D. Capillaries

267. Standard limb lead 1 of the ECG represents cardiac potential differences as they occur between which two limbs?
A. Left arm and left leg
B. Right arm and right leg
C. Right arm and left arm
D. Right arm and left leg

268. Under normal circumstances, what is the major factor determining the cardiac output?
A. Stroke volume
B. Heart rate
C. Rate of venous return

269. Which enzyme affects the intermolecular transfer of amino groups within the myocardium and may increase as a result of myocardial infarction and liver damage?
A. Serum glutamic-pyruvic transaminase (SGPT)
B. Serum glutamate decarboxylase
C. Serum glutamic-oxaloacetic transaminase (SGOT)
D. None of the above

270. Diastole begins with the onset of which heart sound?
A. First
B. Second
C. Third
D. Fourth

271. What is the neurotransmitter at the motor end plates (neuromuscular junctions) between nerve and striated muscle?
A. Norepinephrine
B. Acetylcholine
C. Neostigmine
D. Physiostigmine

272. Calcium ions trigger contraction of muscles by binding to what?
A. Actin
B. Tropomyosin
C. Troponin
D. Melanin

273. The organ of Corti is found where?
A. Inner ear
B. Outer ear
C. Eyeball
D. Testes

274. Stimulation of the parasympathetic nerves excites the papillary sphincter, thereby decreasing the papillary aperture; this process is referred to as what?
A. Miosis
B. Mydriasis
C. Epistaxis
D. Astigmatism

275. A sensory nerve ending that responds to stimuli originating from within the body regarding movement and spatial position is called what?
A. Exteroceptor
B. Interoceptor

C. Proprioceptor
D. Neurocepturs

276. What is considered to be the most vital part of the entire brain and mediates the following reflexes?

- Blinking
- Swallowing
- Vomiting
- Coughing

A. Medulla oblongata
B. Cerebellum
C. Hypothalamus
D. Pons

277. Most of the nonessential amino acids derive their alpha-amino groups from which of the following?
A. Glutamate
B. Pyruvate
C. Oxaloacetate
D. Sucrose

278. Which two amino acids have sulfur containing side chains?
A. Lysine
B. Cysteine
C. Arginine
D. Glutamate
E. Methionine

279. Urea is synthesized where?
A. Kidney
B. Liver
C. Intestines
D. Gallbladder

280. A fluid into which normal body cells can be placed without causing either swelling or shrinkage of cells is said to be what?
A. Hypertonic
B. Isotonic
C. Hypotonic
D. Osmotic

281. Which of the following solutions has an osmotic pressure different from all the others?

A. 1 M glucose
B. 1 M sodium chloride
C. 1 M potassium nitrate
D. None of the above

282. Which of the following mechanisms explains how a single input signal to many neurons, lasting less than one millisecond, can be converted into a sustained output signal lasting many milliseconds?

A. Inhibition
B. Peripheral resistance
C. Synaptic delay
D. End-plate delay

283. Which muscle has a longer refractory period?

A. Ventricular muscle
B. Atrial muscle
C. Both are the same
D. None of the above

284. The average resting membrane potential of nerve and skeletal muscle fibers of mammals is what?

A. (+) 85 millivolts
B. (-) 85 millivolts
C. (-) 45 millivolts
D. (+) 45 millivolts

285. The following factors can cause what to happen to the enamel of developing teeth?

- Vitamin deficiency (A and D)
- Fluorosis
- Congenital syphilis
- Injury or trauma to the mouth
- Inadequate calcium intake

A. Hypoplasia
B. Hypermineralisation
C. Hypomaturatuon
D. All of the above

286. Iron, copper, iodine, manganese, cobalt, and zinc are all considered to be what type of minerals?

A. Major minerals
B. Trace minerals
C. O non-essential ions
D. None of the above

287. Avidin has a high affinity for which vitamin?

A. C
B. D
C. Riboflavin
D. Biotin

288. Which of the following vitamins act as a coenzyme in a fatty acid production and in the oxidation of fatty acids and carbohydrates?

A. C
B. Biotin
C. Cobalamin
D. D

289. What vitamin is important in the prevention of some visual disorders, especially cataracts?

A. D
B. Biotin
C. Ascorbic acid
D. Riboflavin

290. Which of the following is the active form of vitamin D?

A. Cholecalciferol
B. 25-hydroxycholecalciferol
C. 1,25-dihydroxycholecalciferol
D. Ergosterol

291. Which vitamin is essential for the synthesis of prothrombin in the liver?

A. Ascorbic acid
B. A
C. D
D. K

292. Which vitamin is essential for the metabolism of protein, fats and carbohydrates, normal blood formation, and neural function?
A. Vitamin B12
B. Ascorbic acid
C. Vitamin B6
D. Riboflavin

293. Pantothenic acid is what type of vitamin?
A. B
B. C
C. D
D. A

294. Which of the following enzymes is inactivated by phosphorylation of a specific serine residue?
A. Phosphorylase
B. Phosphorylase kinase
C. Glycogen synthetase
D. Enolase

295. What do all of the following have in common?
A. Phosphoenolpyruvte
B. Carbamoyl phosphate
C. Acetyl phosphate
D. Creatine phosphate
E. 1,3-diphosphoglyceric acid
Answer = they all are energy rich phosphate carriers.

296. What reaction do all of the following enzymes catalyze?
A. Pyridoxal phosphate (PLP)
B. Pyridoxamine phosphate (PMP)
C. Transaminase
Answer = they catalyse the reversible transfer of an amino group from an alpha amino acid to an alpha keto acid, especially alpha keto glutaric acid. Such processes are essential to metabolism.

297. Which enzyme is involved in bone mineralization, hydrolysis of phosphoric esters, and functions optimally at pH 9.3?
A. Creatine phosphatase

B. Alkaline phosphatase
C. Hyaluronidase
D. Acid phosphatase

298. The following signs are indicative of a deficiency in what?

- Lack of vigor and stamina
- Weakness
- Mental depression
- Poor resistance to infection
- Impaired healing of wounds
- Slow recovery from disease

A. Fats
B. Proteins
C. Hormones
D. Alcohol

299. The major site of amino acid degradation in mammals is where?

A. Kidney
B. Pancreas
C. Liver
D. Brain

300. Which of the following is a naturally occurring derivative of tryptophan found in platelets and in cells of the brain and the intestine?

A. Heparin
B. Serotonin
C. Histamine
D. Adrenaline

301. Which of the following is the best known stimuli for increasing the rate of thyroid-stimulating hormone secretion of the anterior pituitary?

A. Exposure to heat
B. Exposure to cold
C. Exposure to stress
D. All of the above

302. Which of the following pituitary hormones is under predominant inhibitory control by the hypothalamus?

A. Growth hormone
B. Antidiuretic hormone
C. Somatomedin
D. Prolactin
E. Thyroid-stimulating hormone

303. Which disease causes both extracellular and intracellular dehydration to develop?

A. Addison's disease
B. Diabetes
C. Hyperparathyroidism
D. None of the above

304. Ammonia is formed where?

A. Liver
B. Pancreas
C. Kidney
D. Brain

305. The kidneys regulate hydrogen ion concentration principally by increasing or decreasing the concentration of what in the body fluid?

A. Bicarbonate ion
B. Sodium ion
C. Ammonium ion
D. Calcium ion

306. The countercurrent theory is used to explain the functioning of what part of the kidneys?

A. Bowman's capsule
B. Distal tubule
C. Loops of Henle
D. None of the above

307. The following substances are all normal constituents of what fluid?

- Water
- Urea
- Sodium chloride

- Potassium chloride
- Phosphates
- Uric acid
- Organic salts
- Pigment urobilin

A. Blood
B. Urine
C. Serum
D. Bile

308. Which of the following are absorbed in the main segments of the loops of Henle?

A. Sodium and chloride
B. Potassium and water
C. Sodium and water
D. Potassium and chloride

309. The following signs and symptoms are indicative of what disorder?

A. Yellow discoloration of the skin and mucous membranes and sclerae of the eyes
B. Nausea
C. Vomiting
D. Abdominal pain
E. Dark urine

Answer = Jaundice

310. Where is the major site of production of acetoacetate and 3-hydroxy butyrate?

A. Stomach
B. Liver
C. Kidney
D. Lungs

311. Secretin is produced by cells that line which portion of the GI. tract?

A. Stomach
B. Duodenum and jejunum
C. Esophagus
D. Liver

312. Insulin is secreted by which cells?
A. Alpha cells of the Islets of Langerhans
B. Beta cells of the Islets of Langerhans
C. Gamma cells

313. All of the following can be categorized as what?
A. Pepsinogen
B. Chymotrypsinogen
C. Trypsinogen
D. Procarboxypeptidase
E. Proelastase
Answer = zymogens

314. Chylomicrons are synthesized where?
A. Small intestine
B. Liver
C. G.I. tract
D. Kidneys

315. What two gastrointestinal hormones are mainly responsible for acting on the following organs?
A. Stomach
B. Pancreas
C. Small intestine
D. Large intestine
E. Gall bladder
F. Liver
Answer = secretin and cholecystokinin

316. Which structure monitors the oxygen content of the blood and assists in regulating respiration?
A. Carotid body
B. Hypothalamus
C. Medulla oblongata
D. Pons

317. Which of the following is a proteolytic enzyme that dissolves fibrin?
A. Thrombin
B. Fibrinogen

C. Plasmin
D. None of the above

318. What is the name of the naturally occurring mucopolysaccharide that acts in the body as an antithrombin factor to prevent intravascular clotting?
A. Thrombin
B. Fibrin
C. Heparin
D. All of the above

319. Which enzyme causes fibrinogen to change to fibrin?
A. Enterokinase
B. Plasmin
C. Thrombin
D. Thromboplastin

320. Which of the following substances is found in all cells and is released in allergic, inflammatory reactions?
A. Heparin
B. Histamine
C. Glucose
D. Adrenaline

321. Which structure secretes the hormones progesterone and estrogen?
A. Adrenal cortex
B. Pituitary
C. Corpus luteum
D. Testes

322. Norepinephrine is synthesized naturally in what area?
A. Adrenal cortex
B. Adrenal medulla
C. Anterior pituitary
D. Pancreas

323. Which of the following is a life-threatening condition caused by partial or complete failure of adrenocortical function;
A. Addison's disease
B. Cretinism

C. Cushing's syndrome
D. None of the above

324. What steroid hormone produced by the adrenal cortex regulates sodium and potassium balance in the blood?
A. Aldosterone
B. Epinephrine
C. Vasopressin
D. Insulin

325. What causes the type of apnea which can occur after hyperventilation of an anesthetized patient?
A. Decreased oxygen tension
B. Increased carbon dioxide tension
C. Decreased carbon dioxide tension
D. Increased nitrogen tension

326. Which of the following is believed to be the basic stimulus for exciting the respiratory center?
A. Increased pH
B. Decreased pH
C. Decreased carbon dioxide concentration
D. None of the above

327. Which enzyme below catalyzes below catalyzes the transfer of carbon dioxide from the tissues into the blood and then to the alveolar air?
A. Enolase
B. Aldolase
C. Carbonic anhydrase
D. None of the above

328. The following clinical signs are indicative of what physiological state?
A. Reduced cardiac output
B. Circulating insufficiency
C. Tachycardia
D. Hypotension
E. Restlessness
F. Pallor
G. Diminished urinary output

H. Diminished glomerular filtration
I. Muscular weakness
Answer = shock

329. Antidiuretic hormone (vasopressin) is secreted by the cells of which organ?
A. Hypothalamus
B. Anterior pituitary
C. Adrenal cortex
D. Pancreas

330. Which of the following is a metabolic disorder owing to a deficiency of antidiuretic hormone?
A. Nephrogenic insipidus
B. Diabetes insipidus
C. Neither of the above
D. Diabetes mellitus

331. The rate of secretion of parathyroid hormone is controlled almost entirely by what?
A. Plasma phosphorus ion concentration
B. Plasma calcium ion concentration
C. Plasma potassium ion concentration
D. Urine calcium ion concentration

332. Calcitonin is secreted by which of the following cells?
A. Alpha cells
B. Beta cells
C. Parafollicular cells
D. Sertoli cells

333. Almost all secretions by the pituitary are controlled by signals transmitted from which of the following:
A. Cerebrum
B. Medulla
C. Hypothalamus
D. Pons

334. The following symptoms are characteristic of what disease?
A. Polyuria
B. Polydipsia

C. Weight loss
D. Polyphagia
E. Hyperglycemia
F. Weakness
G. Acidosis
H. Glycosuria
Answer = diabetes mellitus

335. The measurement of the amount of heat directly generated by any oxidative reaction (e.g., evaporation, radiation, conduction, convection) is defined as which one of the following:
A. Direct calorimetry
B. Indirect calorimetry
C. None of the above
D. Centrifugation

336. What is the name of the disorder that results from the incomplete metabolism of tyrosine, in which abnormal amounts of homogentisic acid are excreted?
A. Alkaptonuria
B. Phenylketonuria
C. Hyperammonemia
D. Cystinuria

337. In proteins, the alpha-carboxyl group of one amino acid is joined to the alpha-amino group of another amino acid by what type of bond?
A. Hydrogen bond
B. Hydrostatic bond
C. Peptide bond
D. Carbon-bond

338. The major site of cholesterol synthesis is where?
A. Liver
B. Pancreas
C. Appendix
D. Lung

339. The degradation and oxidation of fatty acids occurs where?
A. In the cytoplasm

B. In the mitochondria
C. In the nucleus
D. In endoplasmic reticulum

340. Prostaglandins are synthesized from what?
A. Saturated fatty acids
B. Unsaturated fatty acids
C. Carbohydrates
D. Hormone insulin

341. B-hydroxybutyric acid and aminoacetic acid are both called what?
A. Ketone bodies
B. Urate bodies
C. Transaminase intermediates
D. Calcium crystals

342. What are the following symptoms indicative of?
A. Ketonuria (ketones in urine)
B. Loss of potassium in urine
C. Fruity odor of acetone on the breath
Answer = ketosis

343. Which enzyme listed below is found in grains and vegetables and is involved in the hydrolysis of starch to maltose?
A. Alpha-amylase
B. Beta-amylase
C. Trans ketolase
D. Hydrolase

344. The arrangement of sugars into D- and L- configurations is based upon their resemblance to which monosaccharide?
A. Glyceraldehyde
B. Dihydroxyacetone
C. Glycine
D. Glucose

345. Another name for Coenzyme Q is what?
A. Adenyl cyclase
B. Ubiquinone
C. Biotin
D. Enolase

346. Aerobic glycolysis yields which of the follcwing?
A. Pyruvic acid
B. Lactic acid
C. Acetic Acid
D. Homogentisic acid

347. In what anaerobic process do all of the following enzymes participate?
- Hexokinase
- Phosphoglucose isomerase
- Phosphofructokinase
- Aldolase
- Triose phosphate isomerase
- Glyceraldehyde 3-phosphate dehydrogenase
- Phosphoglycerate kinase
- Phosphoglyceromutase
- Enolase
- Pyruvate kinase

A. Glycolysis
B. Lipid metabolism
C. Fat catabolism
D. Kreb's cycle

348. Lactose is hydrolyzed to which of the following by the enzyme lactase?
A. Galactose and glucose
B. Glucose
C. Glucose and fructose
D. Fructose and galactose

349. Glucose 6-phosphatase is found most abundantly in which of the following organs?
A. Kidney
B. Liver
C. Intestine
D. Brain

350. Glucose released by the liver into the blood during muscular activity is taken up primarily by what two organs listed below?
A. Skeletal muscle

B. Heart
C. Brain
D. Kidney

351. The rate of glycolysis is primarily controlled by the level of activity of which enzyme?
A. Enolase
B. Aldolase
C. Phosphofructokinase
D. Hexokinase

352. Denaturing agents such as urea and guanidine hydrochloride disrupt which kind of bonds?
A. Covalent
B. Noncovalent
C. Hydrogen bond
D. Ionic bond

353. The major effect of acidosis on the body is what?
A. Increased respiration
B. Increased heart rate
C. Depression of the central nervous system
D. Decreased liver function

354. Which of the following is considered to be the normal hemoglobin?
A. Hemoglobin A
B. Hemoglobin C
C. Hemoglobin F
D. Hemoglobin S

Brain Diet and Self Assessment

1. **Name six highly distinctive and biologically crucial properties of enzymes?**
2. **A substance that alters the rate of an enzymatic reaction by interacting with the enzyme at a site other than the active site is called what?**
3. **Define km value of an enzyme.**

4. **What is the hallmark of competitive inhibition?**
5. **The first law of thermodynamics states what?**
6. **What is the pH of saliva?**
7. **Define isotope.**
8. **Tyrosine is a precursor of what two hormones?**
9. **What is the major bile salt?**
10. **What is the normal plasma concentration of glucose, calcium, and phosphorus?**
11. **What hormone acts to stimulate and to regulate the production of erythrocytes and is therefore able to increase the oxygen-carrying capacity of the blood?**
12. **Sixty-five percent of the total quantity of iron in the body is present in what form?**
13. **What two proteins are the oxygen carriers in vertebrates?**
14. **How will the following situations effect the release of oxygen from oxyhemoglobin?**
    A. Increase in arterial PCO_2
    B. Decrease in arterial PO_2
    C. Increased temperature
    D. Increase in arterial hydrogen ion concentration (pH)
15. **What process are all of the following involved in?**
    A. Calcium
    B. Fibrinogen
    C. Platelets
    D. Prothrombin
    E. Tissue thromboplastin

Answer Key to MCQs in Physiology and Biochemistry

1	B	2	B	3	C	4	B
5	B	6	B	7	D	8	E
9	A	10	E	11	C	12	C, B
13	B	14	C	15	B	16	C
17	A, C	18	B	19	C	20	B
21	C	22	B	23	C	24	D
25	B	26	B	27	D	28	D
29	B	30	C	31	D	32	B
33	C	34	B	35	D	36	C
37	B	38	D	39	A	40	C
41	B	42	C	43	C	44	C
45	D	46	C	47	C	48	A, D
49	C	50	C	51	C	52	B
53	C	54	B, C	55	C	56	A, C
57	B	58	A	59	D	60	D
61	A	62	B, C	63	E	64	C
65	D	66	C	67	C	68	C
69	C	70	B	71	B	72	B
73	C	74	A	75	C	76	C
77	C	78	D	79	C	80	D
81	A	82	D	83	D	84	E
85	C	86	B	87	C	88	D
89	B	90	B	91	D	92	B
93	C	94	B	95	C	96	B
97	C	98	D	99	B	100	B
101	B	102	B	103	A	104	B
105	D	106	B	107	C	108	D
109	C	110	B	111	B	112	B
113	D	114	A	115	A	116	C
117	E	118	B	119	B	120	B
121	C	122	C	123	A	124	C
125	C	126	B	127	C	128	C
129	C	130	B, C	131	C	132	B
133	A	134	B	135	A	136	D
137	B	138	C	139	B	140	C

141	D	142	C	143	D	144	C
145	F	146	E	147	C	148	A
149	B	150	C	151	C	152	D
153	B	154	E	155	C	156	B
157	B	158	D	159	A	160	B
161	C	162	B	163	D	164	B
165	C	166	B	167	D	168	C
169	C	170	B	171	D	172	C
173	A	174	C	175	E	176	C
177	C	178	B	179	C	180	B
181	C	182	C	183	D	184	C
185	D	186	B	187	D	188	C
189	C	190	D	191	C	192	A
193	E	194	B	195	A	196	C
197	D	198	B	199	C	200	D
201	D	202	B	203	C	204	D
205	B	206	C	207	C	208	B
209	C	210	A	211	C	212	C
213	A	214	D	215	B	216	B
217	C	218	C	219	A	220	C
221	C	222	C, D	223	D	224	D
225	B	226	C	227	B	228	C
229	C	230	D	231	B	232	C
233	C	234	C	235	A	236	A
237	B	238	C	239	B	240	B
241	A, C	242	C	243	D	244	C
245	C	246	C	247	B	248	E
249	B	250	D	251	D	252	B
253	C	254	C	255	D	256	B
257	B	258	C	259	B	260	E
261	C	262	B	263	C	264	A
265	B	266	B	267	C	268	C
269	C	270	B	271	B	272	C
273	A	274	A	275	C	276	A
277	A	278	B, E	279	B	280	B
281	A	282	C	283	A	284	B
285	A	286	B	287	D	288	B
289	D	290	C	291	D	292	A

293	A	294	C	295	—	296	—
297	B	298	B	299	C	300	B
301	B	302	D	303	B	304	C
305	A	306	C	307	B	308	C
309	—	310	B	311	B	312	B
313	—	314	C	315	—	316	A
317	C	318	C	319	C	320	B
321	C	322	B	323	A	324	A
325	B	326	B	327	C	328	—
329	A	330	B	331	B	332	C
333	C	334	—	335	A	336	A
337	C	338	A	339	B	340	B
341	A	342	—	343	B	344	A
345	B	346	A	347	A	348	A
349	B	350	A	351	C	352	B
353	C	354	A				

8

Dental Materials

COEFFICIENTS OF THERMAL EXPANSION

Tooth	11.4	
Silicate	7.6	0.7 x the tooth
Dental amalgam	25	2.2 x the tooth
Porcelain	4.1	
PMMA resin	81	
Elastomers	150-220	
Inlay wax	350	
Conventional composite resin	32	3.1 x the tooth
Unfilled resin	92	
Direct filling gold i.e. gold foil		1.3 x the tooth
Gold alloy		1.9 x the tooth
Microfilled resins		5.3 x the tooth

COMPRESSIVE STRENGTHS: (1 Mpa = 145 psi)

ZnO-eugenol	7 mpa
Agar	0.245 mpa
Alginate	49.8 psi, 0.34 mpa

COMPRESSIVE STRENGTHS: (1 Mpa = 145 psi) *(Contd.)*

Direct filled resin	62 mpa
Composite resin	235 mpa
Investment gypsum bonded	2.5 mpa
Zn- phosphate cement	68.7 mpa
Silicate	180 mpa, strongest cement
Glass inomer	140 mpa
Porcelain	331 mpa
Dentin	350 mpa
Low Cu alloys	310 mpa
High Cu alloys	510 mpa
Unfilled resins	69 mpa

Enamel has higher MOE, lower MO resilience and high PL than dentin.

HARDNESS NUMBERS : KHN

Enamel	343
Dentin	65
Amalgam	90
Silicate	65
Glass inomer	60
Direct filling gold	70
Macrofilled resin	55
Soft inlay gold	50
Microfilled resin	25
Unfilled resin	15
Porcelain	463

HARDNESS NUMBERS : KHN (*Contd.*)

Cast gold	95-120
Zn phosphate cement	36
Gypsum type II	7.1
Gypsum type III	24.6
Gypsum type IV	51.8
Emery	2000
Sand	800
Diamond	7000
Austenite	600
Martensite	230-600
Gold alloys	VHN
Type I	50
Type II	90
Type III	120
Type IV	150
Pure gold	BHN =25
Burs	VHN
Steel burs	800
Tungsten carbide	1650-1700

STRESSES DURING MASTICATION

Incisors		9-25 kg
Canines		14-34 kg
Premolars		23-46 kg
Molars	90 – 200 lbs	41-91 kg
Average	170 lbs	77 kg

Sublimation is process of changing of solid to gas directly

Latent heat of fusion is energy released when liquid changes to solid form.

Contact angle is angle formed by the tangent to adhesive with the surface of adherend. **For complete wetting, it should be zero. Surface energy of adherend should be maximum** for complete adhesion.

Fluorides decrease the surface energy of enamel and dentin, so retain less plaque.

Surface energy is force of attraction between outermost atoms of a substance.

Mandatory properties of a dental material are —

- High modulus of elasticity
- High modulus of resilience
- High proportional limit.

Strength = is maximum **stress** required to fracture a material.

Stiffness: **resistance** to elastic deformation, is determined by MOE.

Toughness = **energy** required to fracture a material.

Resilience = capacity to absorb **mechanical energy** without plastic deformation / amount of energy absorbed by a structure when it is stressed not to exceed its PL. It should be small for metal- ceramic restorations.

Modulus of resilience = **energy** required to stress a structure to its proportional limit. Gold alloys have the lowest.

Sag resistance: ability of a metal alloy **to resist** plastic and creep flow under its own weight during porcelain firing and soldering.

Ductility = ability of a material to withstand a permanent deformation under **a tensile load** without fracture.

Elongation is the measure of ductility or the **degree of plastic deformation** prior to fracture.

Malleability = ability of a material to withstand **a compressive load**. Gold is the most D and M material and silver is second.

Creep = the **time dependant** plastic deformation of a material, under a constant force at a temp near its melting point.

Static creep = under constant stress.

Dynamic creep = under fatigue type/variable stress. Eg dental amalgam.

Hue = *color* of an object.

Chroma = strength/**degree of saturation** for a particular hue.

Value = **brightness/ darkness** of an object. It is the most imp criteria for selecting a shade.

Elastic limit = proportional limit = yield strength (EPY), it is the greatest stress to which a material can be subjected without a permanent deformation.

Modulus of elasticity = rigidity = stiffness, shear modulus is 40 % of Young's modulus.

Flexibility = is the strain which occurs when the material is stressed to its PL.

Brittle materials have tensile strength very less than the compressive strength.

Brittleness is the opposite of toughness.

% elongation is the measure of ductility and is related to permanent strain at fracture.

HARDNESS

Brinell hardness no.	Hard steel ball Can not be used with brittle materials or which exhibit elastic recovery
Rockwell HN	**Conical diamond point** or steel ball, Not for brittle materials
Vickers HN	Modified for elastic recovery materials Diamond having a **square based pyramid** Used for brittle materials eg tooth
Knoop HN	Not for elastic recovery materials **Rhombic diamond**

Strain hardening/ work hardening/ cold working: slip of the molecules along the slip- planes due to stresses; metal becomes stronger and harder; decrease in ductility, and corrosion resistance,

Strength of rolled sheath is greater in the transverse direction than in the direction of rolling.

Annealing: causes reversal of cold working.

Occurs in three stages viz recovery, recrystallization, grain growth.

It occurs in **wrought metal only**.

GYPSUM PRODUCTS

GYPSUM—calcination in open air at 110-130° C → beta-form (hemihydrate form)

GYPSUM— 110-130° C in autoclave or 0.5 % sodium succinate in autoclave or 30 % $CaCl_2$ in open air. → alpha – form

Particle size is the chief factor to determine the amount of gauging water required.

Effect of temperature on ST of gypsum

0-50° C	No/little change
> 50° C	Increased
100° C	No reaction occurs ie no setting

Most effective method to control ST= add retarders eg gums, gelatin, they adsorb on hemihydrate surface and decrease its solubility, and growth of crystals.

Solubility of hemihydrate is 3 times > dihydrate

Setting expansion (SE)= 0.06-0.5%, chemical decrease SE.

EFFECTS OF CHEMICALS ON ST

Chemical	Conc./action	ST
NaCl	< 20%/accelerator > 20%/retarder	Decrease Increase
Na_2SO_4	< 12%/accelerator > 12%/retarder	Decrease Increase
K_2SO_4	2-3% /accelerator	Decreases
Borax	Retarder	Increases

Most commonly used accelerator = K_2SO_4

Most effective retarder = borax

STRENGTH

Factors affecting strength are :

1. Increased W/P ratio= decreases strength, increases porosity.
2. Increased spatulation= Increased strength
3. Chemicals= decreased strength

Effects of Increased W/P ratio:

- Increased porosity, ST, Tensile strength
- Decreased compressive strength, SE (setting expansion).

IMPRESSION PLASTERS

Type	Manufacture	W/P ratio	Nomenclature
TYPE I	Heating $CaSO_4$.2 H_2O at 120° C in an open vessel.	0.5-0.6	Impression plaster
TYPE II	Heating Ca SO_4.2 H_2O at 120° C in an open vessel.	0.5-0.6	Model plaster eg POP

IMPRESSION PLASTERS (*Contd.*)

TYPE III	Autoclaving under steam pressure at 120-130° C	0.33	Dental stone/ class I stone, **hydrocal** Eg used for denture casts.
TYPE IV	Heating in boiling 30 % $CaCl_2$ sol or $MgCl_2$ or At 140° C with Na Cl or organic acid in autoclave.	0.24	Dental stone high strength, i.e. **densite**/class II stone/**die stone,** used for dies for inlays.
TYPE V			Dental stone high strength and high expansion

Balanced stone = in which ST is established by adding both accelerator and retarder.

Hardeners —

1. Gypsum hardening solutions
2. Low W/P ratio = best method
3. 2% borax **solution** = forms Ca- tetra borate on the surface.

When a gypsum cast is placed in water, its linear dimension decreases by 0.1% for every 20 min.

At 70 % humidity = gypsum absorbs water from atmosphere and reaction starts.

W/P ratio = type I = 0.6-0.7, and type II = 0.2

IMPRESSION COMPOUNDS

- type I = true compound
- type II = tray compound for primary impression

Flow = a maximum flow of 6% at mouth temperature and a minimum flow of 85% at 45° C is permissible.

Linear contraction of compound from mouth temperature to room temperature 25° C = 0.3-0.4 % and

Volume expansion = 1.38-2.29%

ZOE PASTE

ZnO + eugenol = **chelation** process

Water is essential for the reaction.

Reaction is **autocatalysed**.

ZOE reaction is **never completed.**

Accelerators = water, acetic acid, Zn – acetate, high temperature

Water is the best accelerator eg humidity.

Stoichiometric ratio = 0.25 gm/ml

It has two ST = initial, final ST

ST is decreased by =

- increased ZnO/E ratio
- small ZnO particle size
- accelerators
- moisture eg saliva
- increased temperature eg in oral cavity
- increased mixing time (MT)

Rctarders ie increased ST by

- Boroglycerine
- Cool slab and spatula **(best method)**

Compressive strength =7 mpa

Dimensional stability = <0.1 % shrinkage may occur.

Impression can be *preserved indefinitely,* as there is no relaxation or any other cause of warpage.

HYDROCOLLOIDS

Are lyophilic sols.

2 components = dispersed phase, dispersion medium.

dispersed phase forms MICELLES.

Reaction is a **physical effect** in reversible HC and **chemical** in **irreversible** HC.

Gelation temperature, GT= at which sol form changes to gel form.

Liquefaction temperature, LT= at which gel form changes to sol form.

Hysteresis = difference between GT and LT

Syneresis =loss of water from gel surface by evaporation. Shrinkage occurs by this process.

Imbibition = sorption of water till water is restored, if gel is lacking in water.

AGAR: physical reaction, depends on temperature.

Main component is water.

Is an organic hydrophilic colloid.

Its GT = 37° C; 36-42° C

Its LT = 60-70° C

Borax = increases strength of the gel., increases viscosity of the sol, but retards the setting of gypsum so the cast is soft.

To prevent it, 2 % K_2SO_4 is added as a **plaster hardener** in impression mat.

Compr strength =0.245 mpa, 35.6 psi

Reversible and irreversible HC have a common property that inaccuracies in completed impression can be caused by fracture of fibrils during gelation.

Gel strength: stresses should be applied rapidly, otherwise flow will occur due to disturbing of the network of fibrils,

Brush heap structure of fibrils is formed.

ALGINATE: chemical reaction, cross-linking occurs.

- Potassium alginate

- **Reactor** = $CaSO_4$
- **Retarder** = sodium tri polyphosphate
- Reactor first reacts with retarder
- Compressive strength = 49.8 psi
- W/P =40 ml/ 15 gm
- Thickness of the gel between tray and tissues should be 3 mm./ 3/16".
- Agar can be placed in the mouth for 10 min and it shows no distortion. But alginate if for > 2-3 min. shows distortion.
- Alginate can't produce surface details as accurately as agar, also cast **with alginate is of inferior quality,** so not used for FPD impression.
- **Cold water**/ altering the temperature of water is the **best method** to increase the ST.
- For every 1° C rise in temperature, the ST decreases by 6 sec.
- It should not be placed in the mouth for long, b'coz distortion may occur. But agar can be held for up to 10 mins.

Japanese alginates contain: = soluble and insoluble carbonates (instead of a phosphate), triethanol amine alginate, and $CaSO_4$.

ELASTOMERS: are **hydrophobic**

Types

1. Polysulphides
2. Condensation polymerising silicones
3. Addition polymerising silicones (**best**)
4. Polyethers

(A) Polysulphides: cross-linking reaction, polymerisation occurs by condensation.

Vulcanisation: it is the process of changing the rubber base product or liquid polymer to a rubber like material in **presence of sulphur.**

PbO_2 = **oxidising** agent, helps on chain lengthening,

Reaction is **exothermic**

Retarder = oleic acid

(B) Condensation polymerising silicones

Catalyst = stannous octoate

Reaction is called as room temperature vulcanisation (RTV).

Ethyl alcohol is the by – product of its reaction and so contraction occurs due to its evaporation.

(C) Addition polymerising silicones

Catalyst = platinum salt

It has **no by-products**, so it is v. much stable dimensionally.

These are more stable dimensionally than hydrocolloids.

If cast is poured immediately after removal from mouth, crater like pits are formed in the cast, **due to release of H_2** gas, **so cast should be ɔoured after 15-30 mins.**

RESINS

- Initiator = benzoyl peroxide
- Inhibitor = hydroquinone, O_2
- Plasticizer = butyl acrylate

effects of plasticizer

1. Increases solubility of polymer in monomer
2. Decreases brittleness of polymer
3. Decreases softening or fusion temperature
4. Decreases strength and hardness of resin

Esters of methacrylic acid

PMMA is the hardest in this series.

MMA has a B.P = 100.8 C

21 % polymerisation shrinkage occurs when MMA is polymerised.

But when PMMA and MMA are mixed, the shrinkage is 7 %, (P/M ratio= 2:1)

Composition: P/L ratio = 3:1

	Component	+ Conc.	+ Action
Monomer (liquid)	MMA		
	Hydroquinone	0.006%	Inhibitor
Polymer (powder)	PMMA		
	Dibutyl phthalate	8-10%	Plasticizer
	Ethyl acrylate	5%	Increases solubility of PMMA in MMA
	Benzoyl peroxide		Initiator
	Glycol dimethacrylate	1-2%	Cross-linking agent

Cross linking agents = cause greater resistance to crazing

Curing = a. at 160° F for 9 hrs.

b. 65° C for 90 min = thick portions

c. 100° C for 60 min = thin parts

Cold cure acrylic =

Activator = dimethyl p-toluidine (0.75%)

Initiator = benzoyl peroxide (2%)

Residual monomer = in C.C = 3-5%

In H.C = 0.2-0.5%.

Fit of C.C appliance is better than HC, b'coz of absence of curing stresses.

Linear shrinkage = 0.2-0.5 %

Processing shrinkage = 0.53 % HC; 0.26 % in CC.

Resin **shrinks towards the area of greatest bulk,** i.e. towards ridge part of denture, so tensile stresses occur in thinner region ie palate, and misfit. R/L posterior teeth are pulled towards each other and so increased VDO.

Denture repair is preferred by CC, b'coz HC tends to warp the denture.

Relining: a low curing temperature is used to avoid distortion of denture.

Heat generated is proportional to bulk of the resin, so ridge is stronger than palate.

DIRECT FILLING RESINS (TYPE I)

Acrylic resin is the softest of all restorative materials, KHN=15

Peroxide-amine polymerisation can be **inhibited by** – cavity varnish, eugenol, O_2.

Resins with **high degree of color stability** are activated by **sulfinate system.**

COMPOSITE RESINS (TYPE II)

Chemical cure = benzoyl-peroxide –tertiary amine system

Contain fillers= 70-80%, decrease coeff of thermal expansion.

Coupling agents = vinyl silane

Light cure resins

1. UV light cure = benzoyl peroxide-benzoin methyl ether system
2. Visible LC = benzoyl peroxide – diketone sysem

Size of fillers

- Conventional = 1-100 μ
- Microfilled = 0.04-0.06 μ
- Hybrid = 1-5 μ

Glazing agent = dilute solution of BIS-GMA

Strontium- glass filled BIS-GMA resin is used in class II cavities as it has **maximum wear resistance**.

Acid etching = 33-50 % o-phosphoric acid = for 60 sec. (Recently = 15-30 sec) – Longer in primary teeth.

Washing = 45 sec

Drying = 15 sec

10-20 micron deep tags are formed

Surface area increases by 200 times.

. It is purely a **mechanical bond**.

Ca $(OH)_2$ base is applied to protect dentin.

Solid solutions: eg Ag-Pd alloys. The system is not mechanically separable and has **only one phase.**

Interstitial solid solution = eg steel ie carbon – in – iron.

Eutectic system : components are having partial solid solubility but complete liquid solubility, e.g. Ag - Cu.

It has no solidification range, but **solidify at a constant temperature.**

Brittle b'coz *no slip* can occur.

Do not appear in alloys of < 8.8 % Cu.

Peritectic system eg Ag- Sn.–limited solid solubility of the 2 metals.

DENTAL AMALGAM

Particle size = 25-35 microns

Small average paticle size preferred as it :

- It produces more rapid hardening of amalgam.
- Greater early strength
- Larger particles get pulled out during carving, and voids cause corrosion.

Components and their effects on –

	Compr str.	Expansion	Hardness	Creep/ flow	Tarnish	ST	%
Ag	↑	↑	—	↓	↓	↓	65
Sn	↓	↓	↑	↑	↑	↑	29
Cu	↑	↑	↑	↓	↓	↓	6
Zn	↓	↑	—	—	—	↓	1

↑ Increase ↓ Decrease

Effect of Ag is reverse to that of Sn.

It is the only dental material whose marginal leakage decreases with age and it is due to accumulation of corrosion products.

Ag-Sn + Hg→Ag Hg + Sn Hg + Ag Sn + voids
(α+β) γ1 + γ2 + (β + γ) + V

γ 2 phase is **the weakest phase.**, least corrosion resistant, hardness is 10 % of gamma-1 phase, higher creep. Hexagonal.

Gamma – 2 phase is **most anodic,** gets disintegraed afer loosing electrons; most corrosive;

Solubility of Ag in Hg is much less than Sn , so gamma –1 phase precipitates earlier than gamma – 2.

Gamma – 1 : **matrix phase**, BCC in structure,

In **high Cu alloys**, gamma –2 is eliminated, but neta= Cu Sn and epsilon = Cu_3Sn appear.

Functions of Zn

- Deoxidiser and **scavenger**
- Abnormal/ *delayed expansion* in **presence of water**, due to formation of H_2 gas, in 3-5 days , is up to 400 microns.

Types

1. Low Cu alloy (lathe - cut) = Ag-Sn is *peritectic*
2. High Cu alloy ie Cu is > 6 % by wt.
   - *Admixed alloy* = Ag Sn = Ag Cu, It has copper 9-20 % = eutectic.
   - *Single composition alloy* = Ag-Sn-Cu in 60-27-13 % and Cu = 13-30 % wt.

Dispersant / dispersion amalgam : ie **admix alloy** in which Ag-Cu acts as a dispersion hardner.

Bulk of the restoration contains **original unreacted particles** surrounded by reaction products.

More the unreacted particles, more is the strength.

Lathe – cut alloys require 10 times condensation pressure than spherical alloys for producing same tensile strength.

Spherical powder require lesser Hg- content.

Sterling silver: used for inlays in deciduous teeth. Ag = 92.5 %. Cu = 7.5 %

Amalgamation

Solubility of Ag in Hg is = 0.035 %,

Solubility of Sn in Hg is = 0.6 %

Strengths

Type	Compr str	Compr str	Tensile str
↓ After →	I hr	7 days	24 hrs
Low Cu	145 mpa	343 mpa	60 mpa
Admix	137 mpa	431 mpa	48 mpa
Single composition	262 mpa	510 mpa	64 mpa

Marginal breakdown is the **most common defect** in an amalgam is mainly due to creep.

Creep is least in Single composition alloys.

Tensile strength is very less and so fracture occurs in the isthmus region.

Mercury content : 45-55% is adequate.

At 54 % of Hg = compr strength is 240 mpa.

At 59 % of Hg = compr strength is 125 mpa.

Hg content in finished restoration should be comparable to original M/A ratio. (approx. 50 %)

Less Hg required for spherical alloys.

Rate of hardening : minimal 1 hr compressive strength should be 80 mpa.

Hg : alloy ratio =

For lathe cut = 50 % Hg,

For spherical = 40 % Hg

Mercuroscopic expansion

- Oxidation of gamma – 2 → Sn + Hg
- Sn → corrosion products
- Hg + gamma → gamma – 1 + gamma – 2; it results in unilateral expansion which causes protrusion of restoration from the margins and fracture.

Condensation pressure = 3-4 lbs

Contraction = 20 micron/cm is acceptable

Corrosion products are **mainly the oxides and chlorides** of Sn, and **sulfides** of Ag and Hg.

Diameter of condenser point = ≥ 2 mm

PURE GOLD

Most noble material, most malleable material, has FCC structure.

DIRECT FILLING GOLD: 4 types

1. **Foil**: 25 micron thick, used esp for external surface of restorations.
2. **Electrolytic / mat gold** : used for **interior bulk** of restoration, is an alloy of *Au and Ca* (0.1-0.5 %); CALCIUM.
3. **Powdered gold**: less chair time, as each pellet has 10 times more metal than gold foil. It is *degassed* by only alcohol flame.

It is mainly used in class III and V cavities.

Condensation pressure = 15 psi

On semi cohesive gold = NH_3 gas is adsorbed.

Diameter of condenser point = 0.5-1.0 mm (more for amalgam)

Tensile strength = 500

BHN = 25

Density = 19.3 g/cm^3

Linear contraction of nole metal alloys = at least 1.25 %

Specific-gravity = 19.32

On cold working of gold ie atomic attraction;

- Tensile strength = 134 mpa → 225 mpa
- BHN = 25 → 58
- Yield strength = 0 → 214 mpa
- Proportional limit = 10

CASTING OR GOLD ALLOY: TYPES

I.	Soft	VHN 50
II.	Medium	VHN 90
III.	Hard	VHN 120
IV.	Extra hard	VHN 150

FUNCTIONS OF DIFFERENT COMPONENTS

1. Au : tarnish resistant, noble metal
2. Pd : makes Ag non-tarnishing, increases strength and stiffness, increases fusion temperature, decreases coeff of TE, **whitening** effect, 1% Pd is required for every 3% Ag.
3. Ir: found in grain refined alloys, decreases grain size and so increases Y. strength, more homogeniety, better tarnish resistant,
4. Zn: **oxygen – scavenger** from the surface of Ag.
5. Cu: acts as **main hardner** of the alloy, decreases the corrosion resistance, reddens the alloy, helps in **age- hardening** of the alloy.
6. Ag: decreases red effect of Cu, decreases fusion temperature, causes green discoloration at margins of porcelain— Pb is added.
7. In Sn, Fe: help in bonding with porcelain via oxide film, increases the hardness.

TYPES

Type I	Soft	For small inlays eg. on lateral surfaces of tooth.
Type II	Medium	Inlays subjected to moderate stresses eg thick FPD, and on occlusal surfaces.

TYPES (*Contd.*)

Type III	Hard	Inlays subjected to high stresses eg thin FPD, and jackets etc..
Type IV	Extra hard	Inlays subjected to very high stresses eg RPD saddles.
Metal ceramic	Hard and extra hard	Used with porcelain

White golds : Au > 50%

Low golds : Au = 42-55 %, which is < that in type III and IV golds, is used for crown and bridges.

Yellow colored alloy : Au = 42 %,

Yellow gold : Au >60 %

White precious metal alloy : Pd- dominated.

Pd-Ag alloy: very small Au content.

Karat : part of pure gold in the 24 parts of alloy.

Fineness : parts per thousands in the pure gold.

Pure gold = 1000 fine, i.e. fineness is = 10 times the % of gold in the alloy.

Firing temperature: 1030° C / 1900° F

Linear casting shrinkage of the pure gold = 1.67 %

HEAT TREATMENT: ie a metal is elevated to a temperature above room temperature and held there for a length of time.

(1) Hardening heat treatment = or age hardening :

ie after a solution heat treatment , heating to produce precipitation of a second phase.

- Alloy is first subjected to softening heat treatment to relieve all the strain hardening.
- Then, the casting is kept at aging temperature of 200-450° C for 15-30 min. ie cooling slowly.
- Now, it is water quenched.

It increases hardness, strength, PL, MO Resilience.

It decreases ductility, elongation, degree of plastic deformation.

(2) Softening heat treatment or solution heat treatment

Quenching the alloy in water from a temperature of 700° C ie soaking of alloy at high temperature to produce the solid solution and then quenching.

- Casting is kept at 700° C for 10 min.
- Quench in water.

So a **solid solution** is formed as **ordering of the phases is prevented.**

It decreases hardness, tensile strength, PL.

It increases ductility.

Tarnish: due to formation of thin **films of oxides, chlorides**, sulphides. It is a **surface discoloration** on a metal or a slight loss of luster or surface finish.

Alloys with noble metal content < 65 % usually tarnish.

Corossion: is deterioration of a metal by reaction with its environment, e.g. O_2 and Cl_2 cause corrosion of Ag amalgam, and esp sulfides cause corrosion of alloys having Ag.

Anode: ie metal which gives electrons and gets disintegrated.

Chromium is the best example **of passivity** as an oxide film is formed on the surface.

Sprue: should not be attached at right angles but at 45 degree angle. Correct angle of sprue **prevents turbulence** of the metal.

Sprue pin diameter should be greater than the thickest part of wax pattern.

Liner ≥ 1 mm thick is used (Asbestos).

After investing, *one hour* is allowed for setting of the material before wax elimination.

INLAY CASTING WAXES

TYPE A	Hard, low flow	Not used
Type B	Medium	For direct technique
Type C	Soft	For indirect technique

COMPONENTS

1. Paraffin wax = main component, 40-60 %, gives moldability.
2. Gum dammer = increases smoothness and luster, resistance to flaking and crazing, and toughness of wax.
3. Carnauba wax = increases glossiness and decreases flow.
4. Candel wax = used in place of carnauba wax.
5. Ceresin = gives toughness and carving characters.

Properties –

1. Residue = Should be < 0.1 % wt. when heated to 500° C.
2. Flow = Maximum flow at 37° C = 1 %,
   Minimum flow at 45° C = 70 %
3. coefficient of thermal expansion = 350×10^{-6}/ °C
4. thermal conductivity is = low
5. linear change in dimensions = < 0.6 %

INVESTMENTS

Gypsum bonded	650° C	For conventional gold alloys eg. Inlays, crowns etc.
Phosphate bonded	732-982° C	For porcelain and metal ceramics.
Silica bonded	1090-1180° C	For base metal alloys eg RPD

Casting pressure required with phosphate – bonded investment is greater than with silica – bonded, **b'coz of less permeability.**

Gypsum bonded : 3 types –

Type I = uses thermal expansion to compensate casting shrinkage, used for casting the inlays and crown.

Type II = uses hygroscopic expansion , for inlays / crowns.

Type III = used for partial dentures of gold alloys.

EXPANSIONS

Normal setting expansion = (NSE) = 0-0.6 %

Thermal expansion (TE) = 1-1.6 %

Hygroscopic expansion (HSE) = 1.2-2.2 %

Compositions

Binder = 25-45 %,alpha – hemihydrate of gypsum, provides strength and rigidity, heated to < 700° C, (to < 650° C if carbon is present.)

Refractory = silica, regulates TE

Modifiers = boric acid, Na Cl, regulate ST and SE, prevents shrinkage of gypsum if heated above 300° C.

Forms of silica

1. alpha- quartz → at 575° C → beta- quartz.
2. Alpha –cristobellite → at 200-270° C → beta- form
3. Tridymite → at 117° C → first inversion → at 163° C → second inversion

- HSE = 6 times the NSE
- HSE occurs when **water of hydration is replaced** by water of immersion and so it prevents the confinement of the growing crystals by the surface tension of excess water.
- HSE can be controlled by amount of water added and time of immersion in water.

Wax elimination : by boiling water – but gypsum gets dissolved, loss of surface details.

- By heat : <650° C, for TE. It is better to start burn-out while investment is still wet as water repels the wax out.
- If HSE is used : heat < 480° C only for > 1 hr.but at low heat; **back pressure porosity** can occur due to incomplete elimination of wax.
- During burnout, expansion of wax is greater than investment, which may cause cracks in investment.
- Some metals dissolve gases while molten, release gases when solidify – **pinhole porosity.**

- Lost wax technique
- Flux helps minimizing the porosity, increase fluidity and prevent oxidation.

Cements

Type I cements = fine grains – used for porcelain fitting

Type II cements = medium grains – used for *insulating bases* and orthodontic band cementation.

Zn – silicophosphate cement= translucent – used for cementation of porcelain – jacket.

Cu, Ag, Hg salts are added to cements – for bacteriostatic/ bactericidal properties.

ZOE – has *palliative* action on pulp. Has excellent initial sealing capacity.

Type IV ZOE is used for IRM eg in rampant caries.

GI- adhesion, biocampatible, anticaries (ABC), translucent

Esthetic cements – GI, silicate. Both are translucent, and attacked by oral fluids.

Function of cement bases: to encourage recovery of pulp, and protect it from other insults.

Before condensation of permanent restoration, the strength of cement base should be more than 0.5 mpa-1.2 mpa.

PORCELAIN

Tempering of porcelain: increases thickness of peripheral/ skin porcelain and so decreases the compressive stresses in the skin and prevents cracks.

Mechanical retention: rough surface by air abrasion, **ka textured metal,** increased surface area,

Chemical bonding: by oxides of In, Sn, cleaning by HF acid decreases the bond strength.

Tin oxide coating Platinum is better b'coz it : helps decreasing the metal coping thickness.

Due to high MP of alloy, we can't use gypsum- bonded investment, so use phosphate or silica bonded invesment.

WROUGHT GOLD ALLOYS

Wire is the main form in which it is used,= for RPD clasps, it is type IV alloy.

Type I = high precious metal alloy, contains > 75% precious metal

Type I wires are not age hardenable; fusion temperature = 955° C

Type II = low precious metal alloy, contains > 65% precious metal; fusion temperature = 871° C

P-G-P wires = Pt-Au-Pd

P-S-C wires = Pd-Ag-Cu

Cu= ability of alloy to age hardening.

Ag = decreases the fusion temperature, balances color of Cu.

Ni = strengthener, decreases ductility and tarnish resistance.

Pd, Pt = increase fusion temperature, give fine grain structure,

Zn = as oxygen scavenger,

Value of PL = 2/3 rd of tensile strength.

SOLDERS

Solder : a filler, has lower fusion temperature than the parts to be joined, fusion temperature of the solder **should be at least 50-100° C lesser than** the parts to be joined.

It should have MP in 28-56° C of solidus temperature of the metal units.

Flux : displaces gas layer and tarnish film, protects surface from oxidation.

Flux = borax + boric acid.

Borax = 55 %, sodium perborate is better,

Boric acid = 35 % - it decreases the fusionpoint.

Silica = 10 %, gives viscosity and toughness.

Anti flux = confines the flow of solder eg Pb pencil, rouge.

Types : hard, soft

Solders above 650 fine should not be used where considerable stress is involved.

Cu = increases the melting range.

Ag = narrows the melting range, more free flowing, greater adherence to the metals.

Gap between the parts to be soldered should be = 0.13 mm / 0.005"

Soldering investment : same as quartz investment, also investment with low NSE is better than higher.

Maximum strength is attained if soldered parts are cooled slowly for 5-7 min. and then quenched. Total bench cooling causes brittleness.

BASE METAL ALLOYS

Vitallium/ Haynes stellites/ stellite alloys: Co: Cr = 70 : 30

Cr = **passivating effects**, solid solution hardening.

Ni = decreases strength, fusion temperature, but increases the ductility.

Mn, Si = oxygen scavengers.

B = dec xidiser.

Be = reduces fusion temperature

C = carbides increase strength, but excessive produce brittleness.

Tensile strength = > 700 mpa

% elongation = 1-12 %, minimum required = 1.5 %,

Work hardens easily, so difficult adjustment of clasp arms. Use less undercut than Au.

Mixture of oxygen and acetylene gas is used to melt them.

Casting shrinkage = higher, 2.3 %,

Investment used = **silica bonded**, b'coz of higher fusion temperature, it also has higher thermal expansion,

BURS

Cross cut bur = rough cutting at ultra high speed, but at low speed ie at 10000 rpm, which is better than plane straight bur.

A negative or **zero rake angle** is desirable

A **clearance angle** should be small to give additional bulk at the cutting edges.

PROPERTIES OF ORTHODONTIC WIRES

Large elastic deflection is desirable. High working range is required.

Low constant force is desirable.

Stainless steel: ie when Cr > 11 %.(12-30 %), C < 1.2 %

Ferritic = alpha form. BCC, good corrosion resistance, has no Ni, not work hardenable and heat hardenable,

Austenite form = gamma form, FCC, **highest corrosion resistance,** 18 :8 SS,(18 Cr, 8 Ni, 0.15 % C), **not heat hardenable** but cold work hardenable.

Property of easy work hardening is the characteristic of austenite SS.

Cementite = Fe_3C

Pearlite = lamellar composition

Gamma = alpha + Fe_3C (eutectoid reaction)

Martensite form gives hardness, strength, BCT

Austenite → at 120-220° C → Martensite

Of all the elements added to steel, only Co decreases the hardness.

Soldering temperature for orthodontic silver solder = 620-665° C

Elgiloy = CoCr Ni, wrought alloy

Nitinol = NI, Ti, 55% ; 45%, shape memory, large deflections, can't be soldered or welded.

(DENTAL MATERIALS IN DETAILS)

STRUCTURE OF MATTER

Latent heat of fusion = ie when L changes to S; 1 gm of water = 80 cals of heat; the temp is ka fusion temperature.

Sublimation = ie when S changes to G.

Primary bond = chemical in nature eg Ag + O_2 → is primary bonding.

Secondary bond = physical in nature; gold + O_2 → is secondary bonding.

Linear coeff of thermal expansion = is inversely proportional to MP.

Crystalline solids have low internal energy.

Non - Crystalline solids have high internal energy.

Glass transition temperature = the temperature at which there is an abrupt decrease in thermal expansion coeff and is an indication of formation of short range ordering, e.g. glass, resins.

Adhesion ie b/w molecules of 2 different substances eg adhesion of denture to saliva to mucosa.

Cohesion ie b/w molecules of same substances.

Surface energy = ie energy at surface of solid is greater than in its interior. Greater is the SE, greater is the adhesion.

When primary bonding is involved = the adhesion is ka **chemisorption.**

Wetting = If low surface energy of substance, then less wetting

Presence of halogens may prevent wetting eg teflon.

Contact angle = ie the angle formed by adhesive and adherend at their interface.

Larger CA = poor wetting, less spreadability of the liquid.

Wettability of enamel and dentin **decreases after topical Fluoride** use; so it retains less plaque due to decreased SE.

High SE surface energy of many restoration materials → more plaque → more marginal caries.

P and F sealants decrease the SE and wetting and so less caries.

PHYSICAL PROPERTIES OF DM

Stress = F/ A ie internal force generated in the body by external force/load.

Applied force is perpendicular to the body in case of tensile and compressive stresses, but is parallel to the surface of the object in case of shear stress.

Elastic limit = is the greatest stress from which the body returns to normal.

Proportional limit = is the greatest stress, at which the stress – strain curve degresses from a straight line.

Yield strength = is the stress to produce a particular plastic deformation. (EL = PL = YS)

Modulus of elasticity = connotes rigidity / stiffness of a material.

Maximum flexibility = is the strain when the material is stressed to its PL.

Resilience = is the internal energy ie amount of energy absorbed by a structure. It is associated with springiness.

Strength = is the maximum stress required to fracture a structure.

Toughness = the energy required to fracture a material.

Ductility = denotes the tensile strength; **wire may be drawn** under a tensile load. It decreases with increase in temperature.

Malleability = ie under compression, **sheaths can be formed**. It increases with increase in temperature.

eg. GOLD is the most D and M material; Ag is 2nd; Pt is 3rd ductile; Cu is 3rd malleable.

Creep = time dependent plastic deformation when a constant force is applied to a metal held at a temperature near its MP.

Color = visible range of eye = 400 – 700 nm

Cone cells of retina = for color vision

Eye is most sensitive to light in green – yellow region and least sensitive at either extremes.

Hue = property associated with **COLOR** of an object, e.g. Red, green etc.

Value = the lightness / darkness of a color; ie different **shades.**

Chroma = ie the degree of **saturation** of a particular hue.

Metamerism = objects appear of 2 different shades under 2 different sources of lig.ıt. So, color matching should be done under 2 or more light sources; one of them should be DAYLIGHT.

Color matching should be done in a light source which contain a sufficient near UV component ie (300 – 400 mili micron).

Thermal diffusivity of a material is more imp than its thermal conductivity.

Enamel is stronger under compression in a direction parallel to enamel rods than perpendicular to rods.

Dentin is considerably stronger in tension than enamel (51.5 mpa as cp 10.3 mpa).

Modulus of resilience of enamel is less than dentin in compression and so dentin is better able to absorb impact energy.

Enamel on cusps is stronger than on sides.

BIOLOGICAL CONSIDERATIONS =

Microleakage = except systems based on polyacrylic acid and dentin bonding agents, none of the restorative material provides adhesion to tooth.

Acid etching has decreased chances of microleakage.

Smear layer is 5 – 10 micron thick. It prevents bonding of dental adhesive to tooth.

GYPSUM PRODUCTS

Gypsum = calcium sulphate dihydrate

Principle constituent of dental plaster and stone = calcium sulphate hemihydrate.

When calcium sulphate dihydrate is heated at 110 – 130° C, i.e. **dry calcination**; then calcium sulphate hemihydrate is formed; if gypsum is heated open to air, then beta – hemihydrate is formed ie POP.

If heated under pressure in an autoclave (at 120 – 130° C, 17 psi, 5 – 7 hrs), then alpha – hemihydrate is formed ie dental stone.

Improved stone = formed by boiling gypsum in 30 % $CaCl_2$ and then autoclaved in p.o. 0.5 % sodium succinate = **densest particles** are formed.

Difference b/w plaster and stone = crystals of plaster are spongy, irregular, porous, require more water, less strength.

When calcium sulphate dihydrate is mixed with water, heat **(3900 cals)** is evolved so it is an EXOTHERMIC REACTION.

Needle like crystals are formed ka **SPHERULITES**.

Calcium sulphate hemihydrate is 4 times more soluble in water than dihydrate.

W/P ratio = high W/P = longer ST; weaker gypsum product.

For Type I plaster = 0.5 – 0.75
For Type II plaster = 0.45 – 0.50
For Type III stone = 0.28 – 0.30
For Type IV stone = 0.22 – 0.24
For Type V plaster = 0.18 – 0.22

Loss of gloss = ie excess water is taken up in forming the dihydrate leading to loss of gloss. It is approx 9 min.

Control of ST = impurities decrease ST; finer particles decrease ST; more W/P increases ST; longer and rapid mixing decreases ST (crystals are broken with mixing which increases the no. of nuclei.)

Temperature of water if > 50° C, it decreases the ST,; as temperature approaches the 100° C, no reaction occurs.

Most effective and practical method of control of ST = adding retarders and accelerators.

Accelerator = decrease the ST eg NaCl.

Retarders = increase the ST; act by forming an absorbed layer on hemihydrate to decrease its solubility and upon gypsum crystals to decrease their growth. Eg glue, gelatin, gums.

NaCl = accelerator if < 2%; retarder if > 2 %

$Na_2 - SO_4$ = accelerator if < 3.4 %; retarder if > 3.4 %.

Most common accelerator is $K_2\ SO_4$ > 2 –3 %

Gypsum / dihydrate = acts as accelerator as no. of nuclei increases.

Increase in MT and speed of mixing = accelerator.

Retarder forms a coating on the surface of hemihydrate particles and prevent it from going into solution, e.g. citrates, acetates, borates.

Setting expansion = occurs when hemihydrate changes to dihydrate. During growth, the crystals intercept each other and outward thrust leads to expansion.

It is 0.06 % - 0.5 % linear. In p.o. 4 % K_2SO_4, the SE decreases from 0.5 % to 0.06 %.

If equivalent volumes of hemihydrate, water and dihydrate are compared, the volume of dihydrate is less than the volume of Hemihydrate + water by – 2.37 %.

So actually, a **volume contraction occurs during setting**.

Control of SE = most effectively by CHEMICALS.

Hygroscopic SE = is a physical process. If setting occurs under water — then SE is more than double as compared to in air; is due to additional crystal growth.

Strength

Dry strength = 2 x the wet strength.

Increase in W/P ratio = increase porosity, decrease in dry strength.

Increase MT = it increases the strength upto a limit for approx 1 min. of mixing; but by overmixing, crystals get broken and less interlocking occurs so less strength.

Accelerators and retarders = decrease both wet and dry strength.

Alpha – hemihydrate ie stone = is stronger

Beta – hemihydrate ie POP = is weaker

TYPES

TYPE I = impression plaster, in	is POP with modifiers	For impression; for a final wash impression, construction of full denture
Type II = **model plaster,** Hydrocal	ie dihydrate is calcined under steam pressure; it is stronger; requires less W/P; increased strength	To fill the flask in denture construction
Type III; **Dental stone**; class I stone	3000 – 5000 psi; stronger	For making casts in denture making

TYPES (*Contd.*)

Dental stone high strength, Type IV; class II stone / densitc / improved stone	Good strength / hardness / SE due to cuboidal particles and decreased surface area	For making tooth dies for inlays / bridge
Dental stone, high strength, high expansion; type V	Decreased W/P; increased SE to 0.3 %.	Used for alloys eg base metal which have more casting shrinkage than traditional noble metals.
Synthetic gypsum	Can be prepared from waste products of H_3PO_4 also	

Care of cast

Dry cast should not be placed in water as it is soluble. It should be placed in water – saturated with $CaSO_4$;

If placed in running water = linear dimensions decrease by 0.1 % for every 20 min.

If increased temperature to 90 – 110° C, then shrinkage occurs due to loss of water of crystalisation;

IMPRESSION MATERIALS

Mech of setting	Inelastic materials	Elastic materials
Set by chemical reactions/ irreversible	Plaster; ZOE	Alginate, polysulfide, polyether, silicone
Set by temperature change/reversible	Compound wax	Agar
For edentulous	POP; impression compounds, impression pastes	
For dentulous	Elastic hdrocolloids	

(A) Impression compounds

Are noncrystalline materials; aka **modelling plastics**. Use for edentulous ridges, ka *type I* compounds.

Tray compounds = aka *type II* compounds, its main use is for **border molding** of secondary denture tray.

Properties =

1. **Low thermal conductivity** = so inside softens last, uniform softening is required, it should be thoroughly cooled before it is taken out or distortion of impression by relaxation of stresses may occur.
2. Flow = for better impression, it should be < 6% at mouth temperature, and should not be < 85% at 45° C;
3. Distortion = cast should be poured immediately or with in 1 hour or changes occur due to relaxation of the stresses.

(B) ZOE impression pastes

Used as a secondary / corrective impression material, inelastic, for edentulous mouth.

Chemistry = it is a **chelation** reaction.

1. Hydrolysis of ZnO occurs ie WATER IS ESSENTIAL FOR REACTION.
2. zinc hydroxide combines with eugenol to form a CHELATE and WATER IS A REACTION PRODUCT. This chelate then crytallises to gain strength.

Accelerators = **zinc acetate dihydrate** which is more soluble than ZnO and supplies Zn^{++} more rapidly.

Also calcium chloride is an accelerator.

Acids eg acetic acid, is more active accelerator than water, as it increases speed of zinc hydroxide formation.

High temperature and humidity = accelerator

Composition

Tube I	% AGE	FUNCTION
ZnO	87 %, maximum	
Fixed vegetable/ mineral oils	13 %	Plastisizer; decreases irritant action of eugenol
Tube II		
Eugenol/oil of clove	12 %	Decreases the burning sensation
Gum polymerised rosin	50%, maximum	Speed of reaction; smoothness
Filler/silica	20 %	Gives body to the mix
Lanolin	3 %	
Resinous balsam	10 %	Increases flow
Calcium chloride	5 %	Accelerator, ST controls

Type I = aka hard paste

Type II = aka soft paste

Initial ST = 3 – 6 min.

Final ST = 10 min for type I pastes; 15 min for type II pastes.

Control of ST

1. Zinc acetate / water = decrease the ST
2. Cool slab and spatula = increase the ST
3. Increased humidity and temperature = decrease the ST.
4. Increased MT = decrease ST
5. Olive oil / mineral oil = decrease the ST
6. Oral heat and saliva = decrease the ST

Flow = should be adequate to avoid compression of tissues.

Dimensional changes = is < 0.1 % shrinkage ; so impression can be preserved INDEFINITELY without any shape changes due to stress relaxations.

ZOE REACTION IS NEVER COMPLETE – the eugenol may leach out.

ZOE pastes of non – eugenol types which contain more plasticizers eg petrolatum to decrease sticking to oral tissues.

Non-eugenol pastes = set by **saponification** reaction. This reaction is not affected by temperature and humidity.

Elastic impression materials = reversible HC

Suspensions / emulsions = if particle size is large and can be seen by naked eyes or through a microscope.

Suspensions = ie solids in liquids. (SL)

Emulsions = ie liquid in liquid. (LL)

True solutions = have a single phase.

Colloid and suspensions = have 2 phases ie dispersed phase and dispersion medium

Dispersed phase forms MICELLES, which forms a **brush – heap** structure in which dispersion medium is held by capillary attraction.

Aerosol = ie liquid or solid in air.

Lyosol = ie solid, liquid and gas in liquids.

HC impression materials are solids in liquids = **ie lyophilic**

Organic colloids = are lyophilic.

Metallic dispersions = are lyophobic.

Gelation temperature = ie at which sol changes to gel.

Liquefaction temperature = ie at which gel changes to sol.

Hysteresis = is the difference b/w Liquefaction temperature and Gelation temperature, the LT is > GT. (LT-GT)

It is a physical process by temperature.

Irreversible HC = ie sol changes to gel by **chemical action** eg alginates.

Properties

1. Compressive strength should not be < 35.6 psi.
2. Low rate of loading = it increases the flow / permanent deformation, so impression should be removed RAPIDLY from the mouth.
3. Most of the volume of gel is water. So it shows the phenomenon of **syneresis and imbibition.**
4. Relaxation of gel is never complete.

(C) AGAR

Is a reversible HC impression material.

Agar is a **sulfuric ester of galactose** polymer.

Composition

Components	% age	Functions
Agar	8 – 15	Basic
Water	balance %	**Principle component**
Borate	0.2 – 0.5	Strength
Sulfates	1.0 – 2.0	Accelerator
Thixotropic material	0.3 – 0.5	
Hard wax	0.5 – 1.0	

Borax = increases the strength by increasing density of micelles. It is **an excellent retarder of setting of gypsum products**, which is a disadvantage of pouring cast in agar impression material.

Also, surface of cast prepared in HC impression material has HIGH CONC. OF RESIDUAL HEMIHYDRATE and SYNGENITE and a SOFT CAST SURFACE as compared to surface of cast at glass surface.

TO PREVENT IT, immerse the impression in a solution with accelerator for setting of gypsum, prior to filling or a plaster hardener eg sulfates.

Manipulation = to convert the gel in sol, the boiling water for 10 min. is the best way.

At high altitudes, **propylene glycol** is added to the water to bring 100 C BP of water.

For re - liquefaction, 3 more minutes are required for boiling / reuse.

Circulate cool water at 18 – 21° C for not less than 5 minutes.

Laminate technique = put alginate in tray and agar in prepared tooth.

Rapid cooling generates the stresses near the tray when the gelation first occurs. So **water at 20° C is best than the ice water** for changing sol to gels to avoid stress development.

Remove the impression with a jerk to avoid distortion.

Dimensional stability = by syneresis and imbibition.

In air, syneresis leads to shrinkage due to loss of water. Imbibition leads to overexpansion.

To **store the impression, best is 2 % K_2SO_4** or 100 % relative humidity to prevent the dimensional changes.

Surface hardness = of the cast can be increased by treating the surface of the impression by **hardening solutions befor pouring** the cast, i.e. K_2SO_4, $Zn\ SO_4$, $MnSO_4$ etc. the best is 2% K_2SO_4. It acts as accelerator for the setting of gypsum.

Surface of the cast = best surface if setting is allowed in 100 % relative humidity. The cast should be removed within a reasonable period of time b'coz overtime leads to chalky surface.

Impression can be **disinfected** by = iodophores, bleach or glutraldehyde.

(D) ALGINATE

Chief ingredient = soluble alginate; a linear polymer of sodium salt of anhydro – beta – d – mannuronic acid. Salts eg of Na, K and triethanolamine alginate are used in dental impression materials.

Alginate + water → SOL → gel. It is a **chemical reaction.**

Composition =

K – alginate	15 %	Chief ingredient
$CaSO_4$	16	**Reactor**; increases shelf life and dimensional stability
ZnO	4	**Filler**, controls ST of gypsum
Potassium titanium fluoride	3	**Accelerator** for gypsum; gives hard cast surface
Diatomaceous earth	60	Filler, maximum % so provides strength, stiffness, smooth surface
$NaPO_4$, sod. phosphate Dedusting agents	2	**Retarder**; Increase density of powder

Retarder = it reacts with $CaSO_4$ first than alginate to prevent reaction of $CaSO_4$ with alginate for sometime which has to take place in mouth only, e.g. sodium tri - poly – phosphate.

Reactor = is calcium sulphate as it gives calcium ions. $CaSO_4$ is more insoluble than $CaCl_2$ and supplies Ca^{++} at a slower rate – so reaction is retarded to give ample working time.

Do not inhale the powder as silica is present, which is damaging to lungs.

15 gm of powder and 40 ml of water is required at normal room temperature for 3 – 4 min for gelation.

Japanese alginate = uses triethanolamine alginate + CARBO-NATES (instead of phosphates) + $CaSO_4$.

Gel structure = fibrils are held together by **primary bonds**; are cross linked complex / polymers giving a **brush heap structure** through Calcium ions. It contains unreacted particles and water. Changes in dimensions occur by loss of this entrapped water.

Properties

1. Compressive strength should not be < than 37 psi., it should be > 0.245 mpa, or 35.6 psi. According to ADA, it should be > 0.343 Mpa.

2. Overmixing decreases the strength = by breaking the fibrils.
3. Gelation time is = 3 – 4 min at 20° C.
4. Setting time = **of type I** = 60 – 120 sec; of **type II** = 2 – 4.5 min. it is best regulated by AMOUNT OF RETARDER in manufacturing. But in clinics, it is best regulated by using COLD WATER for mixing, by W/P ratio and by MT.
5. Best method is = temperature of water, esp in summers.
6. Setting in mouth is faster than thc outside, b'coz the temperature inside the oral cavity is higher than the air esp in winters.
7. Permanent deformation of alginate is slightly HIGHER than the reversible HC.
8. Mixing time = 45 – 60 sec.
9. Thickness of gel b/w tray and tissues should be = 3 mm. However, more thickness of alginate is not recommended b'coz then sagging of the material takes place and so change in dimensions can occur.
10. Impression should not be removed from the mouth for at least 2 – 3 min. after gelation.
11. Reversible HC materials show no deleterious effects even when they are held in the mouth for 10 min. but, alginates should be removed from the mouth after 2 –3 min. as prolonged placement causes DISTORTION.
12. **For surface details** = reversible HC and elastomers are better than alginate for details.
13. It should be stored in 100 % relative humidity to avoid change in dimensions, **best is to pour the cast immediately.**
14. **Disinfection of the impression** can be done by dipping in = NaOCl for 10 min, or glutraldehyde solutions.
15. Duplication of cast = is best done by reversible HC materials. Their water content is higher.

ELASTOMERS: 5 types

1. Polysulfide
2. Condensation polymerising silicones (outdated)
3. Addition polymerising silicones

4. Polyethers
5. Visible light cure polyether urethane dimethacrylate. It is a single component system.

Silicones and polysulfides are hydrophobic.

POLYSULFIDES

Vulcanisation = or curing or cross linking = is the process of heating the liquid polymer in p.o of SULFUR to form the rubber.

POLYMERISATION reaction is **exothermic.** It is affected by amount of total material, conc. of initiators, moisture and temperature.

Lead dioxide = is most common **oxidising agent** used for cross linking and lengthening the chains.

Chain lengthening predominates first = it increases the VISCOSITY

Cross linking = gives 3D structure and gives ELASTICITY.

CONDENSATION SILICONES

It is alpha – hydroxy – terminated poly dimethyl siloxane.

Cross linking is through = **alkyl silicates** eg tetraethyl orthosilicates in p.o of **stannous octoate** in terminal groups of silicone polymers.

Reaction occurs at AMBIENT TEMPERATURE, so it is ka ROOM TEMP VULCANISATION (RTV); silicones are formed which have 1000 units approx.

ETHYL ALCOHOL is a **by – product** of the reaction = its evaporation leads to contraction of the impression.

Presence of TIN compounds in catalyst = decreases the shelf life of impression material – due to oxidation of Sn compounds,

ADDITION SILICONES

Ka poly vinyl siloxane or vinyl polysiloxane.

Terminal group = vinyl groups

Cross linking through = hydride groups

Activator = platinum salt catalyst

Reaction is = addition type

Bye – products = NIL, but **H_2 gas may be produced** as bubbles on impression surface if ration of vinyl and hydride group is not balanced.

Base and catalyst, both have vinyl silicones.

Base = hybrid silicone

Catalyst = platinum salt + and retarder also.

Scavenger = Pt, Pd ; they remove H_2 gas.

POLYETHER

Curing occurs by reaction b/w aziridine rings.

Is a **copolymer** of ethylene oxide and tetrahydrofuran.

Cross linking and setting is by = aromatic - sulfonate esters.

Cross linking = by cationic polymerisation via the imine – end groups.

COMPOSITIONS
POLYSULFIDE

Base paste	Accelerator/reactor/catalyst paste
♦ Polysulfide polymer	♦ Lead dioxide = dark brown color
♦ Fillers (TiO_2) = for strength	♦ Fillers
♦ Plasticizer (dibutyl phthalate) = viscosity	♦ Plasticizers = liquid vehicle
♦ Sulfur 0.5 %	♦ Retarder = oleic acid or stearic acid = controls ST

CONDENSATION SILICONES

Base paste

- ♦ silicone polymer (is a liquid)
- ♦ fillers = colloidal silica or microsized metal oxide to form paste. Selection of filler is vimp b'coz silicone has low cohesive energy; particle size should be b/w 5 – 10 microns.

ADDITION SILICONES

Base = poly (methyl hydrogen siloxane) + fillers

Catalyst = Pt salts activator + fillers

POLYETHERS

Base = polyether polymer + colloidal silica (as filler) + glycol ether or phthalate (as platicizer)

Calatyst = alkyl aromatic sulfonate + filler + plasticizer

LIGHT CURE POLYETHERS

Polyether urethane DMA resin + photo initiator + photo accelerators + SiO_2 as filler

Silica Filler has refractive index close to resin for maximum depth of cure.

PROPERTIES

Linear coefficient of thermal expansion = 150 – 220 X 10^{-6} / °C.

Setting time = curing may continue for a considerable time eg > 2 weeks for condensation silicone. **Factors affecting** the ST are :

- Increased temperature = decrease ST / WT
- Cool slab = increases the WT
- WT can be altered by base – accelerator ratio for condensation silicones; and by cooling / retarder for addition silicones.
- Oleic acid = increases the WT of PbO_2 cured polusulfide materials.
- Water / moisture = decreases the ST
- Base – accelerator ratio = a good method for curing rate of condensation silicone.
- Curing rate of addition silicones is more sensitive to TEMPERATURE changes than polysulfides.
- Curing rate of polyethers is less sensitive to TEMPERATURE CHANGES than addition silicones.
- Impression should remain in mouth for 6 – 8 min; and should be removed in a jerk to avoid deformation,

Elasticity

- Elastic properties **improve with curing time.**
- Longer the impression is in the mouth, more accurate it will be.
- Recovery is less rapid for polysulfide than the other 3.
- Elastic **recovery is best for addition silicone** and least for polysulfide.

Permanent deformation after strain in compression in increasing order is

Addition silicones < condensation silicone < polyether < polysulfide (maximum).

- Incomplete recovery after deformation is due to = viscoelastic nature of rubbers.
- **Most stable** is = addition silicone and polyethers.

Stiffness increases in that order = as

Polysulfide < condensation silicone < addition silicone < polyether (maximum).

- **Polysulfide has unpleasant odour** and taste and **difficult to clean.**
- Silicones and polyether are CLEANER TO HANDLE.
- Contact dermatitis by polyether; hypersensitivity by polyether catalyst system.

Dimensional changes

- Contraction during the curing is due to = decrease in volume
- **Condensation silicones** = loose alcohol → contraction
- Polysulfides = loss of volatile accelerator → contraction
- Hydrophilic polyether polymer and addition silicones ABSORB WATER → dimensional changes
- Changes in dimension is greater for condensation silicone and polysulfide than for polyether and addition silicones.

Contraction

1. Type I and type III should not contract > 0.5 % after 24 hrs.
2. Type II should not contract > 1.0 % after 24 hrs.

3. Rubber materials are more dimensionally stable than alginate when stored in AIR.
4. **Condensation silicone take much longer** to reach maximum contraction than other 3.

Cast formation

- Cast should be poured within 30 min for polysulfide and condensation silicones.
- These rubbers do not affect the cast surface.
- **Surface is better** with polyether and addition silicones than polysulfide and agar.
- Gypsum solution does not properly wet the surface of the polysulfide and hydrophobic silicones = so a WETTING AGENT is to be used.

Important points

♦ With some polysulfide materials = **voids appear in surface** of impression after some time due to escaping of entrapped air, "so cast should be poured within 30 min or immediately."
♦ With some **addition silicone impression materials** = some pits appear on cast if poured immediately, which is due to escaping H_2 gas, "so **wait for 15 – 30 min** before pouring."

- LESS THE DISTANCE B/W impression tray and master die ie less bulk of the impression material, more accurate impression is obtained. Only 2 – 4 mm thickness is required. This finding is directly opposite to that recommended for HC impression materials.
  It is **difficult to repair a** rubber impression material.
- **Multiple casts** can be obtained with same impression, but – cast will be less accurate if polysulfide or condensation silicone material is used, so there should be < 30 min gap b/w 2 casts with them.
- With polyether, moisture absorption from gypsum leads to distortion of multiple pours.

Hydrophilic vinyl polysiloxanes

A **surfactant** is added which allows the impression to wet soft tissues better and a better gypsum cast is formed. But these are **difficult to electroplate.**

Disinfection = 2 % glutraldehyde for < 10 min to avoid dimensional changes.

SYNTHETIC RESINS

- Polymerisation is **never complete**; the residual monomer affects the M.Wt of the polymer.
- Resin gains strength only after the degree of polymerisation is 150 – 200 units.
- Strength increases with increase in polymerisation till a specific m.wt; after that no increase in the strength occurs.
- **Cross linking** = increases strength
- **Condensation polymerisation** = bye- products are formed. The process repeats itself. Polymerisation occurs by repeated elimination of small molecules, e.g. polysulfide impression material.
- But, **polyurethane is a condensation polymer without any bye–products.**
- **Addition polymerisation** = most of the dental resins are of this type; **no bye products;** no change in composition during reaction occurs.
- Reaction is not easy to control.
- Requisite = p.o. **unsaturated groups**
- Initiator and activator are involved; it is an **exothermic** reaction; a very rapid process;
- Free radical are formed from the initiators. **Benzyl peroxide gives free radicals** at a temperature b/w 50 – 100 °C;
- **Stages** = 4 ie initiation, propagation, termination, chain transfer.
- **Induction / initiation** = the initiator starts **energy transfer** to the monomer molecule; the required energy is 16,000 – 29,000 cals / mole.
- **Propagation** = **heat is evolved**, polymerisation is never complete;
- **Termination** = by direct **coupling** or by exchange of H – atom from one chain to another.

- **Chain – transfer** = active state is transferred from an activated radical to an inactive molecule and a new nucleus for further growth is created.
- In COLD CURE = benzoyl peroxide – aromatic amine system; **activator** is dimethyl - p-toluidine.
- In HEAT CURE = Activator is HEAT.
- In LIGHT CURE = camphoroquinone and an amine react under visible light.

Inhibition of polymerisation = it prevents polymerisation during storage.

1. 0.006 % *hydroquinone*
2. *oxygen* reacts with free radicals and retards the polymerisation
3. so reaction velocity is less if done in *open air* than in sealed tube

Copolymerisation

2 or more different monomers (M) form the polymer (P).

3 types = random; block; graft.

1. Random = different Ms are randomly distributed along the chain.

2. Block = if identical Ms occur in long sequences along the main P chain.

3. Graft = sequence of one of the M are grafted on to a backbone of 2nd M species.

B and G polymers = have improved impact strength.

Plasticizers = decrease the fusion temperature; increase the solubility of polymer in M; **decrease the brittleness** of P ; decrease the strength and hardness.

Its mechanism of action is – by **partial neutralisation** of secondary bonds or intermolecular forces. It is a form of external plasticizer.

Internal plasticizer = a co-monomer helps in co-polymerisation and becomes a part of polymers eg **butyl acrylate**.

MMA

Volume shrinkage = 21 %

BP = 100.8 °C

Heat of polymerisation = 12.9 kcal / ml

PMMA = important features are

- KHN = 18 – 20
- Tensile strength = 59 mpa
- Takes up water by imbibition
- Both adsorption and absorption ie **sorption** can occur = which increases the weight by 0.5 % / week in water. It depends on m.wt of acrylic; so if greater m.wt, then less wt increases by water absorption.
- It is soluble in chloroform / acetone.

Epoxy resin:

- Adheres to metal, glass, wood.
- Cross linking is easily accomplished.

  Epoxy molecule = diglycidyl ether of bisphenol – A.
- Mainly **used as matrix** for composite restorative material (urethane dimethacrylate can be used as matrix).
- Maximum biting force with CD = 1/6th of the natural dentition.

Heat activated resin

Monomer	Action	POLYMER	Action
Pure MMA		PMMA	
Hydroquinone <= .006%	Inhibitor	Copolymer of MMA and ethyl acrylate <= 5%	Increases the solubility
Glycol DMA = 1 – 2 %	Cross linking agent	Dibutyl phthalate 8 – 10 %	**Plasticizer**; add low m.wt beads PMMA to high m.wt PMMA
Activator	Heat	**Initiator** Pigments	Benzoyl peroxide

- If supplied in gel form = it contains a *vinyl resin* in addition to PMMA.
- If as a **solid component** = a **copolymer** of vinyl chloride and vinyl acetate is used instead of PMMA. Their mixing leads to a polymer mixture of PMMA and predominantly vinyl copolymer resin.
- In **injection molding** = **polystyrene** is used. **No trial closure** is required with injection molding technique.
- **Separating media** = tin foil; cellulose lacquers; solutions of alginate compounds; soap; sodium silicate; starch; but the MOST POPULAR is water-soluble alginates (cold mould seal) which gives **calcium alginate film** on the gypsum surface.
- If water gets incorporated in resin = then it affects polymerisation rate and color; denture may craze due to the stresses formed by evaporation of water.
- Polymer : monomer ratio = 3 : 1 by volume.
- More polymer = decreases the reaction time; decreases the shrinkage of the resin.

P – M reaction = 4 stages

1. Polymer settles in monomer; *incoherent fluid mass* is formed.
2. *Stringiness* = M attacks P; stringy and tacky mass is formed.
3. *Dough stage* = M diffuses in P; smooth and dough like mass; moldable. Non tacky. Packing is done in this stage.
4. M disappears by evaporation and further penetration in P; cohesive and *rubber like mass* formed; cannot be molded;

Dough forming time = less time required with increased temperature (put in warm water at < 55 °C, as at more temperature, the rate of polymerisation increases).

Working time = time required b/w stage 2 and beginning of stage 4 ie material remains in dough form. It is **at least 5 min;** it increases with decrease in temperature.

Polymerisation procedure

- Benzoyl peroxide (is **initiator**) = gives free radicals at temperature > 60° C.

- **Free radicals start process** of polymerisation by combining with monomers and giving free radicals further.
- **Rate of polymerisation** is controlled by rate at which free radicals of benzoyl peroxide are released and the temperature.
- Decrease temperature = increases the m.wt of polymer; increases the reaction time.
- Polymerisation reaction = is **exothermic;** heat may help in proper processing of denture;
- **Internal porosity = BP of monomer is 100.8 °C**; which may boil and produce bubbles in the interior of resin, as heat is not conducted away. This porosity is **not present on surface** b'coz exothermic heat is conducted away from surface of resin into the POP, so temperature does not rise. It occurs frequently if thickness of resin **is more than 3 mm.**
- Polymerisation cycle = temperature rise is a function of rate of polymer formation; temperature rise is dependent **on rate of heat evolution.**
- Immediately place flask in water at 65° C for 90 min. to cure THICK AREAS without porosity; then boil for 60 min to cure THIN AREAS; **bench cooling of the flask is the best.**
- If cooled under water; warpage due to differential thermal contraction. So bench cooling for 30 min and cold tap water for 15 min is satisfactory.

CHEMICAL / COLD CURE / AUTOPOLYMERISING RESINS

- Initiator = 2 % benzoyl peroxide
- Activator = 0.75 % tertiary amine (in monomer)
- Free radicals form by a reaction b/w benzyl peroxide and dimethyl – p – toluidine.
- Degree of polymerisation is LESS (as compared to heat cure).
- Smaller the particle size = more rapid is the polymerisation, b'coz of increased surface area and more wetting.
- Color stability is poor b'coz of oxidation of tertiary amine.
- W.T. is shorter (less than HC)
- Polymerisation reaction may begin before dough stage.

- During trial closure = flash may be a cause to increase the VD of denture.
- Transverse strength is = 80 % of heat cure resins
- Injection moulding is better = as no trial closure is required.

Processing of denture

- At room temperature = no processing stresses develop.
- Better fit; more dimensionally stable.
- Polymerisation continues for several hours.
- **3 – 5 % residual monomer** is left; (0.2 – 0.5 % in heat cure)
- **Exothermic reaction** = temperature of bulky areas is higher than surface; so thin areas are not cured as well and are weaker.

LIGHT CURED RESINS

- Is a composite of urethane – DMA, microfine silica; and high m.wt. acrylic resin monomers.
- Acrylic resin beads = as organic fillers
- **camphoroquinone amines** = as **photo- initiators**

IMPORTANT POINTS

- **polymerisation shrinkage** = density changes from 0.94 to 1.19 gm/cm^3 = so volume shrinkage of cold cure is 21 % and for heat cure is 8 %.
- polymerisation shrinkage contributes very little to linear shrinkage; it is **distributed uniformly** over all the surfaces of denture so fit is unaffected.
- **Thermal shrinkage** = is the **chief contributor to the linear shrinkage** phenomenon.
- Linear coeff of thermal expansion = 81×10^{-6} / °C and linear shrinkage of denture material = 0.2 – 0.69 %
- Polymerisation shrinkage in maxillary denture is seen in PALATAL AREA; = resin **shrinks towards the areas of greatest bulk.**
- **Processing shrinkage** = 0.53 % for heat cure and 0.26 % for cold cure; so dimensional stability is more in cold cure;

- Greater shrinkage for injection resin is due to = high processing temperature.
- Increase VD is more in compression molding than in fluid resin / gypsum mold technique.
- So compression molded cold cure resin dentures are = BEST from dimensional point of view.

Porosity

- Internal porosity in thick parts due to vaporisation of monomer = it is NOT UNIFORM.
- **Thick lingual posterior areas of lower denture base is more porous** than thin buccal portion = which is near to metal flask; so heat is dissipated away.
- Lack of homogenous mix at dough or gel stage = some areas will have more monomer, so shrink more = so *localised shrinkage* and VOIDS APPEAR.
- Delay packing till dough stage = mix is more homogenous then; it is related to dough forming time.
- Due to lack of adequate pressure / lack of dough material in packing = bubbles are not spherical; abundant.
- Surface / **subsurface porosities** = are due to **failure to expel air** inclusions.

Water sorption

1. Is due to polar nature of resin; occurs through diffusion.
2. For 1 % wt increase due to water absorbed = the resin expands linearly 0.23 %; **approx 17 days** (ie very long time) **are required** for full saturation of appliance with water.
3. Relieves the internal stresses as macromolecules are forced apart.
4. After several months = HC compression molded denture is = slightly undersized; and CC compression molded denture is = slightly oversized.

Processing stresses = are **tensile** in character. They develop due to variable thickness of denture in different areas, localised polymerisation shrinkage eg around the necks of the porcelain teeth etc.

Crazing = ie relaxation of surface stresses leads to crack formation. It appears in PMMA under tensile stresses only at right angle to tensile stress **due to separation of polymer chains**. Cross linking decreases the crazing considerably.

Physical properties of resins

- Decrease in polymerisation = decrease strength
- Decrease in curing time = decrease strength, stiffness
- strength, stiffness of heat cure > cold cure
- strength, stiffness are less if resin is stressed under water than if it is stressed under air.
- Properties of resin decrease by abrasive and polishing agents which **generate heat** and **lead to warpage** / release of stresses or partial depolymerisation = decrease strength, stiffness.
- strength, stiffness decrease with water sorption.
- **Bulky parts = have more strength.** Exothermic heat is evolved which depends on the BULK.
- Creep rate of CC = increases more rapidly with stresses than for HC.
- KHN = 16 – 18 for CC; 20 for HC.
- During rapair; **a rounded joint is superior** in strength to a butt joint due to lower stress concentration. Repair is preferred with CC, b'coz HC will cause warpage of denture.
- Also, **avoid overflow of monomer** on the denture surface as it may cause crazing and weakening.

Relining = a low curing temperature is required for relines to avoid distortion of denture;

- Rebasing is preferred over relining b'coz with relining, the monomer diffuses before curing and may cause warpage and processing shrinkage of liner.
- Soft / resilient reliners = absorb some energy of mastication – which is slowly released.

- Plasticized acrylic resins are **permanent soft liners**.
- Room Temperature curing chairside silicones = are temporary soft liners.
- 2 – 3 mm liner thickness is recommended.
- Soft liner decreases strength of denture base = by solvent action of silicone adhesive and monomer and by decrease in thickness.
- **Dibutylin dilaurate catalyst inhibits growth of C. albicans** = but it also decreases as the Sn – compound is washed away from the liner.

Tissue conditioners

- Are highly plasticized acrylic resins.
- Powder = PEMA.
- Liquid = butyl phthalate; butyl glycolate in ethanol or alcohol.
- Absorbs energy elastically; but undergo viscous flow under load and change their form with changing contours of soft tissues.
- **With aging = it looses its plastic property** and gains elastic properties.

Denture cleansers

Composition = alkaline compounds + detergents + flavouring agent + sodium perborate.

sodium perborate reacts with water to **give oxygen bubbles**, which help loosen the debris.

House hold bleach ie **hypochlorite should not be used** with metals.

Infection control = best **by ethylene oxide** gas; glutaraldehyde is C/I b'coz **resin can absorb it**.

Resin teeth are made of PMMA + cross linking agent; their strength can be increased by applying 1:1 solution of **methylene chloride** and MMA at the neck of the teeth for 4 – 5 min.

Porcelain teeth = are brittle, craze by thermal shock, sharp sound on contact; keep VD stable as they do not get abraded. Get retained by **mechanical retention only;** abrade the opposing teeth.

Heat vulcanising silicones = are material of choice in terms of strength and color is polychromatic.

RESTORATIVE RESINS

- Direct filling composite resins are based on BIS – GMA or urethane dimethacrylate UDMA.
- Acrylic resins = has no fillers;
- **Powder** = **PMMA** + **benzoyl Peroxide (initiator)**
- Liquid = MMA + **tertiary amine** (N,N – dimethyl – p - toluidine) (as activator)+ **hydroquinone (inhibitor).**
- Amine activated resins = color changes with UV light.
- **Sulfonate/sulfinic acid system** for polymerisation rather than amine – peroxide system = **color stable**, but unstable in p.o. moisture.
- High polymerisation shrinkage = 5 – 8 %
- High coeff of thermal expansion = 7 – 8 times the tooth and so marginal leakage is HIGH.
- Incremental build up of resin = can compensate the polymerisation shrinkage.

Best properties = are of small particle type of resins.

Component	**Unfilled resin**	**Conventional**	**Microfilled particle**	**Small (Best)**	**Hybrid**
Fillers % vol.	—	60–65	20–55	65–77	60–65
Compr str, psi	10,000	36250–43000	36250-50750	50750–58000	43500–50750
Tensile str mpa	24	50–65	30–50	75–90	70–90
MOE, 10^6 psi	0.34	1.16–2.18	0.44–0.87	2.18–2.9	1.02–1.74
Coeff of th. Expansion	92.8	25–35	50–60	19–26	30–40
KHN	15	55	25–30	50–60	50–60

Composite resins = 2 components which are insoluble in each other.

Polymerisation mechanism is ADDITION TYPE through free radical formation.

1. Resin matrix	BIS- GMA, or UDMA monomer; + MMA monomer or TEG-DMA monomer act as DILUENTS to decrease viscosity of resin monomer. DMA monomer allows extensive **cross linking.**
2. Filler (inorganic)	30 – 70 % vol or 50 – 85 % wt; **Decrease the polymerisation shrinkage**; decreases the coeff of thermal expansion; increase tensile strength; compressive str; MOE; abrasion resistance; e.g. ♦ Quartz / glass particles = 0.1 – 100 micron size. ♦ Silica particles of colloidal size = 0.02 – 0.04 micron aka **microfillers.** ♦ Microfills < 5 wt % are added to modify paste viscosity. ♦ **Quartz** = is chemically inert; but are hard, so difficult to polish; **abrades opposite teeth** etc. ♦ Radiopaque filler by glasses of Ba/ Sr/ Zr; mostly of barium glass; but it may leach out in an aqueous medium.
3. Coupling agent	to bond b/w resin and filler; eg **organo- silanes**
4. Activator	**Chemical activated** = 2 paste system ie ♦ Benzoyl peroxide = initiator ♦ Tertiary amine = as activator **Light activated** = ♦ UV light = has limited penetration in resin and tooth; Benzoyl peroxide – benzoin methylether, system. **Visible LC** =

	♦ Photoinitiator = camphoroquinone < 0.25 wt % (Diketone – tertraryarmine system) ♦ Activator/accelerator = amines eg DEAEMA – 0.15 wt %. ♦ 400 – 500 nm; **blue region** of VIBGYOR. ♦ *Inhibitors* = to increase stability of resin. ♦ Light bulb used = **tungsten halogen** type ♦ Optical modifiers/ **opacifiers** = Ti – dioxide and Al – oxide (0.001 0.007 % wt) = to simulate E and D.

Pattern of shrinkage = is different for both types ie

CC = shrink towards centre of bulk of material

HC = shrink towards the light source.

Classification of composites

1. Conventional = 8 – 12 micron
2. Small particle = 1 – 5 micron
3. Microfilled = 0.04 – 0.4 micron
4. Hybrid = 0.6 – 1.0 micron
5. Hybrid = ground / conventional + microfilled (10 – 15 wt %)

Description

Conventional/ traditional/ macrofilled	♦ Large size particles = 8 – 12 microns up to 50 – 100 microns. Filler = ground quartz; radiolucent; 70 – 80 wt % or 60 – 70 vol%. ♦ It increases compressive strength of resin = 4 – 5 × the unfilled resin. ♦ Increase MOE = 4 – 6 × the unfilled resin. ♦ Tensile strength = 2 × the unfilled resin. ♦ Decrease polymerisation shrinkage = to 2 vol %. ♦ Decrease the coeff. of thermal Expansion = to 30×10^{-6} (92 = unfilled resin).

Description (*Contd.*)

	♦ But it is still the 3 × the tooth. ♦ KHN = 55 (KHN = 15 for unfilled resin). ♦ Hardness increases by fillers and cross linking of resin; but they have rough surface due to **selective abrasion** of soft resin leaving behind hard fillers. ♦ It can be used for class II, IV fillings ie **stress - bearing areas** but have poor resistance to occlusal wear.
Microfilled resins	**Filler** is colloidal silica = 0.02 – 0.04 microns size ie 200 – 300 × smaller than average quartz particles. **Smoother surface** on polishing. Prepolymerised C.Rs = 60 – 70% by wt of silane coated colloidal silica is added to monomer, which is heat cured with **benzoyl peroxide initiator;** grinding is done to particle size of quartz in conventional CR, it is aka **organic filler.** **Better surface finish** = so resin of choice for esthetic restoration. Decreases tensile strength = so fracture propagation.
Small particle composite	Filler size = 1 – 5 micron Contain more inorganic fillers = 80 % by wt than conventional CR Fillers are = glasses containing heavy metals esp Ba. **Has best physical and mechanical properties;** Coeff of TE = decreased but 2 x of the tooth.Better surface smoothness = due to small and highly dense and packed filler.s. Radiopaque. Used for **posterior teeth** restoration; for class II, IV ie high stress areas

Description (*Contd.*)

	Not as good as microfilled and hybrid for anteriors.
Hybrid CR	Total fillers = 75 – 80 %; average particle size = 0.6 – 1.0 microns Smaller particle size and greater amount of microfillers = increased surface area and decreased overall filler loading. Properties range b/w conventional and small particle CR = **better than microfilled.** Used in anterior restoration and class IV = smooth surface and good strength; widely used for stress bearing restorations;
Composites for posterior restorations	First generation of conventional CR wear @ 150 micron / yr, on the occlusal surface and give poor results; Recent materials abrade @ 20 micron/yr. (amalgam @ 10 microns/ yr) CR in which filler particles are small, high in conc, well bonded to matrix are the most resistant to wear, CR is the material of choice if the patient has documented allergy to Hg.
Contraindications to CR restorations	Bruxism; in caries active mouth as CR has no anticariogenic properties; also micro-leakage is more with CR. Pulp is insulted by microleakage or by chemicals. CR restorations can be repaired by placing new CR on old but strength is low (only 50 %) due to less monomers and increased cross linking.
Biocompatibility	Polymerised CR are relatively biocompatible b'coz of minimum solubility and no leachable unreacted species.

Description (*Contd.*)

	But uncured CR esp LC material, at floor of cavity = is reservoir of diffusible components which may cause pulp injury. Protective layer of **calcium hydroxide** should be applied to deep cavity. **ZOE should not be used** = as eugenol interferes with polymerisation.
Chemical cure resin	Benzoyl peroxide – tertiary amine system (as initiator - activator) Avoid air inclusion in the mix = b'coz air acts as polymerisation inhibitors and causes **sticky surface**. **Cavity should be filled from the bottom outward.**
Light cure resin	**Incremental filling** is advised which also helps compensate polymerisation shrinkage. **400 – 500 nm** range / **blue light** is used. Source should be held as close as posssible to the resin without touching. The light may cause RETINAL damage. Curing time = 40 – 60 sec. And the thickness of resin should not be more than 2 – 2.5 mm.

Acid etching

- To improve marginal seal and **mechanical bonding** and to decrease marginal leakage.
- Centres / periphery / combination **of enamel rods** get preferentially dissolved.
- Etched enamel has HIGH SURFACE ENERGY.
- Resin tags = go to 10 – 20 microns in enamel microporosity.
- Ortho – H_3PO_4 is used = 37 % conc
- **Conc > 50 % leads to** formation of monocalcium – phosphate – monohydrate which inhibit further dissolution of enamel.

- Etching time = 60 sec initially (recent researches say = 15 sec. is enough)
- Flourosed teeth require LONG ETCHING TIME.
- Drying = for 30 sec, warm air or ethanol rinse help increase thc bond strength.
- **Enamel bonding agents** = are resin – matrix diluted by monomers to decrease the viscosity. Help to **increase the wettability** of enamel. They improve mechanical bonding by resin tags but microleakage at dentin – resin or cementum-resin interface occurs;
- Ideally the adhesive should be HYDROPHILIC to wet the surface and displace the water. So the agent should contain both hydrophilic and hydrophobic agents.
- Hydrophilic = **bonds to Calcium** in HA or with collagen,
- Hydrophobic = bonds to restorative resin.
- **Dentin bonding agents** = to prevent microleakage at D and C margins as it helps in bonding with D and C; act by chelation , **aluminium oxalate** is used for chelation; HNO_3 in oxalate regent acts as **dentin conditioners;** aldehydes used for bonding to collagen ie organic part.

So initial conditioners or primers are =

1. HNO_3 = which remove smear layer
2. EDTA = opens dentinal tubule
3. Maleic acid = **modest etching of intertubular dentin** in which HEMA etc. enter into finely textured primed dentin to provide mechanical bonding.

- **Sandwich technique** = GI placed to line the dentin for adhesion; and COMPOSITE RESIN CR is bonded to GI and enamel as ususal.
- **Bevel** = exposes the fresh enamel; removes the unsupported enamel; provides proper orientation of enamel rods to etchant; increase the surface area and so retention is enhanced; microleakage is decreased.
- **Pits and fissure sealants** = are polyurethanes or BIS – GMA resins; BIS – GMA is polymerised by amine–peroxide system or light cure; physical properties are close to unfilled resins; decrease the caries by 78%.

METALS

METALS are crystalline solids **except mercury** which is a liquid.

ALLOY IS A SOLID MIXTURE OF two or more metals.

During solidification, heat is evolved as liquid changes to solid which is known as **latent heat of solidification / fusion.**

Initially, *super-cooling* occurs at which the crystallization starts, but then heat of fusion raises the temperature to Tf until the crystallization is complete.

Liquids exhibit a tendency toward a **short range order arrangement.**

Internal energy decreases when liquid changes to solid.

On **rapid cooling** = number of solidification centers appear.

On **slow cooling** = single crystal is formed ka **homogenous nucleation.**

Grain boundary = is the region of transition b/w 2 crystal lattices;

Impurities in metal may be found in greater concentration at grain boundaries than in grain proper and is more easily attacked by chemicals.

WROUGHT METALS

Wires are made by drawing a cast metal.

When a casting is plastically deformed, it is no longer a cast metal but becomes wrought metal.

Whisker specimens = are tiny, **single crystal filaments** (2.5 micros in diameter) and have been **used as reinforcing agents** in composite materials.

Whiskers have a nearly perfect lattice structures while polycrystalline materials have lattice imperfections.

Whiskers do not contain dislocations.

Strain / work hardening or cold working = slip occurs in other intersecting planes; point defects increase and entire grain gets distorted. Greater stress is required to produce further slip and the metal **becomes stronger and harder**.

When it occurs at room temperature = ka **cold working.**

. When done at higher temp = ka **forging** in which increase in rate of atomic diffusion may entirely prevent strain hardening.

Strength of deformed metal is greater in transverse section than in the direction of rolling.

Annealing = reverses the effect of cold working. **3 stages** occur = as recovery; recrytallisation and grain growth.

Higher the MP of metal = higher is the temperature required for annealing.

Use the **temperature approx half to that is required to melt** the metal on absolute temp scale (°K).

(a) Recovery = slight decease in Tensile strength; **no change in ductility**.

If deformation is < 3 %, the annealing can cause full recovery. Eg **orthodontic appliances are made by wrought wires**, should be subjected to stress relief anneal.

(b) Recrystallisation = new grains (strain free grains) are formed at grain boundaries or most severely cold work areas; material attains its soft and ductile conditions.

(c) Grain growth = larger grains decrease the strength; excessive annealing forms larger grains (it occurs in only wrought metals)

Cast vs wrought = in cast structure = heat Rx is ineffective in changing the grain size;

Orthodontics bands and wires are wrought structures. Wires should never be annealed into recrystallisation stage; **only recovery heat Rx is required**;

CONSTITUTION OF ALLOYS

Alloys = are 2 or more metals mutually soluble in molten condition; it solidify over a range of temperature;

Phase = is any physically distinct; homogenous; and mechanically separable portion of a system.

Binary alloys = if 2 elements

Ternary alloys = if 3 elements; can be age hardened;

Solid solution = is the **simplest alloy** in which atoms of 2 metals intermingle in a common space lattice and structure is **homogenous** and metals are soluble in each other. Eg gold alloys, Ag-Pd,

Atoms of Ag directly enter into the space lattice of Pd; system is not mechanically separable and has **only one – phase**.

Solvent = that metal whose space lattice persists;

Solute = is the other metal;

Solvent = metal whose atoms occupy > 50 % of total no. of positions in the space lattice;

Most of the metals used in dentistry **are FCC in structure** and solid solutions.

Brass = Cu-Zn

Liquidus temperature = ie at which the **first solid begins to form.**

Solidus temperature = ie at which the **last liquid solidifies.**

Larger the temperature range b/w solidus and liquidus = the greater is the tendency towards **coring**.

Rapid cooling does not give time for proper diffusion.

Eutectic alloys

- Eutectic means LOWEST MELTING;
- Components exhibit **complete liquid solubility,** but limited solid solubility. Eg Ag-Cu system = 71.9 % Ag + 28.1 % Cu.
- There is **no solidification range** ie a **constant temperature** of solidification is there.
- Eutectics are often used when lower fusion temperature is needed eg solders;
- Require least amount of diffusion;
- It is ka **invariant transition**, b'coz it occurs at a single temperature and composition.
- Eutectic structures does not appear in alloys of < 8.8 % Cu.
- **Are brittle** b'coz of the p.o. insoluble phases definitely inhibits slip.
- Has poor tarnish and corrosion resistance;

Peritectic system

1. Limited solid solubility of 2 metals = peritectic eg Ag – Sn system in amalgam.
2. Uncommon in dentistry
3. It is also invariant reaction ie occurs at a particular composition and temperature.
4. **Coring occurs if rapid cooling** occurs; with alpha phase around beta – grains before the diffusion can occur.

Heat treatment = metal heated to a temperature > room temperature but < the solidus and held there for a length of time.

Quenching = metal is **rapidly cooled** from high temperature to less than the room temperature; it preserves at room temperature that phase which is stable only at high temperature.

If quenched = soft alloy

If slowly cooled = diffusion and so **harder alloy**.

Solution heat treatment: if gold casting is heated at less than solidus temperature and held for a length of time, it becomes a **random solid solution.** It is then **rapidly cooled** to room temperature to a soft and ductile material. It is done at 700° C for 10 min and then quenched.

After it, heating to produce precipitation of second phase is ka PRECIPITATION AGE HARDENING HEAT TREATMENT. Eg 775° C for 30 min.

Sterling silver = Ag – Cu alloy; has 7.5 % Cu and 92.5 % Ag; for inlay in deciduous teeth.

CORROSION

Tarnish = surface discoloration; slight loss of surface finish or luster; surface deposits; due to formation of **thin oxide films.** It is often a forerunner of corrosion.

Corrosion = **actual deterioration** of metal by reaction with its atmosphere leads to disintegration. **Chlorides; oxides, sulfides are** corrosion products.

Chemical corrosion = discoloration of Ag **by sulfur** forming the silver sulfide.

Silver sulfide is the **principle corrosion product** of gold alloys.

Aka **dry corrosion** = as it occurs in the absence of water or other fluid electrolytes.

Electrolyte or electrochemical corrosion = aka **wet corrosion**; as water and electric current as a path of transport of current is required.

Anode = Where + ve ions are formed ie metal surface which is **corroding.** Free electrons are produced, so ka **oxidation reaction.**

Cathode = Electrons are consumed ie **reduction reaction.**

Cathode is the primary driving force in the electrolytic corrosion.

Metals which give up electrons and ionise = as anode.

Metals which accept electrons from external circuit = as cathode.

More active metal is anode and more noble metal is a cathode.

Galvanic corrosion or dissimilar metals = ie b/w Ag and Au in opposing teeth leading to sharp pain.

Grain boundaries of heterogenised metals act as = anodes; interiors of grains as cathode. So **corrosion occurs at grain boundaries.**

Solder joints = corrode due to different composition of alloy and solder.

Stress corrosion = stress incorporated esp at grain boundaries. It is characterised by the fact that eventual fracture occurs inter-granularly.

Burnishing / malleting / cold working localises the stress in some parts of the restorations leading to corrosion = so EXCESSIVE BURNISHING IS C/I at the margins of metallic restorations.

Conc. Cell corrosion = aka **crevice corrosion**. It is due to different types of electrolytes in system.

Corrosion at poor oral hygiene site occurs **due to difference** in **oxygen tension** b/w parts of same restoration = greatest activity occurs around the areas with least oxygen eg pits; irregularities etc.

In the pits = material at the base of pit acts as anode (no oxygen gas); and material at the periphery of pit acts as cathode.

So all metallic restorations SHOULD BE POLISHED to remove pits etc.

Protection of corrosion = by using a noble metal covering applied on base metal; but if noble layer gets disrupted then the base metal / anode is attacked rapidly.

Passivating effect = oxidation layer of some metals eg CHROMIUM; a layer of adsorbed oxygen or closely packed chromic oxide gives a passivating effects.

But tensile **stresses and chlorides can disrupt this** coating. So house hold bleaches should not be used to clean cast partial dentures; removable orthodontic appliances; which are alloyed with chromium.

Alloys with < 65 % noble metal content get tarnished; so Au, Pt, Pd should be there with approx 50 % Au.

Low Ag – Cu ratio is better for tarnish resistance.

Silver sulfide is the common corrosion product of gold alloys containing silver.

Pd enriches the surface of alloy with Au and Pd; blocking sulfide formation.

Galvanic shock = post – op. pain which usually occurs immediately after insertion of a new restoration and gradually subsides.

Best method to decrease the galvanic shock = paint an external varnish on the surface of restoration.

AMALGAM

High Cu alloys are better = as **gamma 2 phase is eliminated;** better corrosion resistance.

Arsenic can lead to pulpal damage.

Most obvious method to reduce residual Hg is by = reducing Hg – alloy ratio initially. It is ka **Eames tech**/ minimal mercury technique.

Hg content of finished restoration should be comparable to that of original M/A ratio; usually in order of 50 %.

Lesser Hg is used for spherical alloys.

A mix with M/A ratio = 6:5 ratio would contain 54.5 % Hg.

M/A for lathe – cut alloys = 1:1

M/A for spherical alloys = Hg is 40 %.

Low M/A ratio amalgams cannot be triturated with hand.

Trituration is vimp = as it **removes oxide layer** coated on alloy particles; then Hg wets the surface of alloy particles to proper amalgamation. Particles surface then gets reacted with Hg for amalgamation.

Volumetric proportioning of Hg is the most common dispenser of M/A.

Spherical alloys require less amalgamation time than the lathe cut alloys.

A properly triturated amalgam mix is = **warm** when removed from capsule; coherent, homogenous; shiny luster.

Residual Hg = it ensures **complete continuity of the matrix phase** b/w remaining alloy particles. It helps bonding of increments to each others.

Fresh mix should be made if condensation takes longer than 3 – 4 min.

Moisture = In Zn – containing alloys, leads to DELAYED EXPANSION, due to formation **of hydrogen gas** when Zn combines with water. It begins 4 – 5 days after condensation; and pain is felt after 10 – 12 days.

Ultimate result of moisture contamination = **premature failure** of restoration.

Condensation of alloy is started in the center and is taken towards periphery.

Working point of condenser is greater in size than in Au – restoration (2 mm diameter).

Condensation force = 15 lbs; (6.8 kg) is advocated; **but 3 – 4 lbs**/ 1.4 – 1.8 kg as an average.

With **spherical alloys** = a larger condensation point can be used;

Objective of carving = to simulate tooth anatomy.

Temperature more than 60° C causes the release of Hg, so **avoid increase in temperature** during burnishing / polishing by proper irrigation.

Concentration cell type corrosion can occur in rough surfaced restoration.

Final finish of restoration should be delayed for 24 hrs or more; a wet abrasive powder should be used to avoid increase in temperature/ heat production.

A slight contraction occurs with modern amalgam alloys when they are properly triturated. Normal limit = 20 microns.

Zn – free alloys =used to **avoid delayed expansion.**

Zn – containing alloys = have **better marginal integrity;** longer survival time.

Toxicity = to dental people is mainly by **inhalation**; safe range is = 50 microgm / cubic.meter of air.

Hg has a vapour pressure, VP = 20 mg / cubic.meter of air. (400 x maximum safe level)

Ultrasonic condensation and vacuum cleaning is **not recommended** = so as to avoid Hg – aerosols.

Hg conc is **higher at marginal areas by 2 – 3 %** than the bulk of restoration. So corrosion; sec. Caries; fractures occur at margins.

In low – Cu alloys = Hg is > 55%; showed marginal fracture; surface deterioration etc.; = so poor materials.

If high Hg = gamma – 2 phase is formed which is weaker and corrosion susceptible.

One of the most common amalgam deterioration is = DITCHED restorations.

Marginal discrepancies > 50 microns = secondary caries may occur.

Absence / **sparsity of gamma – 2 phase** from high – Cu alloys gives = SUPERIOR RESISTANCE TO MARGINAL BREAK-DOWN.

Silver amalgam **resists micro-leakage** by = CORROSION MECHANISM. Corrosion products get collected in the crevices with time.

70 % restoration are still Ag – Hg.

Best for large contact bearing surfaces.

Composition = low Cu alloy = Ag 65, Sn 29, Cu < 6%, and Zn.

Then, later Cu was recommended as = 6 - 30 %

Powder = produced by milling / lathe cutting a cast ingot = into irregular particles.

Or by **atomizing the liquid alloy,** producing **spherical particles.**

Hg dissolves the surface of alloy particles to form new phases.

If Zn is > 0.01 % = it is ka **Zn – containing alloy.**

Ag and Sn made the largest part of the alloy.

Ag – Sn system

Sn ; Ag_3Sn, ie gamma - phase	Increases the Sn – Hg phase which is **weakest** component of amalgam; lacks corrosion resistance.	Sn rich alloys display **less expansion** than Ag – rich alloys.
Cu; 4 –5 %; Cu_3Sn	Hardens and strengthens and decreases the brittleness of the Ag-Sn alloys.	
Zn; < 1 %	As **deoxidiser** (main function); as scavenger.	Without Zn, the alloys are more brittle and less plastic amalgam.

During manufacturing, HOMOGENISING HEAT TREATMENT is done for **phase equilibrium** – at a temperature less than solidus and cooled slowly for proper diffusion.

Here, **quenching** leads to beta – phase formation; and slow cooling leads to formation of gamma – phase formation.

Acid treatment of particles makes them **more reactive** = due to preferential dissolution of specific components from alloys.

(A) Spherical particles are made by ATOMISING the melt into fine droplets. If these droplets solidify before hitting the surface, the spherical shape is maintained.

Average particle size = 15 – 35 microns for early strength and rapid hardening. Small particle size requires more Hg due to more surface area.

Bulk of finished restoration contains = **particles of original alloys** surrounded by reaction products.

(B) Admixed powder = is a **mix of lathe-cut and spherical alloys** = it resists condensation better than spherical alloys.

Amalgam of spherical alloy is very plastic = so proximal anatomical contours are undesirable.

Spherical alloys require lesser Hg = as it has less surface area / volume.

Ag – Sn	Beta , gamma
$Ag_2 Hg_3$	Gamma – 1; BCC
$Sn_8 Hg$	Gamma – 2; hexagonal; **weakest**
Cu – Sn	Epsilon

- Gamma – 1 precipitates earlier than gamma – 2, b'coz solubility of Ag is less than Sn in Hg.
- A low – Cu amalgam is a composite in which unconsumed particles are embedded in gamma – 1 and 2 phases.
- Alloy (beta + gamma) +Hg = gamma-1 + gamma-2 + (beta + gamma) + voids is the main reaction.
- Unconsumed Ag – Sn = have a strong effect; ie more unconsumed particles- the more is the strength.
- **Weakest component** is = gamma – 2 phase,.
- Strength of gamma > gamma-1 > gamma – 2
- gamma – 2 phase = least stable in corrosion. Gamma and gamma-1 are stable in oral atmosphere.
- **High – Cu alloys** = 2 types – ie (Cu > 6 wt %)

1. admixed alloy powder
2. single composition powder.

1. Admixed alloys = total Cu content is 9 – 20 wt %.

Has spherical Ag – Cu eutectic alloy + lathe cut – Cu alloy.

spherical Ag – Cu eutectic alloy = 71.9 wt % Ag + 28.1 wt % Cu

Stronger due to Ag – Cu particles which act as strong – fillers.

(Beta + gamma) + Ag – Cu eutectic + Hg = gamma –1 + neta + both types of unconsumed particles.

Gamma – 2 has been eliminated = so Cu concentration should be at least 12 %.

2. **Single composition alloys** = Cu = 13 – 30 wt %

Ag + Cu + Sn = 60 + 13 + 27 wt %.

Phases = beta = Ag-Sn; gamma = Ag Sn; epsilon = Cu_3 Sn; neta = Cu_6Sn_5 sometimes. Gamma –1 = AgHg.

When AgSnCu + Hg = Ag, Sn dissolves in Hg; very litle Cu dissolves.

Ag-Hg (gamma - 1) forms matrix.

Neta crystals get interlocked b/w gamma-1 grains may interlock gamma-1 and increase resistance to deformation.

Ag-Sn-Cu + Hg = gamma-1 + neta + unconsumed alloy; (very little / no gamma – 2 formed here)

Cavity varnishes = decrease the microleakage.

In Ag-Hg fillings = **microleakage decreases** with time. It is due to accumulation of corrosion products there, but it is slower in cases of high – Cu alloys.

Ag-Hg should not expand / contract > 20 microns / cm at 37° C b/w 5 min. to 24 hrs. after beginning of trituration.

When Ag alloy and Hg are mixed = **contraction results** as the particles dissolve and hence become smaller and gamma – 1 grows.

Volume of gamma – 1 is < sum of initial volume of dissolved Ag and Hg (till growth of gamma-1 continues.)

Then gamma-1 crystals grow and impinge on each other and oppose the contraction.

In p.o of sufficient Hg in the mix, **expansion occurs** when gamma-1 crystals impinge.

So manipulation which results in less Hg in a mix; it causes contraction, e.g. in low M/A ratio, high condensation pressures, longer trituration time and smaller sized alloys particles, contraction occurs.

Smaller sizes particles = increased surface area = more Hg consumed = less residual Hg = contraction.

MOISTURE CONTAMINATION

Zn + water = delayed expansion after 3 – 5 days; it may reach 400 microns (4 %); H_2 gas is the cause of expansion.

Some admixed amalgams continue to expand for 2 yrs b'coz of disappearance of gamma – 2 phase.

STRENGTH

1. **Marginal defects** = most common defects in amalgam, are mainly due to fracture of amalgam.
2. Compressive strength = 310 Mpa = 45,000 psi.
3. Compressive strength of high – Cu amalgam is > low – Cu amalgam.
4. 1 hr compressive strength of single composition amalgam is **twice** that of low – Cu amalgam and admixed amalgam.
5. Tensile strength = amalgam is weaker in tension. Low Cu = 48 Mpa; high Cu = 70 Mpa.
6. Strength is a function of volume fractions of unconsumed alloy + Hg containing phases. Low – Cu amalgam have more of stronger alloy particles and less of the weaker matrix phases.
7. **Gamma – 2 phase is weakest** phase of amalgam; decreases the strength; gets formed in p.o. Hg, so use less M/A ratio.
8. Good condensation pressure is required = expressed out the Hg; decreased porosity; gives strength.
9. Patient should not bite for at least 8 hrs (70 % strength is achieved).

Creep = time dependent plastic deformation when a constant force is applied to a metal held at a temperature near its MP.

High Cu – alloy = creep rate = 0.4 %

Low Cu – alloy = 0.8 – 8.0 %

Select an alloy with creep rate of = < 3 %.

Creep increases with increased gamma – 1 phase volume fraction and decreases with increased size particles of gamma – 1.

Presence of gamma – 2 phase = high creep rate.

Very low creep in single composition alloys = is due to absence of gamma – 2; due to presence of neta (Cu_6Sn_5) rods which act as barriers to deformation of gamma – 1 phase.

Corrosion = microleakage causes CREVICE CORROSION.

Build up of corrosion products seal the margins and decrease microleakage (SELF-SEALING).

Gamma – 2 phase is the culprit for marginal failure and active corrosion in low – Cu traditional alloy; but not in high – Cu alloys.

Most common corrosion products are OXIDES and CHLORIDES OF TIN.

Tarnish = black silver sulfides.

A gold restoration in p.o of silver amalgam = corrosion occurs due to **difference in EMF;** free Hg liberated can weaken Au restoration and galvanism can occur.

High Cu amalgam is cathodic i.r.t. to conventional amalgam = so corrosion is accelerated in the latter.

Gamma – 2 phase is most ANODIC, corrosion is increased;

High Cu alloys = less gamma – 2, less corrosion.

High Hg = high corrosion.

DIRECT FILLING GOLD

BHN = 25

Strength increased by cold working.

Lack of surface oxide with gold allows cold welding.

Cohesion occurs from metallic bonding under pressure of compaction.

Classification

1. Foils = sheet (cohesive/non-cohesive); ropes; cylinders; laminated; platinised
2. Electrolytic precipitates = mat; mat foil; alloyed.
3. Powder

Cohesive and non cohesive gold = only the sheet foil is available in both forms;

Non-cohesive gold = has a **protective volatile film eg ammonia,** to prevent premature cohesion which is removed by heating before using.

Preformed foils = made from no. 4 foil which is carbonised/ corrugated.

Platinized foil = is a laminated foil in which pure platinum foil is b/w 2 sheets of pure gold foils ie (Au - Pt - Au); is bonded by CLADDING process during rolling.

Electrolytic precipitates = formed by **sintering** which causes self – diffusion b/w particles.

Mat gold = **electrolytically precipitated** gold. Better for **internal bulk of restoration** due to easy compaction. These foils are recommended for **external surface** ie mat is covered with a veneer of foils. Greater voids are created as powder has larger surface area.

Mat foil = is a sandwich of **electrolytically precipitated gold powder** b/w sheets of no. 3 gold foils.

Alloyed electrolytic precipitates = **with calcium** is **ka electralloy** RV. **Calcium is 0.1%** and it produces stronger restorations by dispersion strengthening.

Powder gold = average particle size = 15 microns; maximum particle size = 74 microns (atomized).

Removal of surface impurities = at 315 – 760° C for 5 mins. Heat treatment / annealing / desorbing is done for best COHESION. Alcohol flame is used; the alcohol should be pure methanol or ethanol.

Condenser = face of condenser has a series of pyramids / serrations.

Size of condenser point = higher forces are required so the points should be smaller in size; 0.5 – 1 mm dia, is the best. Smaller points give more forces of condensation.

True Density = of pure gold is 19.3.

Apparent density = 16 – 19 gm / cc, so true density is not approached due to voids.

DFGs (direct filling golds) are mainly used in = pits/small class I/repair of margins / class III and V restorations. It can not be used for crowns, cusp building or in high stress areas.

CASTING ALLOYS

Coefficient of thermal expansion has a reciprocal relation with MP.

Karat / fineness = parts of pure gold in 24 parts of alloy.

Fineness = gold alloys by the no. of parts per thousand of gold.

Classification of gold casting alloys :

Type	**Gold + platinum**	**VHN**
I, soft	83 %	50 – 90
II, medium	78	90 – 120
III, hard	78	120 – 150
IV, extra hard	75	150

- Alloys with gold < 65 – 75 % get tarnished readily, so **palladium** is **added to make Ag non–tarnishing** in gold alloys.
- Pt, Pd = decrease coeff. of thermal expansion of gold cp. to porcelain to ensure physical compatibility/veneering.
- Melting range of alloy was increased to permit firing of porcelain on gold alloy at 1040 °C.

Classification

Type	**Use**	**In area of**
Type I, soft	Small inlays	Small stresses
Type II, medium	Thick ¾ crowns; abutments; pontics; full crowns.	Moderate stresses
Type III, hard	Thin ¾ crowns; thin cast backings; abutments; pontics; full crowns; denture bases and short FPDs.	High stresses; can be age – hardened
Type IV, extra hard	Denture bases; bars; clasps; long FPDs; RPD frameworks; full crowns.	Very high stresses; can be age hardened by heat treatment.
Metal ceramics, hard and extra hard	For veneering with porcelain; copings; thin walled crowns; short span FPDs; long span FPDs;	

Classification (*Contd.*)

RPD alloys	Cast RPDs; have replaced type IV alloys.

Type I and II are aka INLAY golds.

Type III and IV are aka CROWN and BRIDGE ALLOYS.

Metal ceramic alloys = noble metal alloys and base metal alloys. All can bond to porcelain. Coeff of thermal expansion is compatible to porcelain.

RPD alloys

- Co – Cr alloys = ka **vitallium;** 60 % Co + 25 – 30 % Cr.
- Ni – Cr = **most often** used; relatively easy casting and finishing. Ni – Cr with Be has low enough casting temperature to be successfully cast into a gypsum bonded investment.
- Ni = used to form strengthening phase.
- Zn = acts as **oxygen scavenger.**
- Ag absorbs **oxygen** from air during melting which is rejected during solidification, causing GAS POROSITY in casting = **Zn avoids it**.
- In; Fe, Sn = harden the alloys.
- Ga = compensates the decreased thermal expansion coefficient.
- Removal of Ag = decreases the propensity of **green stains at** margins of porcelain – metal interface.
- Ir, Ru, Rh (100 – 150 ppm) = make the alloy fine grain.
- Cu = **principal hardener**, but gives a red hue.
- Ag = **decreases the reddening effect of** Cu.
- Pd = used in place of Pt; hardens and **whitens the alloy;** increases the fusion temperature; decreases the cost; makes Ag tarnish resistant. 1 % of Pd is added for every 3 % of Ag.
- Cu = added in low gold alloys; at **the expense of Pd**; it decreases the melting range of alloys to permit use of gypsum bonded investment.

- **Softening heat treatment** = aka **solution heat treatment.** Done at 700° C for 10 min; and then quenching. It increases the ductility and relieves the strain hardening.
- **Hardening heat treatment** = 200 – 450° C for 15 – 30 min; increases the strength, hardness, proportional limit, decreases the ductility.

INLAY CASTING WAX

Type I = medium wax = for direct technique
Type II = soft wax = for indirect technique

Composition

Component	%	Property	
Paraffin wax	Main ingredient; 40 – 60 %.	But *it flakes* when trimmed and does not give a smooth, glossy surface.	—
Gum dammer/ dammer resin		Improves smoothness and luster; increases resistance to flaking/ cracking	Increases the toughness
Carnauba wax		Decreases the flow of paraffin wax; contributes to **glossiness** of wax surface more than the gum dammer.	—
Candelilla wax	To replace carnauba wax	Its MP is lower and not as hard as carnauba wax.	—
Ceresin	To replace some part of paraffin wax	Modifies the toughness and carving characteristics.	—

Composition (*Contd.*)

Nitrogen derivatives of higher fatty acids from MONTAN wax	Synthetic waxes; to replace carnauba wax	Give greater uniformity	—

Properties

- When burnt at 500° C, wax should not leave solid residue in excess of 0.1 % of the original weight of specimen.
- Flow of Type I wax = maximum flow at 37° C should be = 1 %
- Both type I, II waxes should have a minimum flow of 70 % at 45° C and maximum flow of 90 %.
- Low thermal conductivity.
- High coeff of thermal expansion = 350×10^{-6} /°C.
- It can expand 0.7 % with 20° C increase in temperature.
- Can contract to 0.35 % when cooled from 37° C to 25° C.
- For type I waxes = a maximum of 0.6 % linear dimensional change is permitted when heated form 25 to 37° C.
- Distortion of wax takes place = due to release of internal stresses; it is ka **elastic memory.** So, the pattern **should be cast immediately.**

Manipulation

- **Dry heat is better** than the water bath as water can get incorporated in the wax.
- Wax cooling under pressure of finger is distorted less as some inbuilt gas trapped inside the wax may cause expansion / distortion.
- The most practical method to avoid delayed distortion is to = INVEST THE PATTERN IMMEDIATELY.
- Softer waxes, having higher flow produce larger castings than harder waxes.

INVESTMENTS

1. Gypsum bonded — for gold alloys
2. Phosphate bonded — for metal ceramics
3. Ethyl silica bonded — for base metal alloys P.D.

Gypsum bonded

Type I	for inlays or crowns; the casting shrinkage compensation is by **thermal expansion** of investment.
Type II	for inlays of crowns; the shrinkage is compensated by **hygroscopic setting expansion.**
Type III	for partial dentures of gold alloys.

Composition : is a hemihydrate of gypsum and a form of silica.

I. **Alpha – hemihydrate (25 – 45 %)** = gives more strength; provides rigidity; serves as binder.

Used for gold – alloys with melting range of less than 1000° C.

All forms of gypsum products shrink after dehydration from 200 – 400° C.

A slight expansion occurs at approx 700° C..

A **tremendous contraction** occurs at > 700° C. It is due to DECOMPOSITION, the **sulfur gases are emitted,** cause shrinkage and contamination.

So, gypsum should not be heated above 700° C; even safer is that do not heat > 650° C. with those products containing carbon.

II. **Silica** = provides refractory; **regulates thermal expansion;** so compensates for the casting shrinkage of gold; and gypsum.

4 forms = ie quartz, tridymite, cristoballite, fused – quartz.

When q, t, c are heated the change in crystalline form occurs at transition temperature.

Alpha – quartz ➔ beta – quartz at 575° C.

Alpha – cristoballite ➔ beta form at 200 –270° C

Alpha – tridymite ➔ beta form at 117 and 163° C.

Density decreases as alpha changes to beta, so **volume increases** and rapid increase **in linear expansion** occurs.

Modifiers

Reducing agents eg carbon, copper = provide a non-oxidising atmosphere in mold when gold alloy is cast.

Modifiers like boric acid, NaCl = regulate setting expansion, ST and prevent most of the shrinkage of gypsum at > 300° C.

(1) Normal setting expansion = NSE

Silica interferes with interlocking and intermeshing of crystals and so outward thrust leads to NSE.

NSE in air = only 0.6 % is allowed.

Purpose of SE = is to **enlarge the mold to partially compensate for casting shrinkage** of gold.

Thermal expansion of wax pattern occurs by = exothermic heat of gypsum setting.

SE of pattern with thin walls is > with thick wall.

(2) Hygroscopic setting expansion = HSE

Occcurs when gypsum is allowed to set under water; HSE > NSE

HSE = 6 × the NSE.

For type II investment = 1.2 – 2.2 % in water.

Factors controlling the HSE

Effect of composition	1. HSE is proportional to silica content. 2. Alpha–hemihyd. gives more HSE than beta-hemihydrate.	Finer the particle size of silica, more is the HSE.
W/P ratio	High W/P =➔ less HSE	
M.Time	Shorter MT ➔ less HSE	

Factors controlling the HSE (*Contd.*)

Time of immersion	Greatest amount of HSE is seen if immersion occurs before initial set. If delayed ➔ less HSE.
Water	HSE is dependent on the amount of added water.

Theory of HSE

Immersion water replaces the water of hydration and **prevents the confinement of growing crystals** by surface tension of excess water.

Water is attracted b/w particles **by capillary action** and separates the particles causing expansion.

Greater the amount of silica / fillers = the more easily the added water can diffuse through the setting material and greater is the expansion.

Thermal expansion

TE of gypsum bonded investment is directly related to amount and type of silica.

Contraction of gypsum is **entirely balanced** if quartz content is > 75 %.

If cristoballite is present, more expansion occurs.

TE for type I investment should be = 1.0 – 1.6 %;

TE for type II investment should be = 0 – 0.6 % at 500° C."

Maximum TE should be attained at temp < 700° C; b'coz above 700° C, contamination occurs.

Chlorides of K, Na, Li eliminate the contraction caused by gypsum and increase the expansion without the p.o. excessive amount of silica.

Boric acid = hardens the set investment but disintegrates with heating and rough surface results.

Silicas do not prevent gypsum shrinkage but counterbalance it .

Chlorides actually decrease the gypsum shrinkage below temp 700° C.

THERMAL CONTRACTION

Investment contracts to less than its original dimensions; it occurs **due to shrinkage of gypsum,** when it is first heated. Beta form changes to stable form.

Strength = after burn out, the strength should not be greater than that required to resist the impact of the metal entering the mold.

Compressive strength should not be less than 350 psi or 2.46 Mpa; after 2 hrs of setting.

Porosity and investment = for escape of air during entry of metal to avoid **back pressure porosity.**

More gypsum crystals in set investment	Decrease porosity
Less hemihydrate	Increase water ➔ increase porosity
More uniform particle size	Increase porosity
Coarse and fine particles	Decrease porosity

PHOSPHATE BONDED INVESTMENT

For metal – ceramic castings. It is **used with high melting alloys** in which high contraction is there and so **greater expansion** is required.

Filler = 80 % , silica in the form of cristoballite or / and quartz = it provides REFRACTORINESS and high TE.

Binder = MgO and a phosphate which is acid in nature eg mono – ammonium phosphate.

Binder and filler are mixed with **colloidal silica suspension.**

Carbon = to produce clean castings and facilitate dig out of castings.

Gold alloys should not be fluxed on **charcoal blocks**, as it may remove trace elements.

A **carbon – crucible should not be** used for melting the alloys.

Expansion can be increased by using **colloidal silica aqueous solution** instead of water.

Thermal shrinkage in phosphate – investment is due to decomposition of the binder and **evolution of ammonia gas.** (In gypsum bonded = the shrinkage is due to transformation of calcium sulfate from hexagonal to rhombic form.)

Silicate bonded investment = is used for construction for high fusing base metal PD alloys. In it, the binder is silica gel.

Investment	TE	HSE
Gypsum bonded	650 – 700° C	
Phosphate bonded	871° C; high heat	482 – 510° C; low heat
Divestment	677° C; 0.6 %	

Porosity

Type	Prevention
Localised shrinkage P	Use reservoir
Suck back P	Proper position of sprue; 45°
Back pressure porosity	Proper thickness of investment for air escape; 6.5 mm.
Micro – P	Slow solidification.
Pin-hole and gas inclusion P	Reducing zone of flame; avoid gas dissolution in molten metal.
Subsurface P	Control the rate of metal entering the mold.

CASTINGS

For acceptable restorations: the **mean opening at occlusal surface** should not be more than 21 microns and at gingival margins, it should not be more than 74 microns.

Compensation of casting shrinkage: by 2 methods:

- Low heat technique = by HSE / NSE of investment
- High heat technique = by TE of investment.
- TE = at 650 – 700° C for gypsum bonded and at 871° C for phosphate bonded investment.
- HSE = at 482 – 510° C.

Master die = most common die material = type IV or V improved stone.

Chief disadvantage of type IV gypsum die = susceptible to abrasion during wax carving.

To decrease the SE of die material to < 0.1 %, the K_2SO_4 can be added as an accelerator and borax as retarder.

Die spacers = are mostly resins; provide the space for the cement; it should be used **within 0.5 mm of the finish line.**

Divestment = is mixed with colloidal silica liquid; it is a gypsum bonded material; not recommended for high – fusing alloys eg metal – ceramic restorations; very **good for conventional gold alloys;**

Electroformed dies = by electroplating the impression material; it becomes high strength, hardness, abrasion resistant.

- **Electroplating bath** used = $CuSO_4$ solution;
- Hydrocolloid impression are difficult to electroplate.
- Electroformed dies with polysulfide rubber are acceptable in silver cyanide bath.
- **Silver cyanide bath is preferred** to acid Cu – bath, as throwing power of silver cyanide bath is better ; and dimensional stability of polysulfide is better.

Sprue formers

- Should be attached at largest cross section / **greatest bulk** = to avoid distortion of the thin areas.
- **Sprue former** should be **directed away** from thin / delicate section of the pattern; as molten metal can abrade / fracture the investment there.
- It should **not be attached at a right angle** to a broad flat surface = as entering metal impinges the mold surface at this point to create a HOT – SPOT; which causes SUCK BACK POROSITY (flared sprue can prevent it.)
- Sprue should be at 45° to the proximal wall for good casting.
- Its length should be adequate so that the tip of the wax pattern is with in 6.5 mm of the open end / top of the ring for gypsum –

bonded investment; and 3.25 mm for phosphate bonded investment, so as to allow proper escape of gases.

- Molten alloy should flow from thick to thin section.
- In indirect spruing = a **reservoir bar** is positioned b/w the pattern and crucible former.
- **Reservoir** = prevents localised shrinkage porosity; pattern area should solidify first and lastly the reservoir.
- **Casting ring liner** = for allowing the expansion of investment material, e.g. **asbestos** but it is carcinogenic. So **aluminium silicate** ceramic material, cellulose paper, ceramic cellulose combination can be used.
- **Thickness of liner** = should not be more than **1 mm**.
- Since the expansion is always greater in unrestricted direction / longitudinal than in the lateral direction; it is desirable to decrease the expansion in longitudinal direction. So the liner should be placed somewhat short of ends of the ring. 3.25 mm gives more uniform expansion and less distortion of the wax.
- **Dry liner technique** = ie liner is fixed with the sticky wax.
- **Wet liner technique** = ie dip the ring in water. Absorbed water also causes semi – HSE. Liner affords greater NSE; offers unrestricted NSE.
- **For HSE;** the filled casting ring is immediately placed in water bath at 37 – 38° C but for TE, the ring is allowed to bench set.
- Investment should be allowed to set for at least 1 hour.
- Investment should not be allowed to dry-out, and should not be placed in 100 % humidity before the burnout.

Heating

If gypsum bonded material = then 468° C for HSE; or 650° C for TE.

If phosphate bonded material = then 700 – 870° C depending on the alloy.

HSE = at 468° C for 60 – 90 min.; esp for complete wax removal.

Ring can be placed at preheated 468° C without the fear of fracture of investment.

But, carbon from wax may be retained which decreases venting of the mold. And may cause BACK – PRESSURE POROSITY.

Also, the door of the furnace should be kept open slightly so that OXYGEN gas enters inside and helps in complete elimination of wax esp with HSE cases.

Investment should be heated SLOWLY = too rapid heating leads to cracking; the cracks go from inside to outside due to non – uniform heating of the surface and central part of the mold.
Safe heating period = 60 min or longer.

Thermal expansion

Ring is placed in furnace at room temperature and then heated to 650 – 700° C.

Ring is **inverted** when placed = so that wax can flow out.

Ring should be **uprighted near the end** of burn out = so that **oxygen** gas can come in contact with it for complete wax removal.

It temp is more than 700° C = **sulfur dioxide** gas is liberated which causes the surface roughness.

Casting machines

Molten metal is forced inside = under 10 – 15 psi air pressure.

Metal solidifies within = 5 – 10 sec.

With centrifugal casting machines = 2 – 5 rotations of broken arm are given; ceramic crucible is used. Pressure at the tip of casting is 30 – 40 psi; which falls to zero at the button surface.

Thinner sections solidify **faster due to faster heat loss;**

Heat transfer is maximum at highest pressure points.

Induction furnace or electric heating casting machines —

- Here, metal is heated in GRAPHITE crucibles.
- Good for use with metal – ceramic restorations.
- Carbon crucible should not be used with PSA alloys, high Pd; Ni-Cr; Co-Cr alloys at more than 1504° C.

Fuel = oxygen – air and acetylene gas.

Zone of flame	Composition	Property	Use
I	Innermost; air + gas;	No heat present	—
II. Green;	combustion zone; oxidising;	Partial combustion of air and gas	Should be kept away from metal.
III. hottest; dim – blue zone	Reducing zone; use it	Gives bright shiny metal surface	It is in touch with the metal during fusion
IV; outer zone	Oxidising; low temp;	Causes oxidation of alloy.	—

At proper casting temperature; molten alloy is **light orange,** and moves with flame.

The temperature is 38 – 66° C above the liquidus.

Flux is added = to minimize the porosity; increase the fluidity; **prevent the oxidation**; eg borax and boric acid (1 : 1).

Boric acid aids in ***retaining the flux*** on the metal surface.

After casting, the **quenching** is done = for molten metal to get annealed for polishing, etc.; investment becomes soft, fractured for easy removal.

Pickling

Sulfuric acid is best for it.

50 % HCl was used but its fumes corrode the lab equipments.

Casing should not be held with S.S tongs in acid as it may cause an electrolytic cell formation and Cu deposition on the casting surface from the acid.

Burn – out of wax

With phosphate – bonded investment

- It is a 2 – stage procedure with phosphate – bonded investment.
- First, at 200 – 300° C for 30 min; second / complete at 700 – 900° C (the casting temperature).
- Gas – permeability of phosphate – bonded investment is LESS than gypsum bonded investment; so casting pressure required is more.
- Recovery and cleaning of casting is difficult, b'coz silica and phosphate binder are not soluble in HCl / H_2SO_4.
- Acid should not be used to clean the base metal alloys; but use SAND BLASTING with **aluminium oxide.**

CAUSES OF DEFECTIVE CASTINGS

- DISTORTION = due to distortion of wax pattern or hardening of investment or more SE.
- **Surface roughness** = are **finely spaced** surface irregularities whose height / width / direction establish a **predominant surface pattern**. It is due to wax rough surface.
- **Surface irregularities** = are **isolated imperfections** eg nodules, which do not characterize the total surface area.
- **Air bubbles** = cause small nodules.
- Best method to avoid air bubbles is = **vacuum investing**.
- *Wetting agent* may help in preventing the air bubbles.
- **Water films** = causes minute **ridges or veins** on casting surface. Wetting agents can reduce it.
- **Too rapid heating** – causes **fins / spines** on casting surface = so **gradual heating** from the room temperature to 700° C in 60 min should be done.
- **Under heating** = lead to **incomplete removal of wax**. Voids and porosity can occur if carbon – residues remain.
- Higher W/P ratio = increased roughness.
- Low W/P = increase air bubbles.
- **Prolonged heating** = leads to release of the **sulfur compounds**; disintegration of investment.

- Casting pressure = if high = then rough surface occurs; so **0.1 – 0.14 Mpa (15 – 20 psi) or 3** – 4 turns of centrifugal machine is enough.
- Bright concavities on surface = due to p.o. flux in the metal.
- Discoloration = by sulfur contamination.

POROSITY

Caused by	**Examples**
Solidification shrinkage	Localised shrinkage porosity Microporosity
By gas	Pin – hole porosity Gas inclusion porosity Sub surface porosity
By entrapped air in the mold	Back pressure porosity

Localised shrinkage porosity	♦ Is due to incomplete feeding of molten metal. ♦ Approx 1.25 % linear contraction occurs when L ➔ Solid. ♦ Occurs **near the sprue casting junction**. ♦ Where a hot spot is created = SUCK BACK POROSITY occurs. ♦ Treatment = by **flaring the point** of sprue attachment ie RESERVOIR; and by decreasing mold – metal temp difference by 30° C.
Micro-porosity	Generally present in fine grain alloy castings, **when solidification is very rapid**.
Pin – hole porosity, Gas inclusion porosity	♦ On solidification of metals, the gases are expelled forming pin – hole porosity. ♦ Larger spherical porosity = if reducing zone of flame is not used.

Sub surface porosity	By simultaneous nucleation of solid grains and gas bubbles at the first moment, that the metal freezes at the mold walls. Can be decreased by **controlling the rate** at which molten metal enters the mold.
Back pressure porosity	♦ Is due to **inability of gas to escape** through investment pores, if density of investment is high, or temperature of casting/ mold is very low. ♦ **Insufficient casting pressure** does not overcome the back pressure. ♦ Casting pressure should be applied for at least = 4 sec. ♦ Mold gets filled and metal solidifies in = 1 sec; but it is soft, so pressure should be maintained for a few seconds. ♦ Insufficient elimination from the mold = **retained combustion products** block pores = so back pressure occurs. ♦ Incomplete casting due to **incomplete wax elimination** is characterised by = ROUNDED MARGINS and SHINY surface, which is due to the strong reducing atmosphere created by carbon mono-oxide gas due to residual wax.
Incomplete casting	Is due to **insufficient venting of mold** = eg back pressure Or due to high viscosity of fused metal is due to **insufficient heating** = To avoid it, the temperature of alloy should be increased higher than liquidus to decrease its viscosity and surface tension and; it should not solidify prematurely

CEMENTS

- Except Ca $(OH)_2$ and resin cements = all other cements reactions are of ACID-BASE TYPE.
- Silicate and GI cements are used in anterior teeth = as both are translucent and anti-caries.
- Average life of silicate cement = 4 yrs.

SILICATE CEMENT

- Powder is a ceramic = silica + alumina + fluoride compounds + Ca – salts ; all are fused at 1400° C.
- Fluoride compounds melt at lower temperature are ka = CERAMIC FLUXES; act as fusing agents.
- Liquid = water + phosphoric acid + buffer salts.
- Gives severe **pulp response.** (pH < 3; after 1 month < 7 ie normal pH is not attained).
- **Anti-caries** = due to p.o. **Fluorides** (approx 15 % of F is present in powder). Fluoride compounds make enamel surface resistant to acid decalcification, decreased acid solubility.
- Fluoride compounds act as ENZYME INHIBITOR preventing the carbohydrate metabolism.
- Plaque associated with the silicate cement has HIGHER CARBOHYDRATE – TO – N_2 RATIO, which shows that metabolism of carbohydrate is inhibited or bacteria are less. So very less / 3 % chances of secondary caries.
- Compressive strength is less than tensile strength; so brittle.
- Severe pulp irritant = so a **pulp – protection** is needed.
- If soluble Fluoride compounds are added to Ag – Hg = it makes Ag – Hg more prone to corrosion.
- Fluoride – releasing Zn – PO_4 cements = very high solubility.

GI CEMENTS / TYPE II : (A = adhesion; B = biocompatible; C = anti-caries)

- Aka **polyalkenoate** cement.
- Setting reaction and adhesion to tooth involve = **ionic bonds.**
- Used for anterior aesthetic restoration in class III and V cavities.

- True adhesive bond is achieved; so **conservative restoration** of eroded areas can be done; no need of mechanical retention; (adhesion to tooth surface is due to PAA), (poly acrylic acid).
- Not recommended for class II, IV restorations as it lacks = fracture toughness and is more susceptible to wear.

Powder	Liquid; polymer; PAA
♦ Calcium – fluoro – alumino – silicate glass	♦ Itaconic acid
♦ but, higher alumina : silica ratio than silicate cement.	♦ Maleic acid
	♦ Tricarballylic acid
	♦ Tartaric acid

- P:L ratios = 3 : 1 by wt.; M.T = 45 sec.; mix should be GLOSSY which shows the p.o. polyacids and help in adhesion.
- Acids in liquid increase the reactivity of liquid; and decrease the viscosity.
- **Tartaric acid** = improves **handling characteristics;** and decreases the tendency of increasing the viscosity with time.
- If PAA is in powder form = mix with water and tartaric acid = gives a water – settable cement; fast setting.
- **Water** is most important constituent of cement liquid. It is **the reaction medium** = it **hydrates** the reaction products.
- **Main** component of GI powder = $SiO_2 > Al_2O_3 > CaF_2$ in concentration.
- Silica gel matrix is formed = it **sheaths unreacted glass particles**.
- **Dominant phase of matrix** = slow forming **aluminium polysalts**, which can be washed / leached away by initial water contact, so protect the filling immediately after placement apply varnish/vaseline.
- Matrix band is applied = to protect the setting cement from the environment during the initial set = for at least 5 mins. Then surface is protected by VARNISH, etc.
- **Adhesion** = occurs by reaction of carboxyl groups of polyacids with **calcium of hydroxy – apatite crystals** of enamel / dentin.

- Bond to enamel is higher than the dentin; due to greater INORGANIC CONTENT OF ENAMEL and its greater morphologic homogeneity.
- P/L ratios influence ACIDITY = so luting cements are more pulp irritating. So **calcium hydroxide protection** should be given.
- Its pulp reaction is greater than ZOE.

METAL MODIFIED GIC

by mixing **spherical amalgam alloy** particles with type II GIC = is ka SILVER ALLOY ADMIX.

Or by bonding Ag particles by fusion to glass powder particles through high – temperature sintering = it is ka CERMET.

Fracture toughness of GI is very low as compared to CR and amalgam.

Flouride release from admix GI > type II GI > cermet GI.

Fissure sealing = GI is used for P and F > 100 microns as GI has high viscosity; so for P and F < 100 microns size, the acid – etch – LIGHT CURE resin is used.

ZINC OXIDE EUGENOL CEMENT

- Is one of the **least irritating** cement. Its pH is 7;
- Type I = for temporary cementation
- Type II = for permanent cementation
- Type III = for temporary fillings and thermal insulating bases.
- Type IV = for cavity liners.
- **Accelerator** of ZOE reaction = zinc acetates, zinc succinate or propionate.
- Water is NECESSARY to initiate the setting reaction.
- Small particle size = rapid setting; high strength.
- Cooling of mixing slab = slow setting.
- Ortho – EBA = increases the strength.
- **Intermediate** / holding type of restoration = is polymer – reinforced ZOE = ie ZOE + 20 – 40 % of polymer particles.

LINERS

- ZOE = is **palliative** to the pulp; decreases the sensitivity.
- Ca $(OH)_2$ = increases **tertiary dentin formation**; helps in pulp capping.

Cavity varnishes = is a natural gum eg copal, rosin or a synthetic resin dissolved in an organic solvent.

- It decreases the post – op. sensitivity; but has low thermal conductivity.
- Decrease the micro-leakage with Ag-Hg.
- Prevents penetration of acids from Zn – PO_4 and silicate cements into the dentin.
- Prevents the entry of corrosion products in the dentinal tubules.
- Varnish should be **confined to dentin** when placing a silicate / silico – phosphate restoration ; as it **inhibits uptake of fluoride** by enamel.
- It should **not be used under** DIRECT RESIN FILLING MATERIALS – as it softens the resins /**prevents proper wetting** of the cavity by the resin.
- Not indicated with **GI cements** = as film decreases the potential of adhesion / biocompatibility.

Liner = is a liquid in which Ca $(OH)_2$ or ZnO is suspended in a solution of synthetic / natural resins; it **decreases microleakage** and so applied to the walls of the prepared cavity.

- Basic component = Ca $(OH)_2$ in solvents.
- PH > 11, i.e. basic; neutralises acids from cements;
- Should **not be left on margins of the cavity**, as it is soluble in oral fluids.
- ZOE should not be used with direct resin materials = as it interferes with polymerisation of resin. Type IV / low viscosity ZOE also has palliative effect on the pulp.
- Have less strength.

GI liners = 2 types ie conventional P/L system and light cure GI liners.

- Ionic bonding with tooth material.
- Thickness should be < 2 mm for proper curing.
- **Primary purpose of GI liners** = as an intermediate bonding material b/w tooth and composite restoration. It acts as a dentin bonding agent and so decreases the gap at gingival margins which gets formed due to polymerisation shrinkage of the resin.
- It releases fluorides also.
- **Sandwich technique** = GI is placed at the base of cavity; and is covered by CR material (compositive resin = CR).
- Etching of GI = is done for 15 – 20 sec only; longer etching destroys the cement.

BASE : it serves as the **replacement of dentin;** gives thermal and chemical insulation.

- Various materials = eg zinc phosphate; ZOE; GI; poly-carboxylate.
- **Minimum thickness** of the base should be > 0.75 mm.
- Minimum strength of the base should be b/w = 0.5 – 1.2 Mpa for amalgam condensation. More strength is required for **gold** restorations; as more pressure is required for gold condensation.
- It should be strong enough that it should not fracture during insertion of restoration or mastication.
- $Ca(OH)_2$ and ZOE act against chemical irritants also.
- Compressive strength at 7 min. / initial set is important = compr. Strength of ZOE (B) is approx 2 times that of $ZnPO_4$.
- For resins = $Ca(OH)_2$ or GI as a base over ZOE should be used. ZOE should not be used with in direct contact with resin materials = as it interferes with polymerisation of resin.
- Cavity varnishes are applied at margins = they reduce the micro-leakage.
- If $ZnPO_4$ is being used as a base = apply varnish before the base; to prevent irritatory effect of acid.
- If ZOE, $Ca(OH)_2$, GI, polycarboxylate is used as base = then apply varnish after base application, so as to help $Ca(OH)_2$ to initiate dentin development; GI to relevant F^- & uptake by tooth tissue; ZOE for palliative effect on pulp.

LUTING CEMENTS

Zinc phosphate = type I for cementation of castings; type II for other uses.

Type I = is fine grained; forms film of < 25 microns thickness.

Type II = film of < 40 microns is formed.

- Powder contains ZnO (basic component) + MgO (modifier / aids in sintering).
- Liquid = phosphoric acid + metallic salts to decrease reaction rate of liquid to powder.
- Water is very imp. = 33 ± 5 %; it influences the rate and type of P – L reaction and **controls ionisation of liquid.**
- **Aluminium is very imp** for cement formation = it helps formation of cohesive products of Zn – Al – PO_4 gels.
- Setting time = 5 – 9 min.
- **Most effective method to increase the setting time** = cool slab.
- Mechanical interlocking occurs = roughness is required .
- Thinner film b/w casting and tooth = better cementing action is there; less water / salivary solubility.
- PH is 2 after 2 min of mixing; which becomes 5.5 at 24 hrs after mixing (still acidic).
- PH is low with thin mixes. (more acid is required)
- Acid may penetrate dentin up to 1.5 mm thick; leading to pulp injury so protect the pulp with required material.

ZINC SILICO-PHOSPHATE CEMENT

- Powder = silicate glass + ZnO
- Liquid = phosphoric acid + water + Zn and Al salts.
- Type I = < 25 microns thickness film for cementing the precision castings.
- **Less vulnerable to oral fluids**; releases the **Fluorides, so anticaries**.
- pH is less, so **pulp protection** is required.
- **Translucent** = so better for cementing ceramic restoration.

Also GI and resins cements are translucent.

ZINC POLYCARBOXYLATE CEMENT

Adhesion to tooth; *fluoride* release is only 15 – 20 % as compared to GI cement.

Liquid = is aqueous solution of PAA **polyacrylic acid** or a copolymer of acrylic acid + unsaturated carboxylic acids. Acid concentration is 40 %.

Powder = ZnO + MgO + SnF_2.

SnF_2 = modifies the setting time; increases the strength; releases the Fluoride.

Bonding to tooth = PAA reacts via carboxyl groups with calcium of HA of the tooth; strength to enamel is more than dentin.

Zinc phosphate is a NEWTONIAN fluid, but ZINC POLYCARBOXYLATE CEMENT is a PSEUDO-PLASTIC.

Minimum pulpal irritation = Same as ZOE. PH of mix is higher than zinc phosphate cement.

Larger size of PAA molecules as cp to zinc phosphate decrease its diffusion through the dentinal tubules.

Remove the smear layer for proper wetting / adhesion = by 10 % PAA for 10 – 15 sec and washing with water. Do not dessicate.

Failure occurs cohesively or cement-metal interface. Failure with zinc phosphate cement occurs at cement-tooth surface.

GLASS IONOMER CEMENT

- High initial water – solubility = due to **rapid leaching** of soluble substance eg Na, F, in high amounts. So protect with vaseline/ varnish after placement.
- It decreases micro-leakage, **releases fluorides** as **anti –caries.**
- **Smear layer** should **not be removed** but left intact to **act as a barrier** to the penetration of tubules by acid of cement, so deep cavity should be **protected by calcium hydroxide.**
- Prepared tooth structure should not be DEHYDRATED or DESSICATED = as it opens up the tubules, increases acid penetration.

- Susceptible to attack by water / oral fluids during initial set; so protect it by varnish / vaseline.

ZINC OXIDE EUGENOL CEMENT

Type I = for temporary cementation = low strength

Type II = for permanent cementation.

PH = 7, neutral; sealing capacity is good = it decreases the microleakage.

Type II cement = (1) alumina in powder and ortho – EBA in liquid are added or (2) adding polymer in ZOE formulation to increase the strength.

RESIN CEMENTS

- Filled cements = resin matrix + inorganic fillers bound through **organo-silane coupling agent**.
- Resin matrix = diacrylate monomers + DMA monomers.
- **Dentin honding agents** = eg organo-phosphonates;
- Polymerisation = by light curing or by initiator-activator system ie by **peroxide-amine** system or by both ie **dual-cure system.**
- Insoluble in oral fluids = all other cements are soluble.
- Fillers = decreases the polymerisation shrinkage; increases strength; decreases the coeff of thermal expansion.
- It is a **pulpal irritant** = so protect pulp by $Ca(OH)_2$.
- **Best time to remove flash** / excess of this cement = immediately after the restoration is seated. In other cements, flash is removed after the setting.
- Time of exposure of light for light curing = > 40 sec.
- **Ceramic brackets** = by mechanical retention and by coating the back of the bracket with **organosilane** coupling agents.
- In dual cure system = first step is by **chemical activation** which is slow giving better working time; the 2nd step is **by light curing** which is rapid.

Table showing properties of different cements

Property	$ZnPO_4$	Zn- silico PO_4	Modified ZOE	Zn-poly-carbox	GI	Resins	$Ca(OH)_2$
Handling	Easy	Difficult	Inferior				
Life	Long		Less				
Pulp irritation	+	+	Minimum	Good; minimum	–	+	Minimum
Adhesion	–	–	–	+	+	-,acid etch	
Anti-caries, F	–	+	–	+, less	+	–	
Oral solubility	+	Low	More	Depends on P/L	Less	Nil	–
Translucency	–	+	–		+	–	
WT				Shorter			
Brittle	+	+	+	+	+	–	
Fracture toughness							
PH	<2at mix, 5.5 at 24 hrs	Less	7	> $ZnPO_4$			>11
Acid-base reaction	+	+	+	+	+	–	–

CERAMICS: 3 types

- high fusing = 1290 – 1370° C
- medium fusing = 1095 – 1260° C
- low fusing = 870 – 1065° C
- **self glazing porcelain** = is better than applied glaze.
- **Water** is also a glass modifier (hydronium H_3O + ions) = which causes slow crack growth in porcelain.
- **Sintering** = process by which particles of porcelain coalesce at high temperature without complete melting.
- **Leucite** = is K – Al – silicate formed from feldspar at 1150 – 1530° C; is used for PFM restorations.
- **Boric acid** = decreases softening point of glass.

Properties

1. Strength = very less; low strength is due to **stress concentration** at scratches; brittle.
2. Low tensile strength = so crack propogation occurs.
3. Sharp line angles in the restoration = create areas of stress concentration.
4. Color matching should be done under the NORTHERN LIGHT from **blue sky** b'coz it contains the most even balance of light wavelengths. And should be done under **2 or more different light sources**.

How to do strengthening of dental porcelain?

A. Introduction of residual compressive stresses

By **ion exchange** = ka **chemical tempering.** Here, sodium containing glass particles are added in molten KNO_3. Then, K replaces Na+; size of K is more than Na which introduce compressive stresses (700 Mpa).

By **thermal tempering** = **most common method.** It is done by rapid cooling /quenching the object when hot and molten/ soft. Core of the product is soft and skin becomes rigid. Core cooling gives surface compressive stresses.

Mismatching the coeff. of thermal expansion = ie **laminate technique**. PFM restoration are better, b'coz coeff of thermal expansion of metal is higher, so metal contracts more on cooling, compressive stresses come in porcelain and strength increased.

B. Interruption of crack propagation = ie by reinforcing the porcelain with a **dispersed phase** which interferes with crack propagation. **Alumina, Al_2O_3** is used in which the cracks can't penetrate. Aluminious porcelains are used for jacket crowns.

Dicor = **mica crystals** grow in glass on heating; but coeff of thermal expansion should be matching of ceramic and dispersed phase eg Zr, Al.

C. transformation of toughening = by a material which changes in crystal structure under stress eg partially stabilised zirconia (PSZ). Energy of crack propagation is used for PSZ transformation. Disadvantage is that refractive index of PSZ is higher than porcelain which scatters light and gives **opacity.**

FABRICATION

- **Condensation** = surface tension of **water is the driving force** in it. Porcelain should **never dry out** unless condensation is complete.
- **Firing** = done at 650° C for 5 min preheated = to eliminate water; then preheated porcelain is fired. **Vacuum firing** decreases porosity.
- **Glazing** = **decreases crack propagation;** increases strength; gives life – like finishing.
- **Cooling** = but **slow cooling** of PFM restorations can increase the coeff of thermal expansion of porcelain and more likely to crack.

Porcelain teeth = are the only type of denture teeth which allow denture base to be rebased; they cause enamel abrasion; are brittle; clicking noise, are held by mechanical retention.

PFM crown = metal increases strength of porcelain and reinforces it.

- Porcelain should be low fusing and should have coeff of thermal expansion **higher than** ordinary porcelain.
- Base metal 1 % in gold alloys form a *surface oxide layer* which helps in BONDING with porcelain (chemical bond).

- Bonding is CHEMICAL; occurs **through oxide layer**.
- **coeff of thermal expansion** of porcelain and metal should be **approx same** to avoid internal stresses.
- Ceramic used has **high alkali content** (soda/ potash) = to **increase the thermal expansion** to a level compatible to metal coping.
- Metallic oxides = are opacifiers.
- A phosphate or ethyl silicate bonded investment and **thermal expansion** for shrinkage compensation is used.
- Degas the casting at = 980° C.
- **Thickness** of opaque porcelain = 0.2 mm
- Translucent porcelain thickness = use to **make bulk**.
- More tooth structure has to be removed for PFM than all – porcelain crown.
- **Tin oxide coating** on Pt – foil also helps bonding of porcelain to metal. It **decreases subsurface porosity** and micro-cracks. It replaces thicker metal coping with a thin Pt – foil giving more space for porcelain.
- Use an alloy which contracts slightly more than the porcelain on cooling to room temperature. It introduces compressive stresses in porcelain and makes it stronger.
- **Pd – Ag alloys** = **no external oxide layer** is formed, so only **mechanical bonding** with porcelain occurs of this metal.
- **Electrodeposition** of oxides of gold layer and then tin layer = increases bonding. The layer acts as **a buffer zone** to absorb stresses due to difference in coeff of thermal expansion b/w metal and porcelain.
- **Glass ceramic crown** = is a material which is formed into the desired shape as glass and then subjected to **heat treatment** to induce **partial devitrification** ie loss of glassy structure. It is ka CERAMMING. It produces mica crystals; interruption of crack propagation and so increased strength.
- **Dicor** = gives natural appearance of color through **chameleon effect.**
- **Etching of porcelain** is done by = **HF acid.**
- 1.23 % APF and 8 % SnF_2 which are topical fluoride agents for caries prevention **should not bc applied** on PFM restorations as they cause = **roughness within 4 mins**.

SOLDERING

- **Welding** = 2 parts of metal are joined together by melting without any intervening metal.
- **Brazing** = metal parts joined by melting a filler b/w them at temperature below the solidus temperature of metal being joined and is > 450° C.
- **Soldering** = metal parts joined with filler metal at temperature below solidus and below 450° C.

Flux = **removes oxide layer** form the surfaces being joined. It has **3 functions** ie protective; reducing and solvent. (RPS)

Borax and boric acid fluxes are mainly used = as type I = protective and type 2 = are reducing.

Oxides on base metal alloys are more stable and **so fluoride** is used to dissolve them = by type 3 fluxes. Fluoride acts as **solvent.**

Minimum flux should be used = otherwise weak joint is formed.

Filler metal

- Should be compatible with the metals being joined.
- Flow temperature of filler should be **approx 50° C less** than the solidus temperature of the metal parts.
- Overheating should be avoided to prevent weakening, of joint by Recrystallisation.

Heat sources

1. Acetylene gas has highest flame temperature and greater heat content than H_2 and natural gases, but there is a temprature difference in flame from one part to the other part by approx 100° C, so positioning of the torch is critical.
2. **Propane and butane** = has highest heat content and **best choice.** Neutral / slightly **reducing zone** is used.
3. Furnace brazing =

Convection = heat transfer through air.

Conduction = heat transfer through furnace structure.

Radiant heat = heat transfer through heating coils.

WROUGHT ALLOYS

Used for orthodontic wires also.

Elastic deflection of wire is = YS / MOE

Maximum force is a function of = YS

Carbon steel = C < 1.2 %.

Ferrite	BCC
Austenite	FCC
Martensite	BCT

Ferrite = is pure Fe; BCC; low solubility of C (0.02 wt %); stable up to 912° C.

Austenite = FCC; stable up to 912 – 1394° C; maximum C solubility is 2.11 %.

When austenite is cooled slowly = then **iron carbide** (Fe_3C) is precipitated out = it gives strength of softer ferrite and austenite phase, it requires diffusion.

If asutenite is **cooled rapidly**/quenched = a diffusionless transformation to BCT structure is formed , ka **martensite**; it is highly distorted, strained, very hard and brittle. It is used to make **cutting edges of the instruments**.

Tempering = martensite **on heating changes** to ferrite and carbides. It **decreases hardness and increases toughness**.

Stainless steel

It is ka s.s if Cr = 12 – 30 %

Cr = **passivating effect,** gives resistance to tarnish /corrosion.

	Cr	Ni	Carbon
Ferrite , BCC	11.5 – 27 %	0	0.2 max.
Austenite , FCC	16 – 26	7 – 22	0.25 max
Martensite , BCT	11.5 – 17	0 – 2.5	0.15 – 1.20

Ferritic = less strong; not heat hardenable; not readily work hardenable; **little used in dentistry.**

Martensite = Can be heat treated; for surgical / cutting instruments; corrosion resistance is less and decreases after heat Rx; ductility decreases:

YS = 492 Mpa when annealed; 1898 Mpa when quenched.

BHN = 230 when annealed; 600 when quenched.

Austenitic s.s = AISI 302; aka 18 : 8 s.s.

- Most corrosion resistant;
- 18 % Cr + 8% Ni + 0.15 % C.
- type 304 has C = 0.08 %.
- most common for **orthodontic wires/ bands.**
- type 316 L has C = 0.03 %; used **for implants.**
- Cold workable and increases strength.
- Ease in forming.

SENSITISATION

If s.s heated b/w 400 – 900° C, the corrosion resistance is lost due to precipitation of **chromium carbide (Cr_3C),** which is most rapid at 650° C.

So passivating effect of **Cr** is lost, **intergranular corrosion** occurs at grain boundaries.

If s.s is cold worked = carbides precipitates **along slip planes** rather than at grain boundaries and so resistance to corrosion is increased eg ortho. wires.

STABILISATION

Ti is added which gets precipitated in place of Cr. The **conc. of Ti** should be = **6 x the conc of carbon**.

Austenite s.s is susceptible to attack by solutions containing chlorine, so **chloride cleansers should not be used** with them.

Properties

- In orthodontic wires, strength and hardness may increase with decrease in diameter, b'coz of the amount of cold working in forming the wire.

- TS = 2100 Mpa
- YS = 1400 Mpa
- KHN = 600
- Property of readily **strain hardening** is a characteristic of austenite SS which is mainly due to phase change from FCC to BCC.
- BCC ferrite/ martensite are ferromagnetic and austenite is non-magnetic.

Solder

Its MP should be less than that of the SS wire. So gold solder cannot be used.

Silver solder should be used to which Sn and In are added to decrease the fusion temperature and improve solderability.

Solder is **anodic to s.s.** = so corrosion

Solder temperature = 620 – 665° C, solidus – liquidus ranges of the solders should be small.

Flux contains **fluorides / KF** to **dissolve the passivating film** of *chromium* while soldering for better union.

Boric acid is more in conc. than in gold solders as it decreases the fusion temperature.

Reducing zone of the flame should be used.

Color should never exceed = DULL RED.

Use as little heat as possible, for least time = to avoid carbide precipitates, loss of strength etc.

Welding = spot welder is used.

Weld spot seen as **nugget** of the resolidified cast structure.

Strength of weld joint decreases by increasing recrystallisation of wrought structures.

Weld joint is **susceptible to corrosion** due to chromium carbide precipitates and loss of passivation.

Elgiloy = are wrought Co – Cr – Ni alloy

- Co – Cr – Ni alloy = contains 40, 20 , 15 % respectivcly and Fe is 15.8 %.

- **Age hardening** = 260- 650° C range ie 482° C for 5 hrs.
- Softening by heat Rx and quenching at = 1100 – 1200° C
- Should never be annealed.
- Ductility = softened is > SS; hardened < SS.
- Properties are nearly equal to = SS

Recovery heat treatment

Stress relief heat Rx at 370 – 480° C for 11 min, after cold working removes residual stresses.

(1) SS = increased MOE; increased YS; decreased ductility; increased modulus of resilience.

(2) Elgiloy = is more responsive than SS. Increase YS; increased corrosion resistance.

(3) **Ni – Ti wires** = contain Ni = 54; Ti = 44; Co = 2 %. It is present in **1:1 stoichiometric ratio**.

- At high temperature = austenite phase = BCC
- At low temperature = M phase = CPH
- **shape memory / superelasticity** are 2 most imp properties of this wire.
- It gives very **light and continuous forces** for tooth movement.
- Austenite on heat changes to M phase; **shape memory/superelasticity** come into play.
- Cobalt = controls the lower transition temperature; which can be near mouth temperature / 37° C.
- Austenite changes to M – phase **under stress** produces superelasticity. Additional strain is due to volume change which results from the change in crystal structure.
- It cannot be soldered / welded.

(4) Beta – titanium alloys

- Can be highly cold worked.
- Heat Rx is not recommended.
- Welding can be done.

- Has excellent corrosion resistance.
- Can sustain high elastic activations.

(5) **Elgiloy** = is wrought Co – Cr – Ni alloys.

- Co – Cr alloy = aka **vitallium**.
- Co – Ni – Cr = **durallium**
- Ni – Cr = **ticonium**.
- Mechanical properties of vitallium, durallium, ticonium can not be improved by heat Rx.
- Alloys with noble metal content < 65 % = usually tarnish.

(6) **PGP wires** = Pt – Au – Pd wires

PSC wires = Pd – Ag – Cu wires

(7) Wrought gold alloys = for RPD clasps; orthodontic appliances; retention pins; superior fracture resistance.

Role of various components —

1. Pd, Pt	Make wire not to melt / recrystallize during soldering. Also ensure a fine grain structure. Sufficient Pt, Pd should be present to increase the fusion temperature of wrought gold alloy.
2. Cu	**Age hardening** of alloy
3. Ag	**Covers the color** of Cu.
4. Ni	Strengthener of alloy; decreases ductility.
5. Large Ni content	Decreases corrosion resistance.
6. Zn	**Scavenger;** removes oxide layer.

Properties

Microstructure is fibrous / has long crystals.

Wrought metal has increased TS and hardness than cast metal.

IMPLANTS

- Subperiosteal = longest history = 54 % success
- Transosteal = only in mandible = 90 % success

- Endosseous = best
- **Polymeric inserts** in the endosseous implants **act as shock absorbers;** acts as **pseudo – PDL.**
- **Osseointegration** = is an absolute requirement for success of implants.

(1) **Austenitic SS implants** = 18 : 8 = Cr: Ni; C = 0.5 %

- Chromium = for corrosion resistance.
- Ni = stabilises austenite structure; do not use in patients allergic to Ni.
- Most subject to crevice and **pitting corrosion.**

(2) Co – Cr – Mo = as 63%, 30%, 5% cast only; for subperiosteal frames;

Very good corrosion resistance; least ductile to all alloy systems.

(3) Ti / Ti – Al – V = 6% Al; 4% V.

Pure Ti is biocompatible

Passivates on contact with oxygen / tissue fluids by formation of oxide layer.

Breach in oxide layer is *self-healing.*

(4) Polymer / composites = for tissue attachment and replacement augmentation.

ABRASION AND POLISHING

Abrasion = is a cutting action, cutting points are not arranged in a regular pattern, e.g. grinding wheel, diamond bur, pumice cup, sand paper, stone.

Material	**Composition**
Emery	Natural oxide of aluminium ka **corundum**.
Al_2O_3	From bauxite
Levigated alimina	Al_2O_3 by **water floatation** process.
Garnet	Silicates of Al, Co etc.; usually coated on paper or cloth.

Material	Composition
Pumice	Highly siliceous material
'Kieselguhr	Siliceous remains of aquatic plants ka diatoms, ka **diatomaceous earth.**
Tripoli	—
Rouge	Is **iron oxide;** impregnated on a **crocus cloth**
Tin oxide	ie putty powder
Chalk	Calcium carbonate.
Chromic oxide	For SS and metals; hard powder
Sand	—
Carbides	Si, B, on wheels / disks
Diamond	**Hardest** and most effective
Zr – silicates	In dental pastes; disks / strips
Crocus disc	For gold finishing; has FeO ie rouge.
Lavigated alumina	For **porcelain finishing**
Al_2O_3 disc	For CR restorations finishing

Abrasive properties: it should be harder than the work it abrades.

KHN of sand	800
Of emery	2000
Of silicone carbide	2500
Of B – carbide	2800
Of diamond	> 7000

Abrasive should fracture rather than becoming dull.

Polishing agents = have smaller particles as cp to abrasive agents.

Important points for revision

- Elastic limit = proportional limit = yield strength, are used as synonyms. **(EPY)**
- Modulous of elasticity = stiffness = rigidity
- High YS; low MOE = means increased flexibility.
- MOE is independent of heat Rx or other mechanical Rx.
- High proportional limit means = more resistance to permanent deformation.
- **Ductility** = is the ability of a material to withstand permanent deformation under **tensile load.** It helps to make wires. It is the %age elongation.
- A wire of a given composition is SUPERIOR to a casting = b'coz porosity is minimised in wire.
- **Malleability** = is the ability of the material to withstand **compressive load;** so sheaths are formed. It is the %age compression.
- To achieve most harmonious match of color = **Value** is most important.
- When selecting a wire for its ability to withstand stress without permanent deformation, consult tables for its = elastic limits.

BHN	**Hard steel ball** is used; is not for brittle materials and for elastic recovery.
RHN	**Conical diamond point;** not for brittle materials and modified for elastic recovery.
VHN	**Square diamond point** = used for brittle materials;eg tooth, gold.
KHN; **best**	**Rhomboid diamond point;** 172.5 degrees and 130 degrees are angles of rhomboid. It is independent for ductility of materials.
BHN and VHN	For gold
RHN	For composite resins

Stresses during mastication

Teeth	Pounds	Kgs
Incisors	20 – 55	9 – 25
Canines	30 – 75	14 – 34
Premolars	50 – 100	23 – 46
Molars	90 – 200	41 – 91

Gypsum

- **Balanced stone** = in which appropriate amounts of accelerator and retarders are added.
- POP = beta form = formed in open air kettle.
- Dental stone = alpha – form = by autoclaving.
- Die stone / densite = by autoclave + 30% $CaCl_2$ solution.

Classification

- Type I = impression plaster
- Type II = model plaster
- Type III = dental stone; hydrocal; class I stone.
- Type IV = dental stone – high strength; densite; class II stone.

- Optimum water / powder ratio of lab dental stones to **pour diagnostic casts** = 28 ml / 100 gm.
- Optimum water / powder ratio of die stones to **pour master casts** = 24 ml / 100 gm.
- Approx setting time of impression plaster = 2 – 4 min.
- Setting expansion is lower in impression plaster.
- **Purpose of calcination** of gypsum = to remove 3/4th of water from the product ie $CaSO_4.2H_2O \rightarrow CaSO_4.1/2H_2O$
- Strength of gypsum is due to = loss of excess water.
- Setting of plaster is the result of = difference in solubility b/w $CaSO_4.2\ H_2O$ and $CaSO_4.1/2\ H_2O$.

- Solubility rate of gypsum product = 0.2 %
- Type IV gypsum = most successful die – material available.
- Excessive monomer leads to excessive shrinkage.
- *Polymerisation shrinkage* of pure methyl methacrylate = 21 %
- But, if P : M ratio = 3:1 by volume or 2 :1 by wt., then polymerisation shrinkage is = 7 % only.
- Acrylic resin is SOFTEST of all restorative materials.

- **Potassium sulphate** = is accelerator of setting in dental stone in any concentration.
- **Borax** = retarder in setting of dental stone.
- Any modifier (accelerator / retarder) added in dental stone = **decreases setting expansion.**
- Zinc acetate is accelerator for ZOE cement.

Impression materials

- Impression compound is placed in mouth at = 45° C
- **Reactor** in alginate = calcium sulfate
- **Retarder** in alginate = potassium / sodium phosphate; oxalate or carbonate.
- **Japanese alginate** = Alginate in japan = triethanol amine alginate, soluble and insoluble carbonates (in place of phosphates) and calcium sulfate.
- Alginates are made **dust free** by adding = GLYCOL.
- Alginate = is the most economical impression material.
- In ZOE impression material = **2 types of setting times** are there.
- **In non – eugenol pastes** = carboxylic acid is used in place of eugenol.
- **Borax in agar** = increases viscosity, increases strength of gel; but decreases setting time of cast poured in it. So impression is first dipped in 2 % K_2SO_4 for 5 min. and then cast is poured.
- Accelerator in polysulfide material = lead peroxide
- Catalyst in silicone = tin octoate

- cross linking agent in Polyether = sulfonate ester.
- Polyether should be poured = immediately.
- Polysulfide and silicones = **wait for 30 min before pouring**; it actually improves the accuracy of the cast.
- TWO-IN-ONE STAGE impression material = elastomers.
- **Most ideal impression material**; an ultimate impression material = addition curing type impression material.
- Polyether impression material = dimensionally unstable in p.o. moisture. It has high MOE ie high rigidity which is not desirable. It absorbs water.
- **Electroformed** dies can be prepared from the impression taken from = polysulfide and silicones.
- Polysulfide impression materials **are not distorted**, b'coz water loss does not occur.
- Dimensional stability of a mercaptan rubber base impression is promoted by uniform thickness of material = 3 mm ie 1/8 inches.
- Optimal thickness of alginate impression = 3/16 inches; 4.76 mm.
- Agar and mercaptan/ polysulfides can be placed for 1 hour before pouring the cast.
- Agar is put in 100 % humidity; mercaptan / polysulfide can be put on bench.
- Minimum time for which silicone impression is held in mouth = 8 min.
- Dimension stability of mercaptan rubber base impression is promoted by = uniform thickness of material; is 1/8 inch; 3.2 mm.

- **Coupling agent** in resins = organo silane, e.g. vinyl silane
- Initiator in resins = benzoyl **p**eroxide (in **p**owder)
- Inhibitor in resins = hydroquinone, oxygen (in liquid)
- Plasticizer in resins = butyl acrylate or dibutyl phthalate; it decreases brittleness.
- Cross linking agent = glycol dimethacrylate
- Accelerator = amine; heat
- In cold cure; the activator is = dimethyl-p-toluidine

- In heat cure; the activator is = heat.
- **Bakelite** = denture based resin polymerised through, condensation reaction.
- **Chemical cure resins** have = benzoyl peroxide – tertiary amine system.
- **UV Light cure** have = benzoyl peroxide – benzoin methyl ether system.
- **Visible LC have** = diketone – tertiary amine system (one liquid system).

Differences b/w UV LC and visible LC

UV	Visible
Hazard = **retinal damage**	No
Warm up time = saveral minutes	No
Curing = 60 sec	30 sec.
Depth of cure = 1.4 mm	2 – 2.5 mm.

- Range of light used = 420 – 450 nm., blue zone.
- **Deciduous teeth have little or no interprismatic substance** in enamel surrounding the rods, so acid etching causes minimally undercut, rough porous pitted surface = up to 200 microns.
- In adult teeth = 10 – 20 microns tags are formed.
- MMA direct filling resins which has a high degree of color stability are activate by = sulfinic acid.
- Enamel bonding agents = low viscosity resins without fillers.

Dentin bonding agents

1. First generation = phosphate esters of BIS-GMA; aka **scotch bond**.
2. Second generation = chlor-phosphate esters of BIS-GMA.
3. Third generation = GLUMA = gluteraldehyde + HEMA. and 4-META.

- Cyanoacrylates = are used as **surgical sutures,** periodontal dressing
- Polyurethanes = are used as adhesives; P and F sealants; maxillofacial prosthesis.
- Dental P and F sealants are composed of = BIS-GMA.

Cements

- Buffering agent in $ZnPO_4$ cement liquid = are Zn and Al.
- Plane ZOE cement **sets in p.o. of water only,** so matallic hydroxide is introduced in powder to provide water.
- Zinc acetate is accelerator for ZOE cement.
- Minimum pressure required for **gold foil condenstation** = 15 psi.
- Cohesive gold type used only as BULK FILLER = is mat gold.
- Annealing through alcohol is preferred for = spherical gold.
- 24 carat gold = 1000 fine; pure gold.
- With powdered gold = use BUTT joint.
- In Currently available cement bases, most helpful characteristic is = low coeff of thermal conductivity.
- In $ZnPO_4$ liquid = metallic acids added act as buffers, e.g. Zn, Al; which bring pH forem 3.5 → 7.
- PH of polycarboxylate cement liquid = 1.7
- PH of calcium hydroxide = 11.5 – 13.
- ZOE cement is least injurious to the pulp.

Types of GI cements

1. Fast setting = d-tartaric acid is added.
2. Water setting = anhydrous Polyacrylic acid in powder.
3. Reinforced = alumina, titanium oxide, zirconium oxide ; increased strength.
4. Miracle mix = amalgam alloy is added.
5. Cermet GI = miracle mix is sintered – so a uniform paste is achieved.
6. Light cure GI = IIMMA is added.

Investment materials

- Investment materials = have at least 60 – 70 % fillers / refractory.
- **Ethyl silicate** = is a binding agent for high temperature investment ie silica bonded.
- When a phosphate bonded investment is mixed with **colloidal silica solution** rather than water = the contraction is eliminated and an expansion occurs.
- **Green shrinkage** = is associated with silica bonded investment materials.

Gypsum bonded	For gold	At 650° C
Phosphate bonded	For metal ceramic	732 – 982° C
Silica bonded	For base metal alloys	At 1090 – 1180° C

- Type I gypsum bonded investment material = uses thermal expansion; 1 – 1.6 %
- Type II gypsum bonded investment material = uses HSE; 1.2 – 2.2 %
- Type III gypsum bonded investment material = uses thermal expansion; used for RPDs; 1.0 – 1.5 %
- HSE = 6 times NSE.
- When HSE technique is used = investment material is heated at 900 °F for 1 hour.
- For TSE = 1200 °F for 1 hour.
- Strength to dental investment for gold is provided by = alpha – hemihydrate of gypsum; as binder.
- Cristoballite shows greater and earlier expansion than quartz.
- Sprue required for RPDs = 8 – 12 gauge round wax forms.
- Sprue = no. 8 or no. 10 = for large patterns; no. 12 = for small patterns; it should not be more than 6 – 7 mm long.
- Most important property when base metal RPD clasp is adjusted = elongation.

Composite restorative material has

- Less setting time,
- Less setting contraction than silicate cement.
- Similar compressive strength
- No fluoride diffusion
- Better color stability
- Unaffected by oral fluids ie no dissolution in oral fluids.

Amalgam

- Dispersed phase – high Cu alloy = has least creep
- **Tarnish** = silver sulfide is formed.
- **Corrosion products** formed are = tin oxide and tin chlorides / tin hydroxides.
- Corrosion of amalgam = sulfides of Ag and Hg (from Boucher's).
- Which of the following is not a criteria for working qualities of Ag-Hg = time of amalgamation/ compressive strength/ consistency/ carving characteristics. The answer is compressive strength.
- Threshold unit volume of Hg = 50 micro gm / cubic m of the air.

Material	Strength	Expan-sion	Hardness	Flow	ST	Tarnish resistance
Ag	Increased	Increase	—	Decrease	D	I
Sn	D	D	I	I	I	D
Cu	I	I	I	D	D	D
Zn	D	I	—	—	D	—
Overtri-turation	I	D				

- Ag – Cu = eutectic (71.9 : 28.1 %)
- Ag – Sn = peritectic
- **Sterling silver** = Ag – Cu = 92.5 : 7.5 %.

- **Copper** = provides property of age – hardening to the alloys; ie solid – solid transformation.
- **Softening heat Rx** = at 700° C for 10 min and quenching. Quenching prevents ordering and atomic diffusion and so **solid solution** structure persists. Ductlity increases.
- **Hardening heat Rx** = 200 – 450° C at 15 – 30 min. but before age hardening, the alloy is subjected to softening heat Rx to relieve all strain hardening.

Gold alloy

Type	Hardness	Used at	Au %	VHN
I	Soft	On lateral surface of tooth and small inlays	83	60
II	Medium	On occlusal surface and inlays and 3/4th crowns	78	90
III	Hard	FPD; crown and bridges	78	120
IV	Extra hard	RPD saddles	75	150

- Gold foil = formed by beating = **best for finishing.**
- **Mat gold** = by electrolytic precipitation; and then sintered; used for bulk filling only; aka **electrolytic gold.**
- **Electroloy** = alloy of mat gold **with Calcium;** Ca increases strength and hardness.
- Goldent / spherical / powdered gold = by **chemical precipitation** and atomisation; used for core and finishing both.
- **Platinised** gold = ie platinum foil in b/w Au foils.
- **Degassing** is done at = 340 – 370° C for 8 – 10 min.
- Mat gold = for bulk
- Gold alloy indicated for RPDs = type IV.
- Gold alloy have higher YS than Cr-Co alloys.
- Cr-Co alloys will deform permanently at lower loads than gold alloys.

- Gold alloy has MOE = 1/2 of Cr-Co alloys.
- For **gold alloys** = tensile strength / BHN = 500.
- And PL = 2/3rd of the tensile strength.
- Cr-Co alloys are more rapidly work hardened than gold alloys.
- All gold alloys can be softened by heating at 700° C for 10 min before quenching in water = **softening heat** Rx.
- Alloys with Cu 15 – 30 % (class III, IV) harden after softening heat Rx if they are heated to 450° C and cooled uniformly to 250° C over a period of 15 – 30 min = hardening heat Rx.
- Cold working process does not alter MOE.
- Wrought gold wire is better than cast gold.
- Cr-Co alloys have lower density than gold alloys.
- Solidification shrinkage of alloy = 1.4 %
- Reduction in its fusion temperature can be done by = Ag.
- Lowest fineness gold solder used should be ≥ 580 fine.
- Solders above 650 fine should not be used where considerable stress is involved.
- Width of gap b/w adj. units to be soldered should be = 0.001"; (0.005" according to Skinner's.)
- Function of flux = prevents oxidation of metals.
- Function of F fluxes = to remove CrO_2 layer.
- Reducing zone / blue of the flame is used.

Steel

- maximum Carbon content of steel = 1.7%; mainly **austenite.**
- Hardening heat Rx = cooling slowly from 450° C.
- Softening heat Rx = quenching from 700° C.

Band materials used in orthodontics

1. Incisors = 0.125 x 0. 003", 004"
2. Canines / premolars = 0.150" × 0. 004"
3. Molars = 0.180 × 0.005 / 0. 006"

9

MCQs in Dental Materials

1. **Abrasives are graded on the basis of:**
   A. Size of the abrasive particle
   B. Fineness of sieve through which they pass
   C. Size of particles generated during abrasion
   D. Atomic weight of the abrasive particles

2. **The abrasive used in sandblasting technique is:**
   A. Rouge
   B. Aluminium oxide
   C. Sand
   D. Zirconium silicate

3. **In diamond bur, the diamond chips are bound by:**
   A. Ceramic bounding
   B. Electroplating with a nickel base matrix
   C. Silica matrix
   D. Tin matrix

4. **Toothbrush abrasion is more related to:**
   A. Stiffness of toothbrush bristles
   B. Abrasiveness of the dentifrice
   C. Brushing technique
   D. Alignment of teeth

5. **Among the different forms of carbon steels, which is the strongest?**
   A. Ferrite
   B. Austenite

C. Martensite
D. All three have same strength

6. **Stainless steel resist tarnish and corrosion due to the formation of passivating layer of:**
   A. Iron oxide
   B. Iron sulphide
   C. Chromium oxide
   D. Chromium sulphide

7. **The most common form of stainless steel used by orthodontists in the form of bands and wires is:**
   A. Ferrite
   B. Austenite
   C. Martensite
   D. Chromium steel

8. **An 18–8 stainless steel orthodontic wire is heated to 650°C looses its corrosion resistance due to formation of:**
   A. Chromium oxide
   B. Chromium sulphide
   C. Nickel oxide
   D. Chromium carbide

9. **A decrease in diameter of the orthodontic wires causes:**
   A. Increased hardness and strength
   B. Decreased hardness and strength
   C. Increased hardness but decreased strength
   D. Decreased hardness but increased strength

10. **Which of the following orthodontic wires has maximum modulus of elasticity?**
    A. Stainless steel
    B. Chromium-cobalt-nickel
    C. Nickel-titanium
    D. β-titanium

11. **Nickel-titanium wires exhibit the phenomenon of superelasticity in which phase?**
    A. Ferrite
    B. Austenite

C. Martensite
D. None of the above

12. Soldering is different from brazing in that:
A. Filler metal is different
B. Filler metal is melted below the solidus temperature of the metal being joint
C. Filler metal is melted above 450° C
D. Filler metal is melted below 450° C

13. The best choice fuel gas for brazing would be:
A. Hydrogen
B. Natural gas
C. Propane
D. Acetylene

14. The setting of all dental cements involve an acid-base reaction except:
A. Silicate
B. Glass ionomer
C. Zinc phosphate
D. Calcium hydroxide

15. The material that serves as a standard of comparision for materials that cause severe pulpal irritation is:
A. Calcium hydroxide
B. Zinc phosphate
C. Silicate cement
D. Resin cement

16. When comparing plaque formed on natural tooth surface with that formed on silicate restoration, the result would be:
A. There is no difference
B. Plaque associated with silicate is less cariogenic
C. Plaque associated with silicate is more cariogenic
D. More plaque forms on silicate restoration

17. When comparing GIC with composites in terms of conservation of tooth structure:
A. GIC is superior to composites
B. Composites are superior

C. both require same degree of instrumentation
D. None of the above

18. GIC bonds to:
A. Enamel
B. Dentin
C. Enamel and dentin
D. Neither enamel and dentin

19. Compared to conventional GIC, the anticariogenic potential of silver alloy admix GIC is:
A. More
B. Less
C. Same
D. Not related

20. If zinc-oxide eugenol cement is to be used as a base in a cavity, the cavity varnish should:
A. Be used before the cement base is applied
B. Be used after the cement base has set
C. Not to be used
D. None of the above

21. During casting, a sprue-former is attached at right angle to the flat surface of the wax pattern. The porosity resulting from such an arrangement is called:
A. Localized shrinkage porosity
B. Hot-spot porosity
C. Suck-back porosity
D. Microporosity

22. All of the following are die materials except:
A. Amalgam
B. Epoxy resins
C. Acrylic
D. None of the above

23. The difference between indirect spruing and direct spruing lies in the presence of:
A. Crucible former
B. Casting ring

C. Reservoir bar in indirect spruing
D. Reservoir bar in direct spruing

24. The presence of casting ring liner promotes:
A. Normal setting expansion + thermal expansion
B. Normal setting expansion + semihygroscopic expansion
C. Thermal expansion + semihygroscopic expansion
D. Normal setting expansion + thermal expansion + semihygroscopic expansion

25. The casting procedure produces a casting with fins. This may be due to:
A. Overheating of the investment
B. Too rapid heating of the investment
C. Underheating of the investment
D. Low W/P ratio of the investment

26. After the casting procedure was completed, an incomplete casting was obtained with rounded shiny margins. This might be the result of:
A. Insufficient casting pressure
B. High viscosity of the fused metal
C. Incomplete elimination of wax from the mould
D. Low W/P ratio of the investment

27. All forms of gold may be desorbed on a electrically heated tray except:
A. Powder gold
B. Mat gold
C. Mat foil
D. Electralloy

28. Which among the following forms of direct filling gold would give the most dense restoration?
A. Mat gold
B. Powdered gold
C. Gold foil
D. Mat gold + gold foil

29. Compared to the gold casting alloys, the physical properties of direct filling gold are:

A. Superior
B. Inferior
C. Nearly the same
D. None of the above

30. The purpose of calcium in electrolytic precipitate gold is:
A. To prevent the surface contamination of gold
B. To improve the handling characteristics of gold
C. To increase the strength of gold
D. To make the gold oncohesive

31. Failure to completely compact each cylinder of gold is called:
A. Stepping
B. Shingling
C. Bridging
D. Discompacting

32. The cohesion between two successively placed layers of direct filling gold:
A. Hydrogen bonding
B. Metallic bonding
C. There is no cohesion
D. Either of the above depending on the form of gold used

33. Eames's technique refers to:
A. A water defluoridation technique
B. A technique to close midline diastema with composites
C. An isolation technique to prevent moisture contamination of amalgam
D. Mixing silver amalgam with minimum quantity of mercury

34. When the alloy particles and mercury are mixed, the oxide layer coating the alloy particles is dissolved by:
A. Chemical reaction with mercury
B. Mechanical abrasion
C. A combination of chemical reaction and mechanical abrasion
D. There is no oxide coating on alloy particles

35. Delayed expansion in zinc containing amalgams is caused by internal pressure exerted by formation of:
A. Zinc suphide

B. Hydrogen
C. Zinc hydroxide
D. Tin sulphide

36. The maximum level of occupational exposure(μg/cubic meter of air) of mercury considered safe is:
A. 20 μg
B. 50 μg
C. 75 μg
D. 100 μg

37. According to the ADA specification no. 1 for amalgam alloys, alloys containing less than 6% copper are designated:
A. Low copper alloys
B. High copper alloys
C. Lathe cut alloy
D. There is no specification in ADA for copper content

38. The formation of silver sulfide corrosion product in gold alloys exemplifies:
A. Dry corrosion
B. Wet corrosion
C. Semi wet corrosion
D. Semi-dry corrosion

39. Cold blend test is used to measure:
A. Malleability
B. Ductility
C. Toughness
D. Hardness

40. If the viscosity of a liquid decreases with increased shear rate, the liquid is said to be:
A. Plastic
B. Dilatant
C. Newtonian
D. Pseudoplastic

41. The temperature of plaster-water combination is raised to 70°C. The effect on setting time would be:
A. Setting time increases

B. Setting time decreases
C. Setting time remains unchanged
D. Setting time may increase or decrease

42. " Green" strength of gypsum refers to:
A. Dry strength
B. Wet strength
C. Combined strength of plaster and stone
D. Strength after 30 minutes of mixing.

43. The addition of an accelerator or retarder to a gypsum product causes:
A. Increase in wet strength and decrease in dry strength
B. Decrease in wet strength and increase in dry strength
C. Decrease in both wet and dry strength
D. Increase in both wet and dry strength.

44. Synthetic gypsum is obtained from:
A. Corals
B. Waste products of the manufacture of phosphoric acid
C. Byproducts of cement
D. Trees

45. If a gypsum cast is to be soaked in water, the solution best suited would be:
A. Mineral water
B. Triple distilled water
C. A saturated solution of calcium sulfate
D. Normal saline

46. The principal ingredient of reversible hydrocolloid impression material by weight is:
A. Borax
B. Agar
C. Water
D. Wax

47. The main modification in the laminate technique used for impressions of reversible hydrocolloid is:
A. Use of only syringe material for impression
B. Replacement of tray hydrocolloid by alginate

C. Replacement of syringe material by low viscosity addition silicones
D. Replacement of syringe material by ZOE paste.

48. The purpose of zinc oxide in alginate is:
A. To increase the viscosity
B. To improve the taste of alginate
C. To act as a filler
D. To impart strength to alginate

49. The deterioration of alginate seen at higher temperature is due to:
A. Disintegration of calcium sulfate
B. Denaturation of sodium phosphate
C. Degradation of potassium titanium fluoride
D. Depolymerization of potassium alginate

50. An alginate impression produced a chalky stone cast. It may be due to any of the following reasons except:
A. Improper manipulation of stone
B. Premature removal of cast
C. Leaving cast in the impression for too long
D. Improper mixing of alginate

51. The limited shelf-life of condensation silicones is due to:
A. Evaporation of ethyl alcohol
B. Oxidation of tin present in the catalyst
C. Degradation of poly (dimethyl siloxane) polymer
D. High reactivity of tetraethyl orthosilicate at room temperature

52. The class of composites which has the best of physical and mechanical properties is:
A. Small particle
B. Hybrid
C. Microfilled
D. Conventional

53. Which of the following properties of metal remain unchanged as a result of work hardening?
A. Hardness
B. Proportional limit

C. Ductility
D. Elastic modulus

54. Mixing of hydrophilic silicones by wearing latex gloves causes:
A. Retardation of polymerization
B. Poisoning of polymerization
C. Acceleration of polymerization
D. No effect

55. Retardation of polymerization of hydrophilic silicones when mixed with latex gloves is due to:
A. Chemical reaction of latex with silicones
B. Sulfur in latex retards setting of silicones
C. Silicones absorb moisture from latex
D. Both (a) and (b)

56. The "mulling" process in amalgamation ensures:
A. Cohesion of the mix
B. Thorough trituration
C. Removal of excess mercury
D. All the above

57. The tarnish film seen in silver amalgam is due to the formation of:
A. Oxides and chlorides of tin
B. Silver sulfide
C. Copper oxide
D. Tin sulfide

Answer Kcy to MCQs in Dental Materials

1. (B) Abrasives are graded on the basis of fineness of the standard sieve through which they can pass. Finer abrasives are designated as powders and graded as F, FF, FFF, etc. or in case of impregnated papers as 0, 00, 000, etc.
2. (C) Rouge is used for polishing gold and noble metal alloys. Aluminiun oxide is used for finishing composites. Zirconium silicate is a consituent of dental prophylactic pastes.

3. (B) Ceramic bonding is used for silicon carbide or corundum based abrasive points.
4. (B) The stiffness of toothbrush bristles is not a factor in abrasion. The degree of abrasion produced by a given dentifrice is the same for either a hard or soft brush.
5. (C) Carbon steel is an iron-based alloy with less than 1.2% carbon. Ferrite is pure iron at room temperature having a body centered cubic structure and is stable upto 912° C. At temperature between 912°C and 1394°C ferrite changes to a face-centered cubic structure called austenite. If austenite is cooled very rapidly, it transforms itself into a body-centered tetragonal structure called martensite. The resulting lattice is highly distorted and strained, resulting in a very hard strong, brittle alloy. Therefore, the cutting edge of carbon steel instruments is martenistic.
6. (C) Stainless steel is an alloy of iron, carbon and chromium(12–30%). They resist tarnish and corrosion due to the formation of a surface layer of chromium oxide.
7. (B) Austenite stainless steel are the most corrosion resistant of the different forms of stainless steel. The two most common forms used are designated as 18–8 stainless steel (18% chromium, 8% nickel).
8. (D) When heated to such a high temperature, chromium carbide is precipitated and passivating effect of chromium is lost.
9. (A) A decreased diameter causes an increase in strength and hardness because of the cold working in forming the wire.
10. (B) Chromium-cobalt-nickel has the maximum modulus of elasticity. Also this wire can be given maximum 90° bends without fracture.
11. (C) The transition of nickel-titanium from austenite to martensite confers two unique properties—shape memory and superelasticity.
12. (D) In soldering, the filler metal is melted below 450°C while in brazing it is melted above 450°C.
13. (C) Although acetylene has the highest flame temperature, the heat content (amount of heat per unit area) is maximum for propane.

14. (D) With the exception of calcium hydroxide and resin cements, the setting reaction of all cements involve an acid base reaction.
15. (C) For materials that are kind to the pulp, zinc-oxide eugenol serves as a standard of comparison whereas for pulpal irritants, silicate serves as a reference.
16. (B) Silicates exert an anticariogenic action by the presence of fluoride which inhibits the metabolism of carbohydrates.
17. (A) GIC produces a true adhesive bond to tooth structure whereas composites rely on mechanical retention.
18. (C)
19. (A) In admix cement, metal filler particles are not bonded to the cement matrix; thus, pathways for fluid exchange are created. This greatly increases the surface area for leaching of fluoride. Conversely, less fluoride is released from cermet than from its type II counterpart.
20. (B) The type of base governs the order of application of base and varnish. For cements that are pulpal irritants (Zn phosphate), varnish should be applied before the cement base. For biocompatible bases (Ca hydroxide, ZOE, GIC or polycarboxylate) varnish is applied only after the cement base has set.
21. (C) In such an arrangement, the entering molten metal impinges the mould surface at this point producing a localized lingering of molten metal after the casting has solidified. This leads to suck-back porosity.
22 (D) Besides the commonly used type IV and V stone, amalgam, acrylic, polyester and epoxy resins may be used as die materials. However, they are not compatible with all impression materials.
23. (C) In direct spruing, the sprue former provides a direct connection between the wax pattern and the sprue base. With indirect spruing, a reservoir bar is placed between the wax pattern and sprue former base. Indirect spruing is generally used for multiple single units and fixed partial dentures. Moreover, the presence of a reservoir bar prevents the localized shrinkage porosity.

24. (D) The casting ring liner provides space for the normal setting and semihygroscopic expansion during the setting of the investment and for the thermal expansion of the investment when the investment is heated.
25. (B) Too rapid heating causes the outer portion of the investment to become hot before the inner portions. Consequently, the outer layers begin to expand thermally without causing the inner layers to expand. This causes the brittle investment to crack from the interior outwardly in the form of radial cracks. These cracks, in turn, produces a casting with fins or spines.
26. (C) If the remnants of wax remain inside the mould then when the molten alloy contacts the wax particles, an explosion may occur that may produce sufficient back pressure to prevent the mould from getting filled. This produces an incomplete casting. The shiny condition of the metal is due to the strong reducing atmosphere created by the carbon monoxide left by the wax residue. Insufficient casting pressure also produces an incomplete casting with rounded margins which are dull rather than shiny.
27. (A) Desorbing is done as a precautionary measure to remove any surface gases and to ensure a totally clean surface. All forms of gold may be desorbed on an electrically heated tray except powder gold which must be heated in an alcohol flame.
28. (C) The most dense restoration is given by gold foil (15.8 gm/cm^3) followed by mat gold + gold foil (15 gm/cm^3), powdered gold and mat gold.
29. (B) Because of the inferior properties of direct filling gold, they cannot be used to encompass a tooth, nor can they withstand masticatory stresses if used to restore cusps.
30. (C) Calcium is added to electrolytic precipitate of gold in the range of 0.1% to produce stronger restorations by dispersion strengthening.
31. (C) Stepping is systematic moving of condenser point over the cylinder of gold foil so that each step overlaps the previous one. Shingling is the layering of gold foil over that which has been previously condensed.
32. (B)

33. (D)
34. (B)
35. (B) The reaction between zinc present in the amalgam and the moisture produces hydrogen as one of the corrosion products which causes delayed expansion.
36. (B)
37. (D) According to ADA there is no specification for content of amalgam alloys.
38. (A) Dry corrosion or chemical corrosion is one in which there is a direct combination of metallic and non-metallic products. Wet corrosion or electrochemical corrosion is one which requires the presence of water or other fluid electrolytes
39. (A) In cold blend test, the material is clamped and bent around a mandrel of a specified diameter. The number of bends before fracture is counted, and greater the number, greater is the ductility.
40. (D) The materials which behave like a rigid body until some minimum value of stress is reached are referred to as plastic. If viscosity increases with increasing shear rate, the liquid is said to be dilatant. A Newtonian fluid is one in which shear stress is proportional to the strain rate.
41. (A) Between 0° and 50°C, there is very little change. Above 50°C, the reaction gradually slows down. As the temperature approaches 100°C, no reaction takes place. At further higher temperature, the setting reaction is reversed, with the tendency for any crystals formed to change to hemihydrate form.
42. (B) Wet or Green strength of gypsum is the strength when the water in excess of that required for the hydration of the hemihydrate is left in the test specimen. When the specimen has been dried free of excess water, the strength obtained is called dry strength.
43. (C) This may be attributed to the salt added as an adulterant and to the reduction in intercrystalline cohesion.
44. (B)
45. (C) Gypsum is slightly soluble in water. If the cast is immersed in running water, the linear dimensions decrease approx. 0.1%

for every 20 minutes of such immersion. In a water saturated with Ca sulfate, there is negligible expansion of gypsum.

46. (C) Although the basic constituent of reversible hydrocolloid material is agar but by weight the main constituent is water.
47. (B) In laminate technique, the tray hydrocolloid is replaced by chilled alginate that will bond with the syringe agar.
48. (C) The composition of alginate is

Potassium alginate (15%)	main ingredient
Calcium sulfate (16%)	reactor
Zinc oxide (4%)	filler
Potassium titanium fluoride (3%)	accelerator for gypsum
Diatomaceous earth (60%)	filler
Sodium phosphate (2%)	retarder

49. (D)
50. (D)
51. (B) The setting of condensation silicones produces ethyl alcohol that accounts for the contraction seen during setting.
52. (A)
53. (D) The surface hardness, strength and proportional limit are increased, ductility and resistance to corrosion are decreased while elastic modulus of the metal remain unchanged as a result of work hardening.
54. (A) Mixing of hydrophilic silicones with latex gloves causes retardation of polymerization. After the impression is removed it will eventually set. Therefore the setting reaction is not poisoned.
55. (B)
56. (A) Mulling involves quick removal of pestle from the capsule at the end of amalgamation, replacing the lid, reinserting the capsule in the amalgamator and turning it on and then immediately off.
57. (B) Tarnish in silver is due to silver sulfide while oxides and chlorides of tin are the chief corrosion products of amalgam.

Reader's Notes

Reader's Notes

Reader's Notes

Reader's Notes